The Science and Art of Yoga in Mental and Neurological Healthcare

The Science and Art of Yoga in Mental and Neurological Healthcare

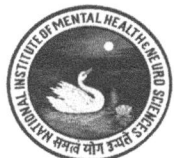 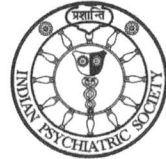

Indian Psychiatric Society Publication

Editors

Shivarama Varambally MD MAMS DSc
Professor of Psychiatry and Head
Department of Integrative Medicine
National Institute of Mental Health and Neuro Sciences (NIMHANS)
Bengaluru, Karnataka, India

Sanju George MBBS FRCPsych
Senior Clinical Psychiatrist and
Professor of Psychiatry and Psychology
Rajagiri College of Social Sciences
Kochi, Kerala, India

TM Srinivasan PhD DSc
Professor
Swami Vivekananda Yoga Anusandhana
Samsthana (S-VYASA) University
Bengaluru, Karnataka, India

Associate Editor

Hemant Bhargav MBBS MD PhD (Yoga)
Assistant Professor (Yoga)
Department of Integrative Medicine
National Institute of Mental Health and Neuro Sciences (NIMHANS)
Bengaluru, Karnataka, India

Forewords

BN Gangadhar
HR Nagendra

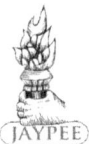

JAYPEE BROTHERS MEDICAL PUBLISHERS
The Health Sciences Publisher
New Delhi | London

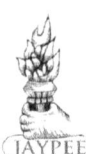 **Jaypee Brothers Medical Publishers (P) Ltd**

Headquarters
Jaypee Brothers Medical Publishers (P) Ltd
EMCA House, 23/23-B
Ansari Road, Daryaganj
New Delhi 110 002, India
Landline: +91-11-23272143, +91-11-23272703
+91-11-23282021, +91-11-23245672
Email: jaypee@jaypeebrothers.com

Corporate Office
Jaypee Brothers Medical Publishers (P) Ltd
4838/24, Ansari Road, Daryaganj
New Delhi 110 002, India
Phone: +91-11-43574357
Fax: +91-11-43574314
Email: jaypee@jaypeebrothers.com

Overseas Office
JP Medical Ltd
83 Victoria Street, London
SW1H 0HW (UK)
Phone: +44 20 3170 8910
Fax: +44 (0)20 3008 6180
Email: info@jpmedpub.com

Website: www.jaypeebrothers.com
Website: www.jaypeedigital.com

© 2021, Jaypee Brothers Medical Publishers

The views and opinions expressed in this book are solely those of the original contributor(s)/author(s) and do not necessarily represent those of editor(s) of the book.

All rights reserved. No part of this publication may be reproduced, stored or transmitted in any form or by any means, electronic, mechanical, photocopying, recording or otherwise, without the prior permission in writing of the publishers.

All brand names and product names used in this book are trade names, service marks, trademarks or registered trademarks of their respective owners. The publisher is not associated with any product or vendor mentioned in this book.

Medical knowledge and practice change constantly. This book is designed to provide accurate, authoritative information about the subject matter in question. However, readers are advised to check the most current information available on procedures included and check information from the manufacturer of each product to be administered, to verify the recommended dose, formula, method and duration of administration, adverse effects and contraindications. It is the responsibility of the practitioner to take all appropriate safety precautions. Neither the publisher nor the author(s)/editor(s) assume any liability for any injury and/or damage to persons or property arising from or related to use of material in this book.

This book is sold on the understanding that the publisher is not engaged in providing professional medical services. If such advice or services are required, the services of a competent medical professional should be sought.

Every effort has been made where necessary to contact holders of copyright to obtain permission to reproduce copyright material. If any have been inadvertently overlooked, the publisher will be pleased to make the necessary arrangements at the first opportunity. The **CD/DVD-ROM** (if any) provided in the sealed envelope with this book is complimentary and free of cost. **Not meant for sale.**

Inquiries for bulk sales may be solicited at: jaypee@jaypeebrothers.com

The Science and Art of Yoga in Mental and Neurological Healthcare

First Edition: **2021**

ISBN: 978-81-948028-1-5

Contributors

Aarti Jagannathan PhD
Associate Professor
Department of Psychiatric Social Work
National Institute of Mental Health and
Neuro Sciences (NIMHANS)
Bengaluru, Karnataka, India

Ajay Kumar Nair PhD
Postdoctoral Research Associate
Center for Healthy Minds
University of Wisconsin
Wisconsin, USA

Ameya Patwardhan MD
Senior Resident
Department of Neurology
National Institute of Mental Health and
Neuro Sciences (NIMHANS)
Bengaluru, Karnataka, India

Arun Thejaus KP MD
Assistant Professor
Department of AYUSH
NITTE University
Mangaluru, Karnataka, India

Bharath Holla MBBS MD PDF
Assistant Professor
Department of Psychiatry and
Integrative Medicine
National Institute of Mental Health and
Neuro Sciences (NIMHANS)
Bengaluru, Karnataka, India

Bindu M Kutty PhD
Professor
Department of Neurophysiology
National Institute of Mental Health and
Neuro Sciences (NIMHANS)
Bengaluru, Karnataka, India

BV Kathyayani PhD
Professor and Principal
College of Nursing
National Institute of Mental Health and
Neuro Sciences (NIMHANS)
Bengaluru, Karnataka, India

Daniel Mintie MSW LCSW
Cognitive-Behavioral Therapist and Teacher
Complementary and Alternative Medicine Program
Georgetown University
Washington, DC, USA

Diya Chatterjee MPhil
Senior Research Fellow
Department of Clinical Psychology
National Institute of Mental Health and
Neuro Sciences (NIMHANS)
Bengaluru, Karnataka, India

Elizabeth Visceglia MD
Assistant Clinical Professor
Department of Psychiatry
Icahn School of Medicine at Mount Sinai
New York, USA

Geetha Desai PhD
Professor
Department of Psychiatry
National Institute of Mental Health and
Neuro Sciences (NIMHANS)
Bengaluru, Karnataka, India

Hariprasad VR PhD
Research Scientist
New Product Innovations
Discovery Sciences Group, R&D
The Himalaya Drug Company
Bengaluru, Karnataka, India

Hemant Bhargav MBBS MD PhD (Yoga)
Assistant Professor (Yoga)
Department of Integrative Medicine
National Institute of Mental Health and
Neuro Sciences (NIMHANS)
Bengaluru, Karnataka, India

Inbaraj G MD
PhD Scholar
Department of Neurophysiology
National Institute of Mental Health and
Neuro Sciences (NIMHANS)
Bengaluru, Karnataka, India

Contributors

Jitender Jakhar MD
Senior Resident
Department of Psychiatry
National Institute of Mental Health and
Neuro Sciences (NIMHANS)
Bengaluru, Karnataka, India

Jyotsna Agrawal PhD
Associate Professor
Department of Clinical Psychology
National Institute of Mental Health and
Neuro Sciences (NIMHANS)
Bengaluru, Karnataka, India

Kankan Gulati MPhil
Senior Research Fellow
Ayurveda, Yoga and Naturopathy, Unani,
Siddha and Homoeopathy (AYUSH)
Department of Integrative Medicine
National Institute of Mental Health and
Neuro Sciences (NIMHANS)
Bengaluru, Karnataka, India

Kaviraja Udupa PhD
Additional Professor
Department of Neurophysiology
National Institute of Mental Health and
Neuro Sciences (NIMHANS)
Bengaluru, Karnataka, India

Kishore Kumar Ramakrishna PhD
Assistant Professor (Ayurveda)
Department of Integrative Medicine
National Institute of Mental Health and
Neuro Sciences (NIMHANS)
Bengaluru, Karnataka, India

Malla Bhaskara Rao DNB (NS) FRCS
Professor
Department of Neurosurgery
National Institute of Mental Health and
Neuro Sciences (NIMHANS)
Bengaluru, Karnataka, India

Matthijs Cornelissen MD
Former Director
Indian Psychology Institute
Puducherry, India

Md Ameer Hamza PhD
Professor
Department of Psychiatric Social Work
National Institute of Mental Health and
Neuro Sciences (NIMHANS)
Bengaluru, Karnataka, India

Michael Berk PhD
Director
The Institute for Mental and Physical Health and
Clinical Translation (IMPACT)
Strategic Research Centre
Deakin University, Australia

Monojit Debnath PhD
Additional Professor
Department of Human Genetics
National Institute of Mental Health and
Neuro Sciences (NIMHANS)
Bengaluru, Karnataka, India

Muralidharan Kesavan MD
Professor
Department of Psychiatry
National Institute of Mental Health and
Neuro Sciences (NIMHANS)
Bengaluru, Karnataka, India

Nagarathna Raghuram MD FRCP
Medical Director
Division of Life Sciences
Swami Vivekananda Yoga Anusandhana
Samsthana University
Bengaluru, Karnataka, India

Narayana Manjunatha MD
Associate Professor
Department of Psychiatry
National Institute of Mental Health and
Neuro Sciences (NIMHANS)
Bengaluru, Karnataka, India

Naren P Rao MD
Additional Professor
Department of Psychiatry
National Institute of Mental Health and
Neuro Sciences (NIMHANS)
Bengaluru, Karnataka, India

Naresh Katla MSc
PhD Scholar
Swami Vivekananda Yoga Anusandhana
Samsthana University
Bengaluru, Karnataka, India

Nishitha Jasti BNYS MSc
Scientist-B (Yoga)
Department of Integrative Medicine
National Institute of Mental Health and
Neuro Sciences (NIMHANS)
Bengaluru, Karnataka, India

Nivedha Mohan Raj BTech
Senior Research Fellow
Department of Neurosurgery
National Institute of Mental Health and
Neuro Sciences (NIMHANS)
Bengaluru, Karnataka, India

P Kaushik MSc
Yoga Therapist
Department of Integrative Medicine
National Institute of Mental Health and
Neuro Sciences (NIMHANS)
Bengaluru, Karnataka, India

Palanimuthu T Sivakumar MD
Professor
Department of Psychiatry
National Institute of Mental Health and
Neuro Sciences (NIMHANS)
Bengaluru, Karnataka, India

Pooja Mailankody MD
Associate Professor
Department of Neurology
National Institute of Mental Health and
Neuro Sciences (NIMHANS)
Bengaluru, Karnataka, India

Pooja More MD
Junior Scientific Officer
Department of Integrative Medicine
National Institute of Mental Health and
Neuro Sciences (NIMHANS)
Bengaluru, Karnataka, India

Praerna H Bhargav MD
Junior Scientific Officer
Department of Integrative Medicine
National Institute of Mental Health and
Neuro Sciences (NIMHANS)
Bengaluru, Karnataka, India

Praveen Angadi MD
Senior Research Fellow
Department of Neurosurgery
National Institute of Mental Health and
Neuro Sciences (NIMHANS)
Bengaluru, Karnataka, India

Rakesh Chander MD
Senior Resident
Department of Psychiatry
National Institute of Mental Health and
Neuro Sciences (NIMHANS)
Bengaluru, Karnataka, India

Ramajayam Govindaraj PhD
Scientist-C
Centre for Consciousness Studies
Department of Neurophysiology
National Institute of Mental Health and
Neuro Sciences (NIMHANS)
Bengaluru, Karnataka, India

Rashmi Arasappa MD
Assistant Professor
Department of Psychiatry
National Institute of Mental Health and
Neuro Sciences (NIMHANS)
Bengaluru, Karnataka, India

Rima Dada PhD
Professor
Department of Anatomy
All India Institute of Medical Sciences
New Delhi, India

Sanchari Mukhopadhyay MD
Senior Resident (Psychiatry)
Department of Integrative Medicine
National Institute of Mental Health and
Neuro Sciences (NIMHANS)
Bengaluru, Karnataka, India

Sanju George MBBS FRCPsych
Senior Clinical Psychiatrist and
Professor of Psychiatry and Psychology
Rajagiri College of Social Sciences
Kochi, Kerala, India

Sathyaprabha TN PhD
Professor and Head
Department of Neurophysiology
National Institute of Mental Health and
Neuro Sciences (NIMHANS)
Bengaluru, Karnataka, India

Shalu Abraham MD
Senior Resident (Psychiatry)
Department of Integrative Medicine
National Institute of Mental Health and
Neuro Sciences (NIMHANS)
Bengaluru, Karnataka, India

Shantala Hegde PhD
Associate Professor
Department of Clinical Psychology
National Institute of Mental Health and
Neuro Sciences (NIMHANS)
Bengaluru, Karnataka, India

Contributors

Shiva Shanker Reddy Mukku DM
Senior Resident
Department of Psychiatry
National Institute of Mental Health and
Neuro Sciences (NIMHANS)
Bengaluru, Karnataka, India

Shivarama Varambally MD MAMS DSc
Professor of Psychiatry and Head
Department of Integrative Medicine
National Institute of Mental Health and
Neuro Sciences (NIMHANS)
Bengaluru, Karnataka, India

Shree Raksha Bhide MSc
Yoga Therapist
Central Council for Research in
Yoga and Naturopathy (CCRYN)
Department of Integrative Medicine
National Institute of Mental Health and
Neuro Sciences (NIMHANS)
Bengaluru, Karnataka, India

Shubha Bhat MSc
Junior Research Fellow
Department of Neurology
National Institute of Mental Health and
Neuro Sciences (NIMHANS)
Bengaluru, Karnataka, India

Shubham Sharma MSc
Yoga Therapist
Department of Integrative Medicine
National Institute of Mental Health and
Neuro Sciences (NIMHANS)
Bengaluru, Karnataka, India

Sneha J Karmani DNB
Consultant Psychiatrist
Aditya Birla Memorial Hospital
Pune, Maharashtra, India

Sowjanya Dumbala BNYS
Senior Research Fellow, AYUSH
Department of Integrative Medicine
National Institute of Mental Health and
Neuro Sciences (NIMHANS)
Bengaluru, Karnataka, India

Sujan MU MD
Assistant Professor
Department of Yoga
JSS Academy of Higher Education and Research
Mysuru, Karnataka, India

Suman Bista MSc
Junior Research Fellow
Department of Integrative Medicine
National Institute of Mental Health and
Neuro Sciences (NIMHANS)
Bengaluru, Karnataka, India

Sumana Venugopal MD
Research Associate
Department of Integrative Medicine
National Institute of Mental Health and
Neuro Sciences (NIMHANS)
Bengaluru, Karnataka, India

Sundarnag Ganjekar MD
Associate Professor
Department of Psychiatry
National Institute of Mental Health and
Neuro Sciences (NIMHANS)
Bengaluru, Karnataka, India

Tarachand Joshi MD
Senior Resident
Department of Neurology
National Institute of Mental Health and
Neuro Sciences (NIMHANS)
Bengaluru, Karnataka, India

TM Srinivasan PhD DSc
Professor
Division of Physical Sciences
Swami Vivekananda Yoga Anusandhana
Samsthana (S-VYASA) University
Bengaluru, Karnataka, India

Umesh Chikkanna MD
Scientist-C (Ayurveda)
Department of Integrative Medicine
National Institute of Mental Health and
Neuro Sciences (NIMHANS)
Bengaluru, Karnataka, India

Urvakhsh Meherwan Mehta MD PhD
Associate Professor
Department of Psychiatry
National Institute of Mental Health and
Neuro Sciences (NIMHANS)
Bengaluru, Karnataka, India

Usha Rani MR MD
Research Officer, CCRYN
Department of Integrative Medicine
National Institute of Mental Health and
Neuro Sciences (NIMHANS)
Bengaluru, Karnataka, India

Vanteemar S Sreeraj MBBS DPM DNB
Clinician Scientist/Assistant Professor
Department of Psychiatry
National Institute of Mental Health and
Neuro Sciences (NIMHANS)
Bengaluru, Karnataka, India

Venkata Lakshmi Narasimha MD PDF DM
Senior Resident
Centre for Addiction Medicine
National Institute of Mental Health and
Neuro Sciences (NIMHANS)
Bengaluru, Karnataka, India

Venkataram Shivakumar PhD
Scientist-D (Psychiatry)
Department of Integrative Medicine
National Institute of Mental Health and
Neuro Sciences (NIMHANS)
Bengaluru, Karnataka, India

Vijay Kumar KG MD
Assistant Professor
Department of Psychiatry
National Institute of Mental Health and
Neuro Sciences (NIMHANS)
Bengaluru, Karnataka, India

Vinod Kumar MD
Research Officer, CCRYN
Department of Integrative Medicine
National Institute of Mental Health and
Neuro Sciences (NIMHANS)
Bengaluru, Karnataka, India

Message From Chairperson

Healthy people make a healthy society, and there can be no two opinions about the transformational potential of health promotion in building a healthy society. Recent clinical, epidemiological and Psycho-Neuro-Immuno-Endocrinological (PNIE) research leaves no room for any doubt regarding the bidirectional relationship between mind and body, and the significance of mind health in determining overall health of a person. Mind-Body Medicine is an evidence-based approach that combines the power of traditional knowledge of yoga and Meditation with modern psychology and medicine and has great potential to evolve as affordable scalable foundation of healthcare truly reflective of the spirit of health promotion, i.e. enabling people to increase control over and to improve their health. It can also be viewed as a useful vehicle to popularize 'mind' interventions and thereby reduction of stigma associated with mind issues. Our national medical association Indian Psychiatric Society (IPS) constituted the Task Force on Mind-Body Medicine in 2019 to respond to these challenges and to harness the opportunities to contribute to public health.

Translation of Mind-Body Medicine into mainstream practice in India faces the challenge of developing suitable training programs and availability of teaching material not only for medical students and practitioners but for the spectrum of healthcare professionals which in this case extends to psychologists, paramedics, practitioners of traditional medicine, teachers of Yoga and Meditation, volunteers and last but not the least, patients themselves. Publication of this book, first of its kind in the Indian context, is not only an opportunity to disseminate scientific knowledge about yoga but is a solid step towards developing source material for training programs.

On behalf of the Task Force on Mind-Body Medicine, it is my pleasant duty to put on record our appreciation and gratitude towards all the contributors of this pioneering work for their effort, which we are sure will inspire several colleagues to not only advance research but to build this movement of "Health for All and All for Health" in the true spirit of health promotion.

Sanjay Phadke MD DPM
Chairperson
IPS's Task Force on Mind-Body Medicine

Message From Publication Committee

The Publication Committee of Indian Psychiatric Society has lately been proactive in providing a vibrant platform for expression of the talent, wisdom and knowledge of its esteemed members. Such a platform provides larger circulation to the insights gained by our fraternity through constant pursuit of expanding the limits of knowledge, especially when it gets associated with the professional expertise of established publishing houses. With this perspective in mind, we are happy to be able to bring out a book on the science and art of yoga for psychiatric and neurological disorders.

Yoga has its roots in Indian soil and psyche. The whole international community acknowledges it and in fact Yoga provides one of our several respectable identities. Simply translated, Yoga refers to the process of union, i.e. union between the mundane and the divine, and union between the *Jivatma* and the *Paramatma*. This book has attempted to provide a glimpse of the union between the science and art of yoga, especially from the perspective of psychiatric and neurological disorders. In fact, it should be our privilege as well as our responsibility to explore various facets of this union and bring it in the public domain. There cannot be a better place and center to explore this dimension than our very own institute of national importance, the National Institute of Mental Health and Neuro Sciences (NIMHANS), Bengaluru, Karnataka, India. This, of-course, is the beginning and the journey has a long way to go before it reaches its ever-evasive destination. Integration of yoga-based therapies into the mainstream, comprehensive and integrated approaches of therapies for alleviation of human sufferings, is extremely important. We congratulate Professor Shivarama Varambally, his editorial team members and esteemed authors for adding not only a book but also a new dimension to the bookshelf of the Indian Psychiatric Society (IPS).

We hope and are also confident that this book shall prove a stepping stone in that direction.

Message From the President

Yoga, which is a gift of ancient Indian wisdom, is a psychobiological endeavor to connect body and mind, individual and universe, and material and divine. We feel proud that our sages made sincere efforts to understand the psychobiological enigma and intricacies of human life and successfully tried to address the problems of multidimensional connect by inventing yoga, which has tools and methods to address simultaneously not only body, but also the psyche and the spirit.

Indian Psychiatric Society (IPS) has always believed in multidimensionality of mental health and addressing its needs comprehensively. We have always included science sessions on Yoga in our academic meetings. Our journal has given sufficient importance to it by publishing research and review articles, and also bringing out one dedicated supplement. It is true that science of psychiatry has developed a common international language but the regional and cultural wisdom is also important, and it is our duty to make sincere scientific efforts to validate and incorporate them in the main stream for the benefits of one and all.

The IPS lauds the praiseworthy scientific endeavors of the National Institute of Mental Health and Neuro Sciences (NIMHANS), Bengaluru, Karnataka, India, in this regard and congratulates the learned editors and authors for their commitments and contributions. We hope that *The Science and Art of Yoga in Mental and Neurological Healthcare* will have a wide readership and influence on clinical practice in India and abroad.

PK Dalal	**Gautam Saha**	**TS Sathyanarayana Rao**
President	Vice-President	Hony General Secretary

Indian Psychiatric Society (IPS)

Foreword

The Department of Integrative Medicine at National Institute of Mental Health and Neuro Sciences (NIMHANS) in its first Avatar as the NIMHANS Integrated Centre for Yoga has been working steadily on applying yoga for mental health disorders. The research conducted in this center for nearly two decades has answered several burning questions. Yoga has formed a convincing place in the treatment of several common and even severe mental disorders, either with or without medications. The staffs have standardized packages, individualized to different illnesses. The mechanisms of action of yoga have also been examined. Yoga brings about neurological changes that are associated with its therapeutic effects.

In this book, the team has gathered very scholarly chapters from internationally known experts in yoga and mental health. This is indeed a treasure that will help all who promote yoga for mental health. The articles are based on available literature evidence, thus making the information highly 'evidence-based'. The efforts are indeed commendable.

I congratulate not just the contributors but also the editorial team. Indian Psychiatric Society (IPS) has always been encouraging on all our yoga-related academic endeavors. I recall the support given by the then Editor of Indian Journal of Psychiatry (Professor TS Sathyanarayana Rao) to bring out a special supplement on yoga in 2013. This effort now to support a book on *The Science and Art of Yoga in Mental and Neurological Healthcare* is yet another example that we thankfully acknowledge. I wish all the users to get the best benefit from this book, and also become enthused to use yoga in the care of individuals with such conditions.

BN Gangadhar MD DSc
Senior Professor (Psychiatry) and Director
National Institute of Mental Health and
Neuro Sciences (NIMHANS)
Program Director
NIMHANS Integrated Centre for Yoga
Bengaluru, Karnataka, India

Foreword

The word "Yoga" was first mentioned in the oldest sacred Indian text *Rig Veda*. The yogic tradition in India can be traced back to the Indus-Saraswati Valley Civilization in Northern India over 5000 years ago. However, it was systematized as a practice by the great sage *Maharishi Patanjali* through his *Patanjali Yoga Sutras*. Earlier, it was considered to be a mystic practice only for saints and sages who were detached from worldly desires. With changing times, this tradition of yoga is now being accepted by a wide majority of people and has achieved worldwide acceptance. Apart from *Patanjali Yoga Sutras* (calling it as *Raja Yoga*), Swami Vivekananda brought out the other three dimensions of Yoga as *Jnana Yoga* based on Upanishadic wisdom base, *Bhakti Yoga* based on *Narada Bhakti Sutras* and *Karma Yoga* using the teachings in *Bhagavad Gita*. From the taboo of a mystic practice, yoga is now considered as a science of holistic living to achieve health and wealth, happiness and bliss, as also efficiency, peace and poise. The benefits of yoga are well recognized, and it has widespread applications to meet the challenges of our modern era including therapeutic indications.

The National Institute of Mental Health and Neuro Sciences (NIMHANS) is pioneer in research pertaining to the field of neurosciences. It is indeed exciting that an "Institute of National Importance" has come forward with evidence to support this age-old Indian tradition. This would be a new beginning in the field of integrative medicine which can help lessen the bridge between modern medicine and traditional systems of medicine in India.

In this book, *The Science and Art of Yoga in Mental and Neurological Healthcare*, the authors have taken great effort to bring forth the scientific evidence of integrated approach of yoga therapy in most of the mental health and neurological conditions. Most of the psychotherapeutic approaches followed in India have been adapted from western literature based on the evidence base. An attempt to have systematic evidence for an indigenous psychotherapeutic approach-like yogic counseling may help in overcoming many hurdles that we face in the field of psychotherapy in India today. It must be noticed that yoga in its entirety is included as a therapy by including even the role of yogic counseling in such conditions.

A section of the book, *"Neurobiological Dimensions"*, has been dedicated to explain in detail the brain correlates and the proposed mechanism of action of bringing balance at all levels by yoga definitely gives the readers a keen interest in knowing Yoga in relation to the neurophysiological changes in the brain and the psycho-neuro-immunological axis (PNI axis). Further on, in section *"Yoga for Clinical Conditions"*, each disorder has been individually described in separate chapters in the light of both yogic knowledge and modern science with a Case Vignette at the end. Each chapter displays a comprehensive compilation of the existing evidence of yoga practices in various disorders, especially the non-communicable diseases (NCDs), which gives an insight into the type of practices that may be of relevance for that particular illness. Interestingly, each chapter also has a part on "Yoga Clinical Insights" which emphasizes the practical challenges and difficulties that the therapist may face while dealing with this section of patients. This is particularly of great value to yoga therapists that will give them a clear picture of what are the Do's and Don'ts in each set of patients.

Apart from explaining the theoretical aspect of yoga, the special yoga practices that have been proven to be effective for various illnesses have been compiled to individual modules for each illness in the Appendix of the book. It has been tabulated with specific details of the *asanas*, the number of repetitions and the time spent in each pose which has been sequenced according to the Yoga experts. Special and advanced techniques including *kriyas*, breathing practices, *pranayama*, meditation, practices of emotion culture, etc., taking into consideration the needs of each age group have been presented accordingly. These modules can provide a template for yoga therapists throughout India and abroad to modify their practices according to the needs of their clients. It can also be evolved as a textbook for medical practitioners.

The last section of the book focuses on Preventive and Health Promotive Aspects of Yoga with chapters on "Yoga for Caregivers", "Yoga for Positive Mental Health", and "Tele-Yoga in Mental Health". The chapter on Tele-Yoga provides the way ahead and makes us realize the immense advantage of technology which is a boon in these days of COVID-19. This online platform for yoga therapy can help in overcoming many hurdles patients face in terms of transportation, supervision and convenience, so that the advantages of this practice can be imparted to a greater audience.

In summary, Yoga, which is an immortal cultural outcome of India, has now become a subject of scientific curiosity paving ways to new discoveries and treatment of various illnesses. The book would definitely be a great addition to the knowledge of integrative medicine and would serve as an important easy to use handbook for yoga therapists dealing with patients suffering from common psychiatric and neurological conditions. The editors should be credited for their efforts to produce a comprehensive manual on collating the knowledge of the Science and Art of Yoga in Mental and Neurological Healthcare.

HR Nagendra PhD
Chancellor
Swami Vivekananda Yoga Anusandhana
Samsthana (S-VYASA) University
Bengaluru, Karnataka, India

Preface

The past few decades have seen a momentous change in the outlook for treatment of neuropsychiatric disorders. The initial optimism in the second half of the 20th century with the advent of new pharmacological agents for psychiatric disorders slowly gave way to an understanding that these agents, while certainly more refined than the earlier drugs, could not really change the long-term prognosis of these disorders and were not devoid of adverse effects either. The biopsychosocial conceptualization of the major psychiatric disorders also emphasized that effective treatment should not be unidimensional. Therefore, multidisciplinary teams and inputs became very important in management of such disorders, and this also brought to the fore the traditional healthcare approaches in which a systemic approach looking at the person as a whole is emphasized. These approaches, which are classified under the rubric of Complementary and Alternative Medicine (CAM), are extensively utilized across the globe, more so in the developing world, for a host of psychiatric and neurological disorders.

Yoga is one of these healthcare approaches, and in the past three decades there has been an increasing volume of scientific evidence to suggest that yoga-based interventions can be effective along with modern medicines and in some cases as a sole treatment. Although yoga originated as one of the six *"darsanas"* or systems of philosophy of ancient India and not as a therapeutic intervention, the application of Yoga to mitigate psychiatric disorders in not new. The *Yoga Sutras* of *Patanjali* introduces Yoga as *citta vritti nirodhah*; practice of Yoga as a means to calm an unruly mind, its rumination and regurgitation of the past and a possible ominous future which destabilizes the body-mind complex and creates many psychiatric problems. Thus, integrating Yoga practices in daily life could bring not just health but open doors to higher levels of creativity and maturity in emotional interaction with one's family, society and the world at large.

In addition to clinical effects, several putative neurobiological mechanisms underlying the effects of Yoga in neuropsychiatric disorders have been demonstrated ranging from neurophysiological measures of autonomic function to changes in neurotransmitter levels and brain imaging parameters. This book, *The Science and Art of Yoga in Mental and Neurological Healthcare*, attempts to bring the reader abreast of these developments and presents a comprehensive as well as practical approach to the use of Yoga as a therapeutic approach in psychiatric and neurological disorders. We view that this book primarily as a manual for the use of Yoga in the care of psychiatric and neurological conditions rather than as a comprehensive textbook.

The initial chapters aim to give the reader a brief introduction to Yoga, the yogic concept of counseling, and the role of Yoga in traditional and modern healthcare in India. The section on Neurobiological Dimensions of Yoga aims to explain the basic concepts which are needed to understand the multilayered effects of yoga in different psychiatric and neurological disorders as well as the various techniques which have been used to unravel these mechanisms. The subsequent chapters on the role of yoga and the current status of evidence in various psychiatric and neurological disorders form the core of this manual and are written by authors who have carried out original research work in the specific area. The final chapters focus on the role of yoga for caregivers of patients with neuropsychiatric disorders, the contribution of yoga to Positive Mental Health (which is critical in these troubled times), and Tele-Yoga, which seems set to occupy a central place in the future of yoga therapy.

Of course, we realize that knowledge is ever-expanding and we are fallible at the best of times. We acknowledge that we may not have covered all the information available and that there may be gaps and deficiencies in this book. We request the readers' forgiveness for the same and hope that within these limitations, this will serve as a guide to professionals in Yoga and Mental Health in their noble quest to help patients and families suffering from mental and neurological disorders.

We are deeply grateful to all the authors and contributors, and we are particularly thankful to Dr Vinay Kumar from the Indian Psychiatric Society (IPS) who was instrumental in bringing out this book in the present form. We also thank all the office-bearers of the IPS, as well as M/s Jaypee Bothers Medical Publishers, New Delhi, India, for making this dream come true. Of course, we owe the greatest debt of gratitude to our Gurus, Professor BN Gangadhar, Professor D Nagaraja and Dr HR Nagendra, who have been the torchbearers in throwing light on the potential of yoga in neuropsychiatric disorders.

Yogena cittasya padena vacam *Malam sarirasya ca vaidyakena* *Yopakarottam pravaram muninam* *Patanjalim pranjaliranato'smi*	I bow down to him who purifies the impurities of the Mind by Yoga, purifies the expression of speech by grammar, and purifies the impurities of the body by Medical Science. He, who is an expert in removing the impurities of the Body, Mind and Speech, to that most excellent of *Munis, Patanjali,* I bow down with folded hands.

Shivarama Varambally
Sanju George
TM Srinivasan
Hemant Bhargav

Acknowledgments

The editors wish to thank the management and staff of M/s Jaypee Brothers Medical Publishers (P) Ltd, New Delhi, India, for their excellent work in bringing this book to light. We particularly would like to thank Dr Savleen Kaur (Development Editor) for her prompt and enthusiastic help in this regard. We would also thank the Indian Psychiatric Society (IPS) and the Publication Committee of the IPS headed by Professor PK Singh for encouraging and helping us to publish the book. Particular thanks are due to Dr Vinay Kumar for his constant encouragement and also inspiring the title of the book. We wish to particularly acknowledge the beautiful and selfless artistic contributions of Dr Nishitha Jasti who has designed the art for the cover page and the section separators in the book. The book would not have been possible without help from National Institute of Mental Health and Neuro Sciences (NIMHANS), beginning with our inspiring Director and Professor BN Gangadhar and extending to the entire administration of the Institute who have been very cooperative. We are deeply grateful to all the authors from the various departments of NIMHANS, Swami Vivekananda Yoga Anusandhana Samsthana (S-VYASA) University, and authors from other institutes in India and abroad, who have contributed their extensive expertise, and completed the chapters within the given time.

We wish to acknowledge the Central Council for Research in Yoga and Naturopathy (CCRYN), Ministry of AYUSH, Government of India for setting up the CCRYN-NIMHANS Collaborative Centre (16-30/2015/CCRYN/CRC/NIMHANS) under which much of the research work covered in this book, has been carried out.

Contents

Section 1: Yoga in Health Care

1. Introduction to Yoga 3
   *Hemant Bhargav, Ramajayam Govindaraj,
   P Kaushik, Nagarathna Raghuram*

2. Basic Concepts of Counseling as per Vedic Literature 13
   *Hemant Bhargav, Nishitha Jasti, Shree Raksha Bhide,
   Kishore Kumar Ramakrishna*

3. From Many to One to Many: The Wheel Completes a
   Cycle for Integrative Approaches in Mental Health 24
   Bharath Holla, Hemant Bhargav, Kishore Kumar Ramakrishna

Section 2: Neurobiological Dimensions

4. Neurophysiology of Yoga 33
   Kaviraja Udupa, Inbaraj G, Sathyaprabha TN

5. Neurophysiology of Meditation 44
   Ajay Kumar Nair, Bindu M Kutty

6. Role of Neuroimaging in Understanding Mental Health Effects of Yoga 51
   Vanteemar S Sreeraj, Venkataram Shivakumar, Vijay Kumar KG, Naren P Rao

7. Role of Transcranial Magnetic Stimulation in Yoga Research 60
   Ramajayam Govindaraj, Jitender Jakhar, Urvakhsh Meherwan Mehta

8. Insights into Mode of Action of Yoga in Mental Disorders:
   A Summary of Biological Evidence 68
   Monojit Debnath, Rima Dada, Michael Berk

Section 3: Yoga for Clinical Conditions

9. General Guidelines for Yoga Therapy 79
   Hemant Bhargav, Shivarama Varambally

10. Yoga Therapy for Depression 87
    Praerna H Bhargav, Sneha J Karmani, Muralidharan Kesavan

11. Yoga for Anxiety Disorders 100
    Pooja More, Rakesh Chander, Narayana Manjunatha, Daniel Mintie

12. Yoga in Obsessive Compulsive Disorder 111
    Sanchari Mukhopadhyay, Nishitha Jasti, Shubha Bhat, Shubham Sharma

13. Yoga Therapy for Schizophrenia 118
    Elizabeth Visceglia, Rashmi Arasappa, Ramajayam Govindaraj

14. Evidence for Efficacy of Yoga in Geriatric Psychiatry 126
    *Palanimuthu T Sivakumar, Shiva Shanker Reddy Mukku,
    Hariprasad VR, BV Kathyayani*

15. Yoga for Childhood and Adolescent Psychiatric Disorders 137
    Shalu Abraham, Rashmi Arasappa, Kankan Gulati, Umesh Chikkanna

16. Yoga for Substance Use Disorders 152
    *Venkata Lakshmi Narasimha, Sumana Venugopal,
    Bharath Holla, Hemant Bhargav*

17. Yoga in Chronic Pain Syndromes 165
    Sowjanya Dumbala, Kankan Gulati, Sundarnag Ganjekar, Geetha Desai

18. Yoga for Low Back Pain 176
    Ameya Patwardhan, Vinod Kumar, Tarachand Joshi, Suman Bista

19. Yoga for Migraine 186
    Usha Rani MR, Sujan MU, Kaviraja Udupa, Sathyaprabha TN

20. Yoga in Parkinson's Disease 197
    Diya Chatterjee, Shantala Hegde, Arun Thejaus KP, Pooja Mailankody

21. Yoga for Epilepsy 205
    Praveen Angadi, Nivedha Mohan Raj, Malla Bhaskara Rao

Section 4: Other Important Aspects of Yoga

22. Yoga for Caregivers 217
    Aarti Jagannathan, Md Ameer Hamza, Naresh Katla

23. Yoga and Positive Mental Health 221
    Jyotsna Agrawal, Matthijs Cornelissen

24. Looking Ahead: Tele-Yoga in Mental Health 228
    *Sanchari Mukhopadhyay, Nishitha Jasti,
    Venkataram Shivakumar, Aarti Jagannathan*

Appendix 1: Yoga Therapy Modules for Common Neuropsychiatric Disorders

1.1 Validated Yoga Module for Depression 241

1.2 Validated Yoga Module for Generalized Anxiety Disorder 243

1.3 Validated Yoga Module for Obsessive Compulsive Disorder 245

1.4 Validated Yoga Module for Schizophrenia 247

1.5 Validated Yoga Module for Bipolar Affective Disorder 249

1.6 Validated Yoga Module for Older Adults 253

1.7	Yoga Module for Attention Deficit Hyperactivity Disorder	255
1.8	Yoga Module for Autism Spectrum Disorder	257
1.9	Validated Yoga Module for Opioid Use Disorder/ Substance Use Disorders	260
1.10	Validated Yoga Module for Somatoform Pain Disorder	263
1.11	Validated Yoga Module for Low Back Pain	265
1.12	Validated Yoga Module for Migraine	267
1.13	Validated Yoga Module for Parkinson's Disease	270
1.14	Validated Yoga Module for Epilepsy	272
1.15	Validated Yoga Module for Caregivers of Patients with Schizophrenia	274
1.16	Tele-Yoga Module for Stress Reduction	275
1.17	Guided Yogic Relaxation (GYR)	276

Index *279*

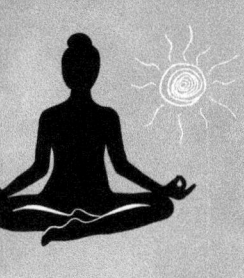

SECTION 1

Yoga in Health Care

1. **Introduction to Yoga**
   *Hemant Bhargav, Ramajayam Govindaraj,
   P Kaushik, Nagarathna Raghuram*

2. **Basic Concepts of Counseling as per Vedic Literature**
   *Hemant Bhargav, Nishitha Jasti, Shree Raksha Bhide,
   Kishore Kumar Ramakrishna*

3. **From Many to One to Many: The Wheel Completes a Cycle for Integrative Approaches in Mental Health**
   Bharath Holla, Hemant Bhargav, Kishore Kumar Ramakrishna

CHAPTER 1

Introduction to Yoga

Hemant Bhargav, Ramajayam Govindaraj, P Kaushik, Nagarathna Raghuram

INTRODUCTION

The term yoga is derived from the Sanskrit word "yuj" meaning to unite; the union of the individual self with the supreme self. Yoga is one among the six major systems of philosophy (*ṣaḍdarśanas*) that emerged in ancient India. These included *Sankhya, Yoga, Nyaya, Vaisheshika, Purva Mimamsa,* and *Uttara Mimamsa*. These are also called as *astika* (orthodox) *darshanas* as they believe the *Vedas* as the authoritative text.

Yoga (along with various physical postures or asanas) that has got recent attention globally, can be traced back to the *Vedic* period. Since then, it has undergone various modifications and what we know as yoga today is vastly different from the way yoga was originally practiced.

Given below is a brief look at the evolution of yoga (**Fig. 1**).

VEDIC PERIOD (2000 BC AND EARLIER)

The word yoga has been used broadly in the *Vedic* literature with different meanings to it. The *Rig Veda*, oldest amongst the *Vedas*, uses the word as "*yunajmi*"[1] which means the fire oblations given to the Gods. Further, the *Atharva Veda* mentions *ashtayoga* and *shatyoga*,[2] i.e., yoga of eight facets and six facets which interpret as acquiring the unacquired. Concepts such as *ahimsa* (nonviolence), *satya* (truthfulness), *asteya* (nonstealing), *brahmacharya* (conduct consistent with Brahman), *tapas* (austerity), *swadhayaya* (introspection), and *ishvara pranidhana* (surrender to higher principle/consciousness) which are all part of *ashtanga yoga* today can be traced back to *Atharva Veda*. Hence, it may be said that different methods employed for self-advancement in the *Vedic* period have contributed to the development of yoga.

PRECLASSICAL PERIOD (1500–700 BC)

Upanishads, which are the essence of the *Vedas*, clearly describe Yoga. For example, *Kathopanishad* defines yoga as: "When the sense organs are controlled and the mind achieves a state of steadiness, this state is called Yoga."[3] However, understanding of Yoga

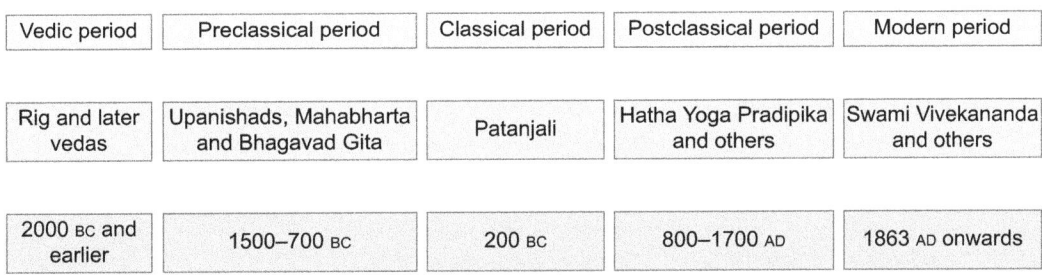

Fig. 1: Evolution of yoga.

in *Upanishadic* literature was more concerned with practices which focused on philosophy and contemplation on the soul (*ātman* or Real-Self).

Bhagavad Gita (BG) discusses yoga extensively. Almost every chapter's name has the term "yoga". But the yoga of Bhagavad Gita is more of a lifestyle and behavioral modification rather than breathing or posture-related practice. The most popular discussions on yoga which are very relevant even in modern times are related to excellence in work, equilibrium of mind, and moderation in activities—excellence in work means doing any work efficiently without attachment toward the fruits of the action (*karmasukauśalaṁ*; BG 2.50);[4] equilibrium (*samatvaṁ*; BG 2.48) of mind,[4] which is a balanced state where adversities and achievements are viewed equally as an enriching experience; moderation means avoiding extremes in eating and fasting, sleeping and waking, activity and rest (*yuktā*; BG 6.17).[4]

CLASSICAL PERIOD (200 BC)

During the classical period, Patanjali compiled 196 sutras (aphorisms) of yoga. Patanjali's view on yoga is known as *Raja Yoga* or *Ashtanga Yoga* or classical yoga. Patanjali begins his treatise by defining the word "yoga" in his second sutra:

योगश्चित्तवृत्तिनिरोधः ॥ २ ॥
yogaścitta-vṛtti-nirodhaḥ
– Patanjali Yoga Sutras 1.2[5]

K Taimni translates it as "Yoga is the inhibition (*nirodhaḥ*) of the modifications (*vṛtti*) of the mind (*citta*)." Swami Vivekananda translates the sutra as "Yoga is restraining the mind—stuff (*citta*) from taking various forms (*vṛtti*)." **Table 1** provides some popular definitions of Yoga according to yogic texts.

The eight limbs of Yoga described by Patanjali are: *yama* (abstinences), *niyama* (observances), *asana* (yoga postures), *pranayama* (breath control), *pratyahara* (withdrawal of the senses), *dharana* (concentration), *dhyana* (meditation), and *samadhi* (absorption). Although Patanjali added physical postures and regulation of the breath to yoga, the sutras do not have any named *asanas* or *pranayama* implying the use of such tools that involve body and breath, for calming the mind only. **Table 2** provides an overview of the eight limbs of Yoga according to Patanjali.

POSTCLASSICAL PERIOD (800–1700 AD)

The *Rishis* (ancient sages) during this period gave yoga a new outlook by giving greater importance to the *asanas, kriyas,* and *pranayama* for cleansing of the body and

TABLE 1: Popular definitions of yoga according to yogic texts.

S. No.	Definition of yoga	Meaning	Reference
1.	Yogaścitta-vṛtti-nirodhaḥ	Yoga is the mastery over modifications of the mind	Patanjali Yoga Sutra 1.2[5]
2.	Samatvam yoga uchyate	Yoga is equanimity of the mind (in success and failure)	Bhagavad Gita 2.48[4]
3.	Manah Prashamanopayah yoga ityabhidhiyate	Yoga is a subtle technique to calm down the mind	Yoga Vashishtha 3:9:32[6]
4.	Yogah karmasu kaushalam	Yoga is excellence in action	Bhagavad Gita 2.50[4]
5.	Duhkha-samyoga-viyogam yoga-samjnitam	Yoga is that which severs the connection with sorrow	Bhagavad Gita 6.23[4]
6.	Yuktahara-viharasya yukta-cheshtasya karmasu Yukta-svapna-avabodhasya yogo-bhavati dukhaha	Yoga is the destroyer of the sufferings for the one who observes moderation in eating, sleeping, recreation, and work	Bhagavad Gita 6.17[4]

TABLE 2: An overview of the eight limbs of yoga according to Patanjali.

S. No.	Limb of yoga	Definition according to Patanjali[5]	Purpose
1.	Yama (PYS:2.30)	Five ethical precepts: *Satya* (Truth), *Ahimsa* (Nonviolence), *Bramhacharya* (Sense organ control), *Asteya* (Nonstealing) and *Aparigraha* (Nonhoarding)	• Individual observances • Control over lower instincts
2.	Niyama (PYS:2.32)	Five individual observances: *Shoucha* (Cleanliness), *Santosha* (Satisfaction), *Tapas* (Austerity or perseverance), *Swadhyaya* (Self-introspection) and *Ishvara Pranidhana* (Surrender to a higher principle/consciousness)	• Promoting higher order • Social and spiritual behaviors
3.	Asana (PYS:2.46)	*Sthira sukham asanam:* An asana is a posture that is steady and pleasant	Achieving stillness of the body
4.	Pranayama (PYS:2.49) prana (breath) and āyāma (restraining, or stretching)	*Tasmin Sati swasa-praswasa-yor-gati-vichhedah pranayamah:* In that state of being in asana or posture, breaking the movement of inspiratory or expiratory breath is regulation of breath	Achieving minimum possible rate of breathing and fluctuations in breath
5.	Pratyahara (PYS:2.54) prati ("against" or "contra") and ahara ("bring near, fetch")	*Sva vishaya asamprayoge chittasya svarupe anukarah iva indriyanam pratyaharah:* Learn to withdraw the mind from physical senses; freed from its ties to outer objects, the mind can arrive at its own real nature	Turning the consciousness inward
6.	Dharana (PYS:3.1)	*Desha-bandhah chittasya dharana*: Locking the mind on an object is focus	Develop an ability to focus the mind
7.	Dhyana (PYS:3.2)	*Tatra pratyaya-ikatanata dhyanam:* Effortless flow of consciousness toward the object of focus is fixation	Expansion of consciousness
8.	Samadhi (PYS:3.3)	*Tadeva artha matra nirbhasam svarupa shunyam iva samadhih:* Then the observer dissolves and the true nature of the object shines forth	Dissolution of observer and deeper insight into one's own nature

mind. This is popular as *Hatha yoga* where "Ha" means the "Sun" and "Tha" means the "Moon". It is described as a set of yogic techniques which focusses on aligning the physical body and energies of an individual in tune with nature. *Hatha yoga* practices aim at harmonizing the biorhythms within the individual (body, breath, emotion, and intellect) with that of the nature. Some popular texts related to *Hatha yoga* are *Hatha Yoga Pradipika, Gheranda Samhita, Hatha Rathnavali, Shiva Samhita, Goraksha Samhita,* and *Siddha Siddhanta Paddhati.*

MODERN PERIOD (FROM 1863 AD ONWARDS)

Yoga philosophy was introduced to the rest of the world by Swami Vivekananda in his historic speech at the Parliament of Religions in Chicago (9th September, 1893). Many yogis like Maharishi Mahesh Yogi, Paramahansa Yogananda, and Ramana Maharshi influenced the Western world profoundly through their spiritual accomplishments and gradually yoga was accepted throughout the world as a secular spiritual practice rather than a ritual-based religious doctrine. In recent times, yoga masters like T Krishnamacharya (and his three disciples, BKS Iyengar, Pattabhi Jois, and TVK Desikachar), Swami Kuvalayananda, Swami Shivananda, Baba Ramdev, Sadhguru Jaggi Vasudev, Guru Sri Sri Ravishankar, and many others have popularized yoga globally. In the last two decades, yoga became immensely popular. Its popularity reached new heights when 21st June was proclaimed as the "International Day of Yoga" in the United Nations General Assembly in 2014, and first International day of yoga was celebrated in 2015.

WHAT YOGA IS NOT?

With the rise in popularity, understanding of the essence of yoga got diluted. Majority of the population started understanding yoga as merely physical. To understand what is not yoga, let's consider this example. Let us assume that there are four people approaching a yoga teacher to learn yoga for various reasons: A young athletic person, a middle-aged person who is morbidly obese, a patient who underwent a surgery a week ago, and an 80-year-old person. Who do we think will perform yoga better? This question has been asked to various audiences (including yoga practitioners) and most of the time the answer was—the young athletic guy. Why do we think so? Let us go back to the definition of Yoga as stated by Maharishi Patanjali: *yogaś-citta-vṛtti-nirodhaḥ* || 2 ||

According to this, yoga is the ability to direct the mind exclusively toward an object and sustain that attention without any distraction. The object can be a concrete one, either external to ourselves or part of ourselves. It can be an area of interest, a concept, or something beyond the level of the senses, such as God.

With this definition in mind, let us ask ourselves the question again. We will then understand the gap between the actual definition of yoga and the yoga we perceive, practice, and teach today. Although there are some practical reasons for us to tweak the definition, especially in a therapeutic context either towards the physical spectrum or mental spectrum, it is important to have the generic comprehensive definition of Yoga in the background, to make it beneficial to humanity without any differences merely based on physical flexibility, age, disease state, etc. as illustrated in the above example.

CLARIFYING THE MISUNDERSTANDINGS

Is Yoga only Asana?

In the entire *Yoga Sutras* of Patanjali, there is not even a single named asana or pranayama, although majority of the public including many yoga practitioners emphasize more on yogasana or pranayama, and consider it as yoga.

Let us understand the two important components of yoga: asana and pranayama, to get more insight into what is not yoga. Let us talk about asana first. Typically, asana is practiced in three steps: (1) attaining the posture, (2) maintaining the posture steadily and comfortably, and (3) releasing the posture. Asana practice involves bodily movements similar to physical exercise. But the key components of this asana practice unlike exercise are alertness without tension and relaxation without dullness or heaviness. Further Maharishi Patanjali explained "asana as steady and comfortable posture." Here, the steps 1 and 3 are not considered asana. Maintenance of steady comfortable posture is asana. It is important to understand why maintaining the posture steadily and comfortably is called asana, in the context of yoga definition. Asana is translated in English as "posture." Posture literally means the position in which one holds their body while standing or sitting and interestingly, the way one holds one's body is determined by their mental attitude. For example, a depressed person stoops and looks down, whereas a confident person looks straight with upright chest. So, there is a causal connection between one's posture and mental attitude. According to neuromuscular physiology, phasic responses are related to movements, whereas tonic responses are related to mental attitude and a sustained mental attitude gives rise to a particular physical posture. The beauty of Patanjali's definition of asana is more appreciable when we understand the connection of a posture and mental attitude. It also throws light on why asana is maintenance of a pose, but not the movements to attain the pose. The logic is quite simple—if mental attitude can shape the posture of a person, then consciously holding a particular pose with steadiness and comfort should also have an impact on one's mental attitude. After all, yoga is shaping one's mental attitude for peaceful living.

Is Yoga only Pranayama?

Similar to asana, pranayama involves three steps: (1) inhaling, (2) exhaling, and (3) holding the breath (after inhalation or exhalation or both). Again, as per definition in Yoga scriptures, inhaling or exhaling slowly is not pranayama. Breath holding, either after inhalation or exhalation or both, is defined as pranayama. To be more precise, pranayama is not even holding of breath using willpower, but an automatic or comfortable conscious suspension of breathing after inhalation or exhalation. Yogic scriptures emphasize the importance of breath suspension because it has a strong impact on the mind, apart from its effect on the body. It is important to understand what happens during breath holding to understand the context in which pranayama fits into the definition of yoga—controlling the mental modifications. During automatic or voluntary suspension of breathing within one's limit, there are increased carbon dioxide levels and decreased oxygen levels at the central chemoreceptors and peripheral chemoreceptors respectively within the brain which triggers the respiratory center for exhalation. As one regulates breathing by holding comfortably, slowly this voluntary training to withstand increased carbon dioxide level and decreased oxygen level leads to calmness of mind. It is this calmness of mind that is targeted through pranayama too, apart from the physical benefits.

Is Yoga Different from Meditation?

The idea of meditation emerges only when one misunderstands yogasana for yoga. When Yoga is practiced as a lifestyle with the purpose of bringing peace in life, meditation is embedded in the broad concept of yoga. But still, the terms "Yoga and Meditation" are widely used in recent times, as most of the people use yoga as a health promoting tool with more focus on the physical components such as asana and pranayama which are easier to do than the other limbs of yoga such as Dharana. So conceptually, yoga encompasses meditation, although in recent times they are viewed as two different phenomena.

Thus, it becomes evident that all the components including the physical practices namely asana and pranayama of *Ashtanga* yoga revolve around this concept of mastering the mind for experiencing peace. Hence, it is needless to say that the different tools that are used to reach the state of mental peace may be an important component of Yoga but they themselves cannot be called yoga. In this context, yoga is a holistic concept which should be seen in its wholesome, with *yama, niyama, asana, pranayama, pratyahara, dharana, dhyana,* and *samadhi* together, and not as a stand-alone. Calling any single component as yoga does not hold true as per the definition of yoga.

▇ ATTITUDE TOWARDS THE MIND IN YOGA PHILOSOPHY

Another important thing to understand is that Yoga, as a discipline, uses skillful techniques to "master" the mind and not to "control" the mind. What is the difference between "controlling" and "mastering"? Controlling means an effortful suppression of the urges of the mind by dealing with the mind directly using ones will power, whereas mastery involves purification and slowing down of the mind using yogic techniques without suppression and with proper understanding of the mind. A Yogi considers the mind like a naughty child and deals with it skillfully using attitudes of both care and strictness, and not just by thoughtless suppression.

YOGA AS THERAPY

Yoga traditionally developed as a technique for accelerating spiritual evolution of human beings. The improvement in physical and mental health is actually a by-product of the yoga practice. But in the last three to four decades, with rapid emergence of noncommunicable disorders (NCDs) such as hypertension, heart disease, obesity, type 2 diabetes mellitus, cancer, mental health disorders etc., yoga therapy has gained importance as a lifestyle intervention. All major NCDs are multifactorial in origin and are deeply rooted in disturbances of lifestyle and biorhythms. Thus, yoga-based lifestyle modification, which adopts a multipronged holistic approach, emerged as an attractive nonpharmacological adjuvant for prevention and management of NCDs. There has been an exponential rise in yoga research in the last two decades and it has focused on assessing the potential role of yoga-based lifestyle in prevention and management of NCDs. Yoga therapy is now regarded in the Western world as a holistic approach to health and is classified by the National Institute of Health as a form of Traditional System of Medicine. Different components of Yoga have been utilized by scientists in a variety of disorders and current evidence shows efficacy of Yoga as an adjuvant or sole treatment for the management of common NCDs such as hypertension, heart disease, obesity, cancer, low back pain, fibromyalgia, bronchial asthma, depression, stress, and schizophrenia.[7]

YOGIC MODEL FOR HEALTH AND DISEASE

According to *Taittiriya Upanishad*,[8] there are five layers of consciousness that define an individual from gross to subtle: (1) Physical layer (physical body: *Annamaya kosha*), (2) layer of subtle energy (*Pranamaya kosha*), (3) layer of emotions (*Manomaya kosha*), (4) layer of knowledge (*Vijnanamaya kosha*), and (5) layer of bliss (*Anandmaya kosha*). Every individual and the whole creation consist of these five layers, in manifest or unmanifest form. The first three are called as lower layers and last two are called as higher layers. All these five layers are not separate compartments but are essentially one continuum of consciousness from gross to subtle **(Fig. 2)**. Each subtler layer encompasses the grosser layer within it and expands beyond as well. The subtler the layer, the more freedom

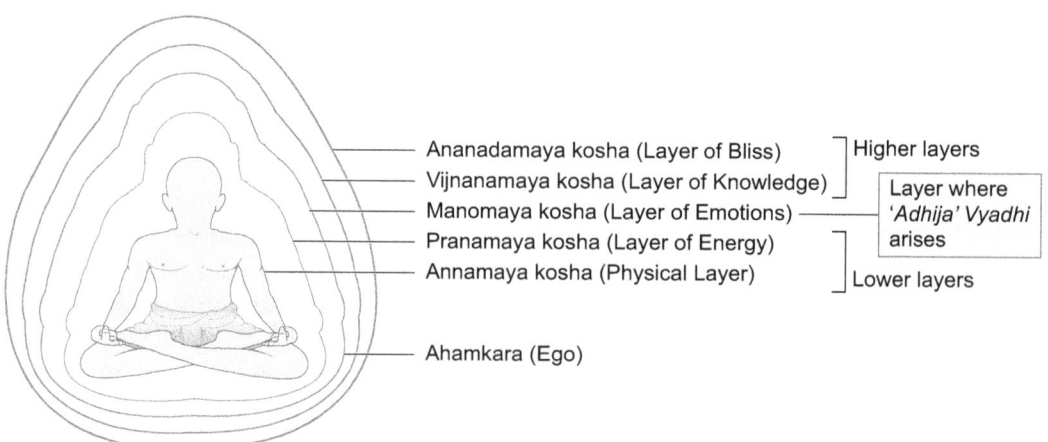

Fig. 2: Five layers of consciousness (Panchakosha model).

it has from the time and space dimensions that govern the physical existence.

These layers of consciousness are manifested in the behavior of individuals. *Annamaya* and *Pranamaya koshas* are manifested by the physical existence and signs of life, respectively. *Manomaya kosha* is manifested by emotions generated due to likes or dislikes toward any stimuli, mainly containing repetitive thoughts which keep tossing in the dimensions of likes and dislikes, without the ability to come to clear decision. Higher layer of *Vijnyanamaya kosha* is manifested when an individual is able to gain clear insight into the situation and is able to take a decision without any doubt. *Anandamaya kosha* is manifested by the actions of creativity and cosmic well-being which are driven by inner bliss and intelligence. The lower three layers (*Annamaya, Pranamaya,* and *Manomaya*) are manifested by default in the behavior of the individual but the manifestation of higher layers of consciousness (*Vijnyanamaya kosha* and *Anandamaya kosha*) depends on how relaxed and calm the lower three layers are. If there is turbulence and unrest in lower layers then higher layers get obscured and their manifestation is blocked. Higher layers are always in tune with the cosmic intelligence, bliss, and harmony. When they are manifested, they naturally bring balance and harmony in the lower layers that are conducive to overall health. Thus, slowing down and relaxation of lower layers are important factors in yoga therapy. So, the key components for a healthy life are: (A) relaxed body, (B) slow and steady breath, and (C) calm mind.

Understanding the Pathophysiology of Disease According to Yoga

Yoga Vashishtha,[6] an ancient yoga text, explains that *Vyadhi* (any illness affecting the physical layer) can be broadly classified into two types based on the underlying cause: (1) Disease due to external factors (*Anadhija Vyadhi*) and (2) Disease due to internal factors (*Adhija Vyadhi*). *Anadhija vyadhis* are caused due to physical factors in the external environment (*Annamaya kosha*) of an individual such as accidents, injuries, infections, and poisoning. *Adhija vyadhis* (*Aa = Avaranam* means covering; *Dhi* = Wisdom/Intelligence), on the other hand, are caused due to imbalances and disharmony in the other lower layers of consciousness (*Pranamaya* and *Manomaya kosha*) of the individual. Some illnesses are caused as a combination of both (Mixed *adhija* and *anadhija vyadhi*) for example, in some cancers, both carcinogen (*anadhija* component) as well as individual genetic predisposition and psyche (*adhija* components) may play a role.

Excluding the diseases caused by external factors such as accidents, infections and so on, majority of the diseases which trouble us in the current century belong to the *Adhija* or mixed category (hypertension, type 2 diabetes mellitus, heart disease, obesity, cancer, and depression) where lifestyle plays an important role. The most important component in modifying the lifestyle is the "Mind" of an individual, as in this era of information where everybody knows what is to be done and what kind of lifestyle should be followed, the most difficult thing is to manage one's own mind! Yogic texts like *Bhagavad Gita* describe that "For him who has learnt the art of managing the mind, the mind is the best of friends; but for one who has failed to do so, his very mind will be the greatest enemy (BG 6.6)." All the eight limbs of yoga, described above, actually are nothing but highly refined tools for managing the mind only.

The yoga-based model of illness explains disease development as follows: *Adhija Vyadhi's* begin as conflict in the layer of emotions (*Manomaya kosha*) which continues for a long time (months and years) in the form of repeated cyclical patterns of deep-rooted emotionally charged thoughts (*chitta vrittis*). These *vritti's* obstruct the higher layers (layers of knowledge and bliss). They manifest as repeated patterns of thoughts which are speeded up, emotionally charged, and are associated with a feeling of distress or uneasiness. These thoughts keep surfacing periodically in the mind of an individual but remain unresolved. Such thoughts are accelerated if the layer of emotions is constricted due to its attachment to lower layers, whereas they reduce when the layer of emotions is relaxed and expanded due to its contact with higher layers. As these thoughts increase in intensity and duration, they cause imbalances to percolate deeper and deeper into the system with each and every repetition. This, over a period of time, either leads to blockages/resistance in the *pranic* (subtle energy) channels or causes excessive uncontrolled flow; thereby disturbing the layer of *Pranamaya kosha*. Imbalances in the *Pranamaya kosha* manifest in the form of irregular and speeded up breathing pattern and overactivity or underactivity (or hypersensitivity or undersensitivity) of physiological functions. If the root cause still persists and accentuates, then slowly the problem deepens down causing electrochemical and biological disturbances in the body finally manifesting as an organic medical illness. Thus, according to the yogic understanding the imbalances in the layers of consciousness due to the phenomena of "speed" and "constriction" are the root cause of disease.

Individuals with high willpower have more powerful *Ahamkara* or sense of "I" ness and thus, they may be able to suppress these imbalances in the layer of emotions and push them down to lower layers more strongly (and develop illnesses such as hypertension, heart disease, diabetes, etc.), whereas individuals with less powerful *Ahamkara* (weak ego) may not be able to do so, and thus, may express the imbalance directly from the layer of emotions and develop psychological disturbances and psychiatric disorders (such as anxiety, depression, or psychosis in that order depending on the levels of weakness of ego). Individuals with moderate levels of *Ahamkara* may manifest it both ways in the form of psychological distress as well as physical pains (e.g., somatoform pain disorders, fibromyalgia, depression with somatic syndrome, etc.).[9] **Figure 3** describes how diseases are caused from yoga perspective and how this can be similar to the conceptualization of disease from modern science perspective.

■ THE PROCESS OF YOGA THERAPY (*PRATI-PRASAVA*)

According to Yoga Vashishtha, diseases due to an "external" cause (*Anadhija Vyadhi*) could be cured by "external" agents such as *mantra* (recitation of specific sound combinations), *aushadhi* (herbs or minerals), and *shalya* (surgery); whereas diseases due to an "internal" cause would require balancing

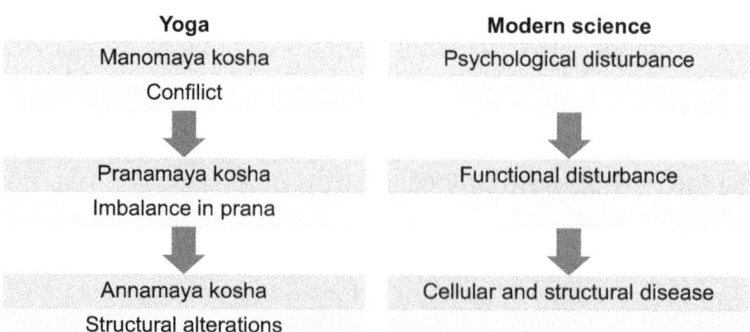

Fig. 3: Overview of the pathogenesis of noncommunicable disorders according to yoga and its understanding as per modern science.

of the internal layers of consciousness. Such balancing would happen by conscious reversal of the imbalance through "slowing down" and "expansion" of the layers in the reverse direction, i.e., from the physical layer to the layer of bliss (*prati-prasava*).[6,9]

This concept is quite relevant in present times where one can see that diseases due to "external causes" such as infections, accidents, injuries, and poisoning have been managed very well by modern medicine as it relies on exploration of the external world through science and technology. However, when we look at disorders which lack any specific "external" cause (e.g., type 2 diabetes mellitus, essential hypertension, asthma, cancers, depression, anxiety, psychosis, etc.) solutions from external means such as drugs, radiotherapy, and surgery are not completely satisfactory. We have achieved some control, but no cure. Ancient Indian sages were scientists who explored the "inner" world and came with the technology of yogic practices to address the "internal" cause.

As discussed earlier, yoga therapy understands NCDs as manifestation of "speed" and "constriction" in the third layer of consciousness which percolates to the lower layers over a period of time and settles down as disease. Thus, the basic approach is to "relax" and "expand". This is achieved by applying the eight-limbed approach of yoga **(see Table 1)** on layers of consciousness with the focus on "slowing down" and "expansion" at each layer (sometimes brief phases of intensity and speed may be required in practices but that is only to break the stagnation and reach deeper levels of relaxation): (1) Physical layer: *asanas* (maintaining the postures with comfort and stability), *shoucha* (cleanliness), and *Tapas* (observing austerity and moderation); (2) Layer of energy: *pranayama* and *kriyas* (regulation of breath); (3) Layer of emotions: *santosha* [(feeling of satisfaction and contentment, *Ishvara pranidhana* (surrender to higher principle in life, thinking about people who have evolved through this path)], *bhajans* (singing devotional songs in groups), *satsangh* (keeping company with people who are devoted to higher principles in life), *dharana* (voluntary focusing of the mind); (4) Layer of knowledge: *Swadhyaya* (introspection into one's own thoughts, behavior and existence) and *dhyana* (gradual involuntary focusing and defocusing with expansion of consciousness); and (5) Layer of bliss: *Samadhi* (merging with the most expanded layer, the layer of bliss, feeling oneness). Thus, the basic approach is to relax deeper and deeper and expand. Another *Vedic* scripture (*Mandukya Karika*) provides an important principle to balance the deeper layers of consciousness. It says "If the mind is sleepy, stimulate and awaken it (using yogic techniques of fast breathing, etc.); if it is too excited calm it down (using slow breathing, *shavasana, yoga nidra*, etc.)." By repeating the same again and again and by thus, keeping the mind in the state of equilibrium, the deeper agitations of the subconscious mind will come onto the surface. Become aware of them and go deeper into relaxation. This principle of "stimulation and relaxation" is also to be taken into consideration while designing the yoga-based lifestyle modifications for management of NCDs.[10]

■ CONCLUSION

Yoga is an ancient science which provides comprehensive understanding about human existence, health, and disease. It provides a model which aims at well-being at all the levels: physical, physiological, psychological, and spiritual. The holistic approach of yoga-based lifestyle may serve as an important adjuvant for prevention and management of common noncommunicable disorders.

■ REFERENCES

1. Müller FM. The hymns of the Rig-Veda in the Samhita and Pada Texts. Trübner and Company; 1877.

2. Sastri K (Ed). Saunakiya Atharvaveda Samhita. Delhi: Madhavapustakalayah; 1975.
3. Chinmayananda S. Kathopanishad: A dialogue with death. Central Chinmaya Mission Trust; 2003.
4. Chinmayananda S. Commentary on Bhagavad-Gita. Mumbai, India: Sai Enterprises; 1992.
5. Saraswati S, Saraswati SN. Four chapters on freedom: Commentary on the yoga sutras of Patanjali. Nesma Books India; 2002.
6. Venkatesananda S. The Supreme Yoga: A New Translation of the Yoga Vāsiṣṭha. New Age Books; 2005.
7. Khalsa SB, Cohen L, McCall TB, Telles S (Eds). The Principles and Practice of Yoga in Health Care. SAGE Publications, Incorporated; 2017.
8. Chinmayananda S. Taittiriya Upanishad. Central Chinmaya Mission Trust; 2014.
9. Nagendra HR, Nagarathna R. Promotion of Positive Health. Bengaluru: Swami Vivekananda Yoga Prakashana. 2001:51.
10. Chinmayananda S (Ed). Discourses on Mandukya Upanishad with Gaudapada's Karika. Chinmaya Publication Trust; 1966.

Basic Concepts of Counseling as per Vedic Literature

CHAPTER 2

Hemant Bhargav, Nishitha Jasti, Shree Raksha Bhide, Kishore Kumar Ramakrishna

INTRODUCTION

Although the current and popular understanding of *Yoga* is to consider it as a practice dealing with body, breath, and mind, there is a substantial knowledge base available in *Vedic* literature which deals with the philosophical aspects of Yoga. Considering the huge demand for trained counselors, this may be particularly useful and relevant in India where there is a need for culturally-sensitive counseling programs. This chapter discusses the fundamental principles which can be applied for the development of a *Vedic* literature-based counseling program.

BASIC CONCEPTS AND PRINCIPLES OF COUNSELING

Many Vedic texts including the *Bhagavad Gita* (BG), *Yoga Vashishtha,* and *Upanishads* are written in the form of dialogues between two people. Typically, there are situations where one person is in a state of psychological crisis and seeks guidance from the other person who is more spiritually evolved, stable and endowed with wisdom. Such situations have been observed in (1) *Bhagavad Gita*: where *Arjuna* was in a state of acute panic and depression, and was unable to perform his duties as a warrior. He was guided by Lord *Krishna* through conversations in a question and answer pattern. This ultimately led to *Arjuna* being able to overcome his psychological disturbances and perform appropriate actions in the war;[1] (2) *Yoga Vashishtha*: where *Rama* was in the state of severe depression with suicidal thoughts and ideas of extreme pessimism about life, and not wanting to take over the charge of his Kingdom as King. He was then directed by his father *Dasharatha* to meet *Vashishtha*, who was a great spiritual master. *Rama* asked *Vashishtha* several fundamental questions about life, disease, and death, and after a long series of questions and answers, he achieved clearer insight and regained the enthusiasm to lead his Kingdom successfully;[2] and (3) *Upanishads: Taittiriya Upanishad*—*Guru* and father, *Varuna*, guides his teenage son *Bhrigu* who suffers from identity crisis;[3] similarly three disciples in similar situations as *Bhrigu* were guided by their *Guru Pippalada* in *Prashnopanishad*;[4] In *Kathopanishad*, a story is narrated where *Yama* answers *Nachiketa's* (his disciple) fundamental questions on death and life after death, etc.[5]

It is important to understand that in these texts, as discussed above, the disciple himself approached the teacher for guidance. It has also been written in the *Bhagavad Gita* that guidance should not be given without being asked for.[1] Thus, the first key principle of *Vedic* counseling is: **(1)** *To counsel only those who seek guidance.*

Secondly, all major Vedic texts follow a pattern where the teacher first allows the disciple to speak his mind. In the *Bhagavad Gita*, the entire first chapter (called *Arjuna Vishada Yoga* or The Yoga of *Arjuna's* Depression) and initial part of the second chapter only deals with *Arjuna* describing his psychological situation and justifying his decision of not fighting the war. Interestingly, his teacher *Krishna* did not interfere when *Arjuna* was speaking. *Krishna* only started speaking when *Arjuna* finished ventilating his feelings.[1] Hence, the second key principle of *Vedic* counseling is: **(2)** *To listen completely with a calm mind, without interfering and without interfering and judging.*

Throughout the *Bhagavad Gita*, it can be observed that *Krishna* offers *Arjuna* choices to choose his path for spiritual well-being and coping. Specifically, in *Chapter 12* from *Sloka 8–12*, *Krishna* gives options to *Arjuna*. The first option he gives is to have a one-pointed focus on the supreme consciousness and surrender all worries to Him (BG 12.8). Then looking at the expressions of *Arjuna*, *Krishna* realizes that this is a difficult task for Arjuna, so he gives him the second option of "*Abhyasa yoga*" or "the Yoga of Practice" (BG 12.9). *Krishna* says, "if one-pointed focus is difficult for you, perform the practice of Yoga regularly, by this you will slowly develop the ability to focus". Further, when *Krishna* feels that *Arjuna* wants an even easier path than this, he says "If you cannot practice the regulations of *Abhyasa yoga*, then just try to work for Me, because by working for Me you will come to the perfect stage" (BG 12.10). Finally, *Krishna* gives an even easier option and states, "If however, you are unable to work in this consciousness, then try to act by giving up all results of your work and try to be self-situated" (BG 12.11). Thus, it can be clearly seen that *Krishna* is giving *Arjuna* different options to choose from different streams of *Yoga*, starting with *Jnana yoga* (Yoga of knowledge), then *Raja yoga* or *Abhyasa yoga* (Yoga of practice), followed by *Bhakti yoga* (Yoga of devotion), and finally *Karma yoga* (Yoga of action). Also, *Krishna* is careful enough to let *Arjuna* know that none of the paths is inferior to the other and even the path advocated by him at the last (*Karma yoga*) is great, and all lead to the same goal. *Arjuna* (being emotional by nature and being driven by actions) chooses the path of *Karma* and *Bhakti*, and he says at the end "My dear *Krishna*, my illusion is now gone. I have regained my memory by your mercy, and I am now firm and free from doubt and I am prepared to act according to your instructions."[1] Hence, other key principles of yogic counseling are: **(3)** *To understand the personality and capacity of the subject and give him/her an option to choose from a variety of directions and* **(4)** *To also let them know that all paths are equally good and will yield the same goal.*

It is very important to note that directions given by the teacher are never forced upon the disciple, and the disciple always has the choice and freedom to decide. Even at the end of the *Bhagavad Gita*, Lord Krishna tells *Arjuna*:[1]

iti te jnanam akhyatam
guhyad guhyataram maya
vimrsyaitad asesena
yathecchasi tatha kuru (BG 18.63)

"*Thus, I have explained to you this knowledge that is more secret than all secrets. Ponder over it deeply, and then do as you wish.*"

The fifth principle of *Vedic* counseling is: **(5)** *Not to expect anything and to give the subject, the freedom to decide.* Many therapists get emotionally involved with their clients and expect clients to always follow the advice given. *Vedic* texts emphasize performing one's actions with full heart without getting attached and without expecting anything in return. Also, to avoid burnout and to retain the ability to help many more patients, it is important that a therapist develops this art of counseling (acting as an instrument of higher consciousness and avoiding the sense of doer-ship) by expanding his consciousness to feel attached to the whole patient population which needs him rather than to a single patient. Hence, the sixth principle of Vedic counseling is: **(6)** *To feel connected to the whole and not to a part*. A specific example is found in the *Bhagavad Gita* (BG 2.70):

*apuryamanam acala-pratistham
samudram apah pravisanti yadvat
tadvat kama yam pravisanti sarve
sa santim apnoti na kama-kami (BG 2.70)*

"*A person who is not disturbed by the incessant flow of desires—that enter like rivers into the ocean which is ever being filled but is always still—can alone achieve peace, and not the man who strives to satisfy such desires.*"

Finally, it is important to observe and understand the psyche of the subject. The fundamental approaches for counseling described here are vital in gaining a complete insight into the mind of the individual according to the *Vedic* philosophy.

Theory of Trigunas

Samkhya philosophy details the evolution, sustenance, and dissolution of creation in terms of *trigunas*.[6] Further, *gunas* in the context of understanding the personality and behavioral tendencies have been lucidly detailed in the *Bhagavad Gita*.[1] *Trigunas* are broad and very inclusive due to their ability to explain most of the behavioral tendencies. These three *gunas* are *sattva*, *rajas*, and *tamas*. The dominance of each *guna* results in characteristic behavior patterns and describes a personality type. A *sattvic* personality demonstrates enthusiasm in performing his duties being indifferent to result of the action. Such people show thorough discernment while not attaching their identity to false pride and material attachments, leading to purity in their thoughts. Their social interactions demonstrate an attitude of oneness among all beings. They prefer *sattvic* food which is juicy, sweet, oleaginous and nourishing in nature. *Rajasic* personalities tend to initiate activities with intense ambition and relentless desires, with the anticipation of fruits of their actions. They perform activities that bring material well-being and fame but otherwise not beneficial to the society at large. Their intellect is impeded due to improper understanding and results in improper discrimination. Due to their attachment to material well-being, they exhibit negative emotional states of fear, anxiety, anger, greed, and so on. They have a sense of superiority in their social interactions. They prefer *rajasic* food that is spicy, sour, salty, hot and pungent, and these tend to cause pain and disease. A *Tamas*-dominant personality is disposed to be lethargic, stubborn, deluded and revengeful in their actions. They host strong negative emotions which distort their intellect completely resulting in delusions and a very poor discernment. They tend to give up all their duties due to inertia and ignorance. Their social interactions and activities are impractical and inflict injury to self and others. They prefer food that is cold, lacks freshness, cooked much before (>3 hours) being eaten, nonjuicy, tasteless, and unhygienic. Besides these three personalities, *Yoga* philosophy mentions a fourth personality type with the mode of spirituality. This dimension (*Gunatita*) describes mental equanimity, detachment to materialism, and a state of all-inclusiveness. Individuals with this trait recognize that play of *trigunas* is short-lived and become detached to them. Thereby, they stay neutral to the extremes of stimuli, remain nonjudgmental in all situations, and they do not get influenced with honor or dishonor. They perform all their duties devoting to a higher principle of life.[1]

In summary, **(7)** *it is necessary to understand these guna-based personality types* because the science of *Yoga* expounds the necessity of transition from the state of *Tamas* to *Rajas*, *Rajas* to *Sattva* and then to *Gunatita*, to experience complete wellness at physical, mental, social, and spiritual planes of existence.

Personalities Based on Yogic Path of Evolution for Coping

The ancient yogic texts provide classification of society into four categories (varnas) based on *gunas* and action (*karma*).[1] The four varnas are: (1) *Brahmana*, (2) *Kshatriya*, (3) *Vaishya*, and (4) *Shudra*. These four varnas are prototypes representing a particular behavioral domain which dominates a personality. For example, *Brahmana* is a person who likes intellectual stimulations, who seeks to understand the mechanisms through which various phenomena in life happen and he seeks to apply this knowledge for social welfare. People who have aptitude toward teaching, research, science, law, engineering or philosophy may fall into this category. Similarly, *Vaishya* has the capacity to plan and organize. They are the ones who execute the ideas in a systematic and structured manner in society; they may also have a liking toward financial matters. In modern times, administrative officers, human resource managers, entrepreneurs, and accountants may come under this category. *Kshatriyas* on the other hand are powerful, competitive, and aggressive. They like challenges, and they protect the weaker sections of the society. They fight for justice. People who have liking toward joining army or police force or sports, etc., may come under this category. *Shudras* on the other hand have liking toward serving people. They form the very base of the social structure.[1] People enjoying professions such as homemaker, chef, doctor, nurse or social worker, or artists, etc., may be considered under this category. It is interesting to note here that there may be a close resemblance between four *varnas* described in *Bhagavad Gita* and "Big Five" personality traits described in modern psychology. The "Openness to experience" is the trait found most commonly in a "*Brahmana*", "Conscientiousness" on the other hand would be found in a "*Vaishya*". Similarly, the trait of "Extroversion" may be dominant in a "*Kshatriya*", and "Agreeableness" may characterize a "*Shudra*", respectively.

Each personality type may find a specific path of Yoga to be more conducive for practice and as a coping strategy. There are four major streams of yoga that are described in the *Bhagavad Gita*: *Jnana yoga* (path of knowledge), *Raja yoga* (path of practice), *Karma yoga* (path of action), and *Bhakti yoga* (path of devotion).[1] *Jnana yoga* is a systematic process to evolution, using the intellect through acquiring higher wisdom. The *Brahmana varna* might find it easy to adopt *Jnana yoga* while practicing the teachings of its essence for their coping. Asking deeper fundamental questions about the existence and contemplating on them may help such a person grow toward positive mental health. *Raja yoga* involves systematic practice of eight limbs of yoga to attain mastery over the mind. This requires immense willpower and might suit *Kshatriya varna*. Nurturing their willpower will help them cope with stressful situations. The practice and philosophy of *Karma yoga* involves performing one's duties for a higher principle of life, without any attachment to the results. This might be appropriate for *Vaishya varna*. They might prefer to work and keep themselves busy, to alleviate suffering. Lastly, *Bhakti yoga* is the path of surrendering oneself to the divine or higher principle of life. This is likely to be conducive to *Shudra varna*, as they find it easy to surrender their emotions to a higher principle of life during hardships.[1] This system of classification allows **(8)** *prescription of specific Yogic philosophical approaches and techniques for coping, to a particular personality type*. Though we may not practically find people falling into such tight compartments of personality classifications in the modern times and most of them may actually have a combination of traits, this kind of understanding may still help in some way to get an idea about one's personality traits and thus, his/her likelihood of following a particular (or combination of) *yogic* path/s.

All the different personality types may have people in the whole spectrum of *trigunas*, manifesting their tendencies in constructive, destructive or neutral ways. The journey according to *Yoga* philosophy is for smooth progression from *Tamas* to *Rajas*, *Rajas* to *Sattva*, and then to *Gunatita* (pathological to healthy, and from healthy to positive mental health). This progression shall translate into better physical and psychological well-being of the individual, and further facilitate peace and social harmony in society.

Five Layers of Consciousness: Panchakosha Model

Taittiriya Upanishad describes five layers of consciousness: (1) *Annamaya kosha* (sheath of physical body), (2) *Pranamaya kosha* (sheath of energy), (3) *Manomaya kosha* (sheath of mind), (4) *Vijnanamaya kosha* (sheath of intellect), and (5) *Anandamaya kosha* (sheath of ultimate bliss).[3] *Chapter 1* provides detailed description of the *Panchakosha* model and its implications in health and disease. **(9)** During counseling, it is important to address imbalances at each of the layers and correct them by using yogic techniques. *Manomaya kosha* should be given the utmost importance as it is here that most of the psychosomatic disorders originate (please read *Chapter 1* for understanding).[7] *Mandukya Karika* provides the basis by which counseling should be done to correct imbalances in *Manomaya kosha*:[8]

"Laye sambodhayet cittam; Vikshiptam samayet punah
Sakashayam vijaniyat samapraptam na calayet" (Mandukya Karika: 3.44)

"When the mind is dull and insensitive, stimulate it. When the mind is agitated and excited, calm it down. Repeat the same again and again and try to keep mind in the state of equilibrium. Deep-rooted stressors will then come into the sphere of awareness giving deeper insight. When the state of equanimity is achieved in the mind, try to sustain it as along as possible without disturbing."

Case vignette given at the end of the chapter will offer a deeper insight into this *Sloka*.

Understanding of the Yamas and Niyamas in Lifestyle

From the above, it can be understood that the practice of yoga does not restrict itself to physical postures. It is also about thoughts and emotions being cultivated, the nature of actions being performed and the interactions with surroundings.[9] In this context, the first two limbs of *Ashtanga yoga*, i.e., *Yama* and *Niyama* are particularly important. According to *Patanjali*, *Yamas* are the five social observances recommended to establish peace and harmony in society. They are: (1) *Satya* (truthfulness), (2) *Ahimsa* (nonviolence), (3) *Asteya* (nonstealing), (4) *Brahmacharya* (self-restraint), and (5) *Aparigraha* (nonhoarding). *Satya* is truthfulness that is to be followed at the level of intentions, speech, and actions for the universal well-being. *Ahimsa* involves cultivating the attitude of being compassionate and nonviolent to others in their intentions, speech, and actions. This naturally unfolds the unconditional love and bliss within and around the practitioner. For the practice of *Asteya* (nonstealing), one needs to be content with whatever one has and refrain taking what belongs to others. *Brahmacharya* (self-restraint) involves practicing restraint at activities of the body, speech, and mind; bringing about moderation in food, sleep, sexual activity, and other activities involving the senses. Practice of *Aparigraha* (nonhoarding) starts by inculcating detachment to the personal possessions that ultimately should diminish the attitude of hoarding. The practice of *Yamas* will naturally cut down the incessant flow of desires and its consequent mental turbulences. *Niyamas* are the five individual observances to promote physical and psychological well-being. These are the directions in which an individual should channelize his/her energies. They are: (1) *Saucha* (purity), (2) *Santosha* (contentment), (3) *Tapas* (penance), (4) *Svadhyaya* (self-examination), and (5) *Ishvara Pranidhana* (surrendering to the higher principle of life). One must observe *Saucha* (purity) of body, mind, and speech by not hosting any negative thoughts or emotions toward self and others. As mentioned above, one must be content (*Santosha*) with whatever one has rather than feeling sad about what one does not. This also further enables one to practice *Asteya*. *Tapas* (penance) involves intense practice of yoga disciplines despite adversities with one's willpower to achieve a higher goal. *Svadhyaya* (self-examination) is where the practitioner reflects on one's own thought patterns, emotions, and stage of learning. This provides a chance to correct negative notional thinking and related vicious emotional cycles which impede the growth of the practitioner. *Ishvara Pranidhana* is surrendering oneself to the higher principle of life. Thereby, devoting all the actions and their fruits to the higher principle which ultimately reduces the sense of despair.[9] The practice of *Yamas* and *Niyamas* makes a huge difference to the practice of the rest of the limbs of yoga, declutters the mind and also improves resilience to endure the odds of life. **(10)** *It stands important to assess the level of practice of Yamas and Niyamas in an individual*, alleviate confusions and promote their righteous practice during the process of counseling.

Understanding of the Doshas and Their Balance

According to *Yoga* and *Ayurveda*, the fundamental doshas; *Vata*, *Pitta*, and *Kapha*, play a very important role in the pathogenesis of disease and restoration of health. These arise from the basic *Panchamahabhutas*: earth, water, fire, air, and space. Air and space together form *vata*; water and fire form *pitta*; and water and earth form *kapha dosha*. Each *dosha* predominance has a characteristic in terms of physique, physiology, and psychology (see *Chapter 3* for more details). *Vata, pitta*, and *kapha doshas* relate to *rajas, sattva*, and *tamas* psychological attributes (*gunas*), respectively in normalcy. *Vata* governs the flow and movement in the body, and displays qualities such as dry, rough, cold, and mobile. *Pitta* is responsible for digestion and metabolism and displays qualities such as heat, sharpness, and acidic. Lastly, *kapha* is responsible for mass, lubrication, and strength of joints in the body. It shows qualities such as moist, sticky, cold, heavy, and static.[10] The vitiation in the levels of these *doshas* leads to illness and restores the balance between them, bringing the individual back to good health. Vitiation takes place generally due to the incompatibility between the *dosha* predominance (*Prakriti*) in an individual, environmental influences and the lifestyle being followed. As it is already known that one's physiological functions (circadian rhythm, digestion, metabolism, reproductive cycle, and so on) significantly influence the psyche of an individual, and are also responsible for many lifestyle disorders,[11] it is very crucial to maintain these physiological functions optimally by maintaining the balance in *tridoshas*. To maintain this balance, a set of practices in terms of diet (*Ahara*), daily and seasonal regimen (*Vihara*) and self-reflection (*Vichara*) are recommended to balance *doshas*. *Vata dosha*-predominant individuals are advised to consume foods that are sweet and sour. They must also have shower with warm water, practice less intense exercises, and sleep for at least 8 hours a day. They must undergo *Basti* (enema) procedure especially during the rainy season. *Pitta*-predominant individuals are advised sweet and bitter tastes. They can have lukewarm or cold-water showers, can practice moderate intensity exercises and sleep moderately up to 6–7 hours a day. They are recommended to undergo *Virechana* (induced purgation) procedure during the Autumn season. *Kapha*-predominant individuals must prefer pungent, bitter, and astringent tastes. They must be advised to have hot water bath, powder massages, and practice high-intensity and dynamic exercises. They are recommended to sleep for 4-6 hours a day. They should avoid daytime sleep. They must undergo *Vamana* (induced emesis) procedure during the Spring season.[12,13] Chapter 3 (Table 2) actually provides some references in ancient yogic texts where yoga practices were prescribed for balancing the *doshas*. Thus, **(11)** *it is vital to understand the composition of doshas and recommend suitable lifestyle accordingly.*

Modes of Consciousness according to Vedas: Wakefulness, Dream, Sleep and Transcendental

The *Mandukya Upanishad* provides details pertaining to different modes of human consciousness.[8,14] It states that the consciousness has four dimensions (wakefulness, dream, sleep, and transcendental) and each one is denoted by a particular sound. Human personalities are characterized by dominance of one or the other dimension of consciousness, which may predispose them to different kinds of physical or psychological disorders. The first dimension, *Vaishvanara Purusha*, is the consciousness which moves out through the senses and illuminates the external world. This consciousness allows sense perception and is denoted by the sound "AAA". It is interesting to note that it is the natural tendency of a human being to produce this kind of sound in the situations where there is intense awareness of the external surroundings or when the physical body is provoked, e.g., in the time of fight, injury or pain. The second dimension is the *"Tejas Purusha"*. It has been described as the consciousness projected in the mental space (dream or imagination). This aspect of consciousness is denoted by the sound "UUU". The third dimension is the *"Prajna Purusha"*. It is the consciousness moving inward and is denoted by the sound "MMM". Humming is a natural sound produced by human beings whenever they perceive joy within (that may arise out of a sensation), for example, when one tastes one's favorite dish there is a natural tendency to close the eyes and produce the humming sound "MMM" as one enjoys the taste and feels the joy within. The *Upanishad* then describes another dimension which is called as the *"Turiya"* or "Trance". This dimension is transcendental and it has been described as the point of origin of consciousness where all the three dimensions described above (AAA, UUU, and MMM) originate and terminate. It has characteristics of all the other three: wakefulness, dream and sleep together, and beyond (a state of wakeful-dreamful-sleep with deeper insights into the existence, very difficult to describe in words!). *Turiya* is denoted by the "Silence" between two *AUM*s which persists in the background even when the word *AUM* is uttered. A useful analogy to understand the relationship is to understand the first three dimensions of consciousness as waves in the ocean and the fourth one as the ocean itself.[8,14] Patanjali further provides subclassification of the first three dimensions where he describes *Vrittis* (agitations of the mind in his *Yoga Sutras*).[9] The first dimension of wakefulness is divided into two subtypes: (1) *Pramana* (right perception through the senses) and (2) *Viparyaya* (wrong perception of the sensory information). The second dimension of the state of "dream" is also subdivided into two types: (1) *Vikalpa* (imagination without touch with ground reality) and (2) *Smriti* (repetition in the mind of what has been experienced in the past as it is). The third dimension of "sleep" was retained as it is by *Patanjali* as the fifth *vritti*. In fact, yoga, according to Patanjali, is defined as a systematic technique that can allow a person to enter into the state of *Turiya* (i.e., *chitta vritti nirodhah*) through transcendence of all the other three dimensions of consciousness described above.

This state cleanses and heals all deep-rooted impressions, habits, fears, and anxiety in the mind. It can make the mind innocent again for fresh learning and perception. This can transform an individual. Once a question was asked to Swami Vivekananda: "What is the difference between sleep and samadhi (trance or *turiya*)?" Swami Vivekananda replied: "When a fool goes into sleep, he wakes up as fool. But when a fool goes into samadhi, he wakes up as a wise man!"[15]

The philosophy mentioned above carries important clinical implications. As per yogic understanding, a particular personality may get excessively attached to one dimension and hence may have difficulties due to the lesser expression of another. For example, a person with excessive attachment to *Vaishvanara purusha* and *Tejas purusha* (AAA-UUU type personality) may have sharp observation but he may suffer from hypervigilance, anxiety, fear, and anticipation which may lead to insomnia (lesser expression of *Prajna purusha* or MMM aspect of personality). Such a person may benefit from practice of *Bhramari pranayama* (humming breath). Similarly, the personality type attached more intensely to *Tejas purusha* and *Prajna purusha* (UUU-MMM type personality) may be excessively imaginative and introvert. They may refrain themselves from social connections and may carry a risk of losing touch with reality, they may also be less active occupationally. Such personalities carry a risk of developing depression or psychosis if the expression of *Vaishvanara purusha* (AAA, outward dimension) is depleted beyond a certain threshold. Theoretically, such people may benefit by loud chanting of the sound "AAA". Thus, according to *Vedic* philosophy, the sign of health is to have balance between dimensions of AAA, UUU, and MMM, i.e., to have perfect harmony in biorhythms. If through *Yoga nidra* or other relaxation procedures, a person is able to stay in the transcendental state of *Turiya*, the amount of time he/she spends in that state is directly proportional to the amount of freedom and mastery the person gets over the first three dimensions of consciousness. Hence, considering the clinical implication of the states of awareness, **(12)** *it is also important to assess the level of attachment to these states of consciousness and prescribe practices accordingly*. **Figure 1** provides the basis of personality traits as per *Vedic* literature and their relationship with psychological variables.

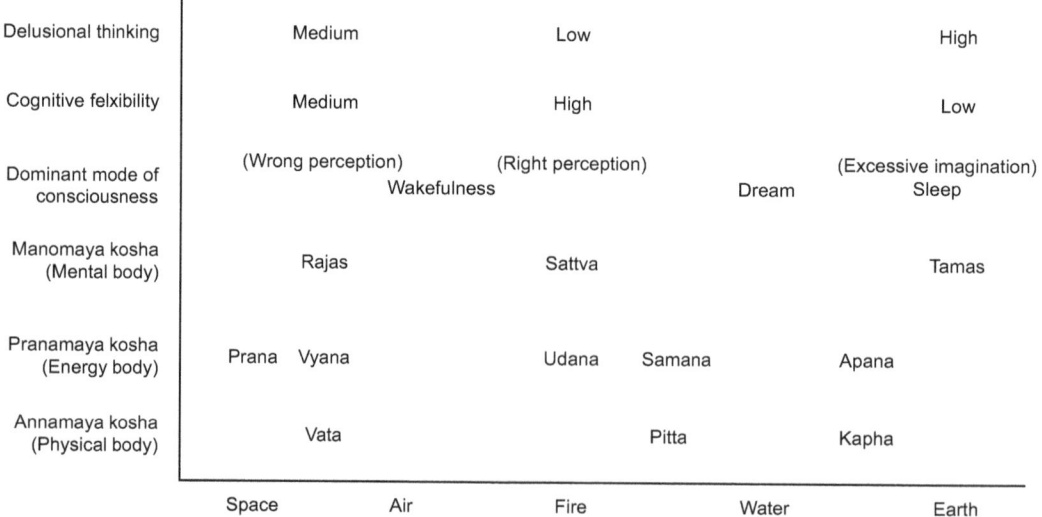

Fig. 1: Basis of personality traits as per *vedic* literature and their relationship with psychological tendencies.

TABLE 1: Important principles of vedic counseling.

Principle no.	Principle of vedic counseling
1.	To counsel only those who seek guidance
2.	To listen completely with a calm mind, without interfering and judging
3.	To understand the personality and capacity of the subject, and give him/her an option to choose from a variety of directions
4.	To understand that all paths of evolution are equally good and yield to the same goal
5.	Not to expect and to give freedom to the subject to decide
6.	To feel connected to the whole and not to a part
7.	To observe composition of *gunas*
8.	To observe dominant personality traits of intellect, willpower, emotion, and action to help decide appropriate direction
9.	To assess the five layers of consciousness
10.	To understand the status of *Yamas* and *Niyamas* for lifestyle correction
11.	To assess *doshas* and advise lifestyle changes to balance them
12.	To assess dimensions of wakefulness, sleep, and dream

CONCLUSION

Vedic philosophy is rich with knowledge pertaining to the human psyche. This knowledge base has the potential to evolve into a systematic holistic counseling program if combined with modern psychotherapy. **Table 1** provides an overview of the main principles of counseling according to *Vedic* literature. More research is warranted to explore this further.

CASE VIGNETTE

A 60-year-old patient, Mr R, a retired bank employee, came for Yoga therapy with chief complaints of bloating sensation in the abdomen and allergies to many common food items which would induce "indigestion" and gaseous distention leading to discomfort, since last 6 years. He also complained of difficulty in sleeping for 3 years. He had suffered from hypertension for 15 years. All basic investigations were carried out and no abnormality was detected. He had tried modern medicine, Ayurveda, and Homeopathy. He would find temporary relief with medications but would again develop same problem after a while. This led him to try Yoga therapy. Given this background, it was decided to understand his psychological state better through counseling sessions.

He was kind and cooperative, and rapport was easily established in the first session. Initially, the counselor focused merely on listening to him. Subject denied any stressors in his life and most of his initial conversations were related to his stomach problems. He was encouraged to open up and talk about other spheres of his life including his work, family, and society. Listening to him, it was observed that he was a Rajas-dominant personality, he was strict and organized in his work, held high determination to achieve what he decided, and he was always punctual and hated when people came late. He did not believe in expressing his stresses and tensions. In fact, he denied presence of any kind stressor in his life at the time of counseling. He had more Kshatriya traits and was willpower dominant. Thus, it was understood that path of Raja yoga or Yoga of systematic practice would suit him the best. The Panchakosha model was explained to him, where emphasis was put on "Pranamaya kosha" imbalances (as patient was reluctant to accept that his problem is purely psychological, and physical investigations were not revealing any abnormality). It was also explained to him that his vital energy or life force (prana or vayu) was out of balance. It had accumulated excessively in the abdominal region and so that part had become hypersensitive. It was explained to him that this "Prana", like physical energy, can neither be created nor be destroyed, but it can be redistributed in the body by doing Yoga practices mindfully. "Wherever awareness goes, prana flows in that direction" and thus, the aim was to obtain uniform distribution of "prana" throughout the body.[13] This approach satisfied the patient. He learnt some useful Yoga practices to be performed for 20 minutes daily and continued doing the same and he complied well with his Yoga practices.

After four sessions of counseling, he started opening up more and shared more personal details. He revealed that he finds it difficult to control his anger and forget things. He revealed that there was a time in the past when he had not spoken to his only son for more than a year. It was the time when his son was studying engineering (10 years ago) and was living in the hostel. He came to know that his son has got addicted to cannabis (ganja), and this was a big shock for him. He had been worrying about his son since then. In an attempt to get his son out of addiction, he brought him back home from the hostel. During that time, there was a big argument between both of them after which they did not speak to each other for a year. The patient said "at that time my son told me—You are the worst father in this world". When he said this, tears rolled down his eyes. Although this incident had taken place 10 years ago, still when he uttered that particular sentence there was sufficient emotional energy to bring him to tears. Such emotions which remain buried within the psyche are like burning coals below the ashes, they remain "alive" for years. They are referred to as "Kashayam" in the above-mentioned Sloka in section "Five Layers of Consciousness: Panchakosha Model". After regular practice of Yoga, the suppressed emotional conflicts started to come to the surface and into the sphere of awareness. Although he is now speaking to his son and everything has settled, still this particular incident went very deep into his Manomaya kosha and the root cause behind this were his Rajasic traits. He had a very strong sense of doership and he expected his son to be really grateful for whatever he had done for him. But with that sentence, everything got shattered in a moment and he was deeply hurt.

Over the next sessions, he was made "aware" (Vijaniyat) about such "alive emotions" in his mind. He was advised to follow the "Yama" of "Santosha" (contentment) and Niyama of "Tapas", i.e., regular practice of Yoga. He was advised to practice deep abdominal breathing, followed by whole body joint loosening, simple Yogasanas which involves twisting of the waist region (Kati chakrasana, Vakrasana, and Bhunamanasana) and then rest in Shavasana. After this, he was asked to "vent his anger out" while exhaling forcefully during Bhastrika fast breathing practice, and then do balancing practices of Nadi shuddhi and Bhramari (humming breath) pranayama. He was asked to perform these practices twice a day (morning and evening before food). Also, Yoga nidra (once a week) and Sattvic diet (freshly prepared, less spicy and easily digestible food) were advised. After 6 months, he reported significant improvement in his symptoms. Anger outbursts reduced; he became more accommodative in his behavior. His ability to digest food improved considerably (though his allergic tendency to certain food items persisted), bloating sensation and associated discomfort disappeared, sleep quality improved and blood pressure was maintained within normal limits with reduced dosage of medications.

REFERENCES

1. Chinmayananda S. Commentary on Bhagavad-Gita. Mumbai, India: Sai Enterprises; 1992.
2. Atreya BL. The Philosophy of the Yoga-Vasiṣṭha. A Comparative, Critical and Synthetic Survey of the Philosophical Ideas of Vasiṣṭha as Presented

in the Yoga-Vasiṣṭha-Maha-Ramayaṇa (Doctoral dissertation). Madras, India: Theosophical Publishing House; 1936.
3. Chinmayananda S. Commentary on Taittiriya Upanishad. Mumbai, India: Central Chinmaya Mission Trust; 2018.
4. Chinmayananda S. Commentary on Prashnopanishad. Mumbai, India: Central Chinmaya Mission Trust; 2018.
5. Chinmayananda S. Commentary on Kathopanishad. Mumbai, India: Central Chinmaya Mission Trust; 2018.
6. Virupakshananda S. Samkhya Karika of Isvara Krsna. Chennai: Ramakrishna Math; 2013.
7. Kavuri V, Raghuram N, Malamud A, Selvan SR. Irritable Bowel Syndrome: Yoga as Remedial Therapy. Evidence-Based Complementary and Alternative Medicine; 2015.
8. Chinmayananda S. Mandukya Upanishad with Gaudapada's Karika. Mumbai, India: Central Chinmaya Mission Trust; 2018.
9. Saraswati SS. Commentary on Patanjali Yoga Sutras. Bihar, India: Yoga Publications Trust; 1976.
10. Pal M. The tridosha theory. Anc Sci Life. 1991; 10(3):144-55.
11. Goyeche JR, Ago Y, Ikemi Y. Asthma: the yoga perspective. Part I. The somatopsychic imbalance in asthma: towards a holistic therapy. J Asthma Res. 1980;17(3):111-21.
12. Ramaiah Ramakrishna B. Healthy life-style prescriptions for different personality types (tridosha prakriti). J Ayurveda Holistic Med. 2014;2(7):30-6.
13. Muktibodhananda S. Hatha Yoga Pradipika. Delhi, India: Sri Satguru Publications; 2012.
14. Rama S. Om the Eternal Witness: Secrets of the Mandukya Upanishad. Dehradun India: Lotus Press; 2008.
15. Vivekananda S. The Complete Works of Swami Vivekananda. Kolkata, India: Partha Sinha; 2019.

CHAPTER 3

From Many to One to Many: The Wheel Completes a Cycle for Integrative Approaches in Mental Health

Bharath Holla, Hemant Bhargav, Kishore Kumar Ramakrishna

■ INTRODUCTION

In this chapter, we will introduce the concept of Integrative Mental Health and the promise it holds for the future of treatment approaches in psychiatry. Integrative medicine (IM) is an emerging field of health care that seeks to combine the best of evidence-informed approaches of conventional and traditional systems of medicine, to provide personalized, safe, and cost-effective treatments, while taking account of the whole person (body, mind, and spirit), including all aspects of lifestyle. Thus, IM approaches tend to be grounded in systems medicine, with network of interacting components that seek to expand medical reductionism to holism.[1]

■ CAUSES OF PSYCHIATRIC DISORDERS: EVOLUTION OF THE UNDERSTANDING

Kenneth S Kendler, a pioneer in psychiatric genetics and nosology, traces the history of the search for causes of medical and psychiatric disorders in a recent article.[2] He posits that up until the latter part of the 19th century, multicausal theories were popular. He cites examples from Robert Burton's natural and supernatural causes of depression (listed in his magnum opus The Anatomy of Melancholy in 1621) to physical and moral (psychological) causes of insanity by Thomas Arnold in 1786 and Jean Esquirol in 1838.

With advances in the microbiological methods, monocausal origins based on germ theory were found for many infectious diseases. This made a dramatic change in the health conditions with effective treatment and preventive methods for communicable diseases. This eventually led to a paradigm shift in the causal thinking of origin of disease to monocausal theories of etiology (*the doctrine of specific etiology*) across all branches of medicine, from the earlier multicausal approaches. In the latter half of the 20th century, however, the deaths due to infectious agents reduced and the world witnessed the emergence of noncommunicable disorders (NCDs) in epidemic proportions. With this re-emergence, western medicine and medical epidemiology completed the full circle by moving the focus back from a monocausal infectious diseases model to the multifactorial chronic disease model. It is in this context that the traditional systems of medicine (such as Ayurveda and Yoga) which focus on lifestyle management, can provide an important contribution to health care paving the way for an IM approach.

Integrative medicine practitioners adopt a multicausal perspective in clinical work and in explanations of psychiatric disorders to patients. They encourage a "this-and-that" strategy in place of a "this-or-that" approach, thereby enabling responsible medical pluralism.

■ AYURVEDA AS SYSTEMS MEDICINE

Āyurveda derives its theories of creation and existence from *sāmkhya* (one among *shad darśanas*—ancient Indian philosophical traditions).³ Yoga is also considered as a form of *sānkhya darśana*.⁴ Therefore, both share common concepts of existence. *Prakṛti* (the unmanifest) consists all elements of existence in the most subtle form and the process of creation starts when *puruṣa* (life) comes into its contact. During creation, the subtler forms of *pañcamahābhūta* [five elements that comprise all substances, viz., *pṛthvī* (Earth), *ap* (water), *tejas* (fire), *vāyu* (air), and *ākaśa* (ether)] with the help of *trigunāḥ*, viz., *rajas* (positive formational energy), *tamas* (negative formational energy), and *sattva* (harmony of rajas and tamas) get themselves organized into the structure of a living organism.⁵

Āyurveda, as per the *vedic* tradition, puts emphasis on the balance of five basic elements of nature through prakriti-based classification of physiological processes and personality as the basis for health. The prakriti-based classification involves three factors (*doshas*): *vata* (air + space), *pitta* (fire + water), and *kapha* (water + earth) and their psychological counterparts, the *gunas (sattva, rajas, and tamas)*. **Table 1** provides the characteristics of different Ayurveda-based prakriti types.

Fundamental concepts of disease causation according to Ayurveda focus on host vulnerability rather than a single causative factor. Generally, balance and harmony of the following factors promotes resilience against any disease according to Ayurveda: *doṣhas* (*vāta, pitta*, and *kapha*), *dhātu* (tissues), *bala* (strength to thrive, viz., inherited from birth, by virtue of time like youth, special regimens to strengthen health enhancement), *kāla* (time, viz., harmony in biorhythms and age), *agni* (digestion and metabolism), *prakṛiti* (inherited constitution based on *vāta, pitta*, and *kapha*), *sattva* (mental strength), *sātmya* (compatibility to varied food and environment), and *āhara* (food habits).⁶

Mental disorders in particular are considered as a result of inability to control emotions and manage a balanced lifestyle. This propels the individual toward imbalances in the *doshas* and *gunas* that become the basis for development of mental disorder. Excessive attachment toward thinking process leads to further derangement of the lifestyle (diet, activity, sleep, and recreation) and biorhythms which cause further disturbances in the mind. This vicious cycle becomes a perpetuating factor for mental health disorders.⁷

In *Charaka Samhita*, during a scientific debate on origin of diseases, an ancient scientist *Śaraloma* presents his view that predominance of *rajas* and *tamas* factors in the *manas* (mind) are the source of all diseases (of mind and body).⁸ It is pertinent to understand the contextual dichotomy while understanding the terms *sattva, rajas*, and *tamas*. These three are known as *gunās* (primordial energy forms) in the context of creation.⁹ Whereas, in the context of *manas*, *rajas*, and *tamas* are called *manodoṣas*, i.e., they are vulnerabilities constantly trying to create disharmony by causing emotional attachment of varied intensities in thought and action.¹⁰ To elaborate, any event that induces gratification is *sukha* and this leads to *iccha* (liking) and *pravṛtti* (action) in the same direction. Similarly, any event that induces *duḥkha* (agony) leads to *dweṣa* or dislike and causes restraint in progressing toward that direction (this repulsive action in the opposite direction is also known as *pravṛti*). *Pravṛtti* in both directions results in *upadha* (drive to emotionally involve in events of life) and is responsible for all types of *duḥkha* (agony) including diseases of the body and mind.¹¹,¹² Relieving oneself from *upadha* is the only and the best way to a healthy state of body and mind.¹² Appropriate way to get rid of *upadha* is to regulate *rajas* and *tamas* (mind forces that drive emotions), i.e., attaining such a balanced and harmonious state of mind where actions are driven by higher goals of universal well-being and not by individual—*sukha, duḥkha, iccha* or *dweṣa*. Such state of mind has been described as *mokṣha* (detached state of mind) or *niṣṭha*.¹³ Yoga is an ideal method of reigning in *rajas* and *tamas*. Yogic techniques help

TABLE 1: Characteristics of different Ayurveda-based prakriti types.

Aspect of constitution	Vata	Pitta	Kapha
Body frame	Thin	Moderate	Heavy
Body weight	Low (difficult to gain weight)	Moderate	Overweight (quick to gain weight)
Skin	Dry, rough, cool, brown	Soft, oily, warm, fair, red, yellowish	Thick, oily, cool pale, white
Hair	Black, dry, kinky	Soft, oily, yellow, early gray, red	Thick, oily, wavy
Teeth	Protruded, big/crooked/gums emaciated	Moderate in size, yellowish tinge, soft gums	Strong, white
Eyes	Small, dull, dry, brown/black	Sharp, penetrating, green, gray, yellow	Big, attractive, blue eyes, thick eyelashes
Appetite	Variable, scanty	Good, excessive, unbearable	Good appetite but can bear hunger easily
Taste that is conducive	Sweet, salty, sour	Sweet, bitter, astringent	Pungent, bitter, astringent
Taste that is not conducive	Pungent, bitter, astringent	Spicy, sour, salty, pungent	Sweet, sour, salty
Thirst	Variable	Excessive	Scanty
Defecation	Dry, hard, constipated	Soft, oily, tendency towards loosely formed stools	Thick, oily, more in quantity, well-formed stools, less frequency
Physical activity	Very active	Moderate	Lethargic (aversion to rigorous physical activity)
Mind	Restless, active, fluctuating decisions	Impulsive, ambitious, intelligent, short-tempered	Calm, slow and steady
Emotional temperament	Fearful, insecure, unpredictable	Aggressive, irritable, jealous	Calm, greedy, attached
Memory	Recent memory good but remote memory poor	Both recent and remote memories are good	Recent memory low but remote memory good
Dreams	Fearful, jumping, flying, running	Fiery, anger, violence, war	Watery, river, ocean, lake, swimming, romantic
Sleep	Scanty, interrupted	Moderate and sound	Heavy, prolonged
Speech	Fast	Moderate speed	Comparatively slow and calculative
Handling finances	Tendency towards excessive and impulsive spending	Moderate, spends on luxuries	Saves money, tendency to spend more on food
Pulse	Thready, feeble, moves like a snake	Moderate, jumping like a frog	Broad, slow, moves like a swan

to withdraw mind from focusing on external objects and to redirect itself internally, thus giving human beings power to channelize their energies toward attainment of *mokṣha* state.[14] This approach to treatment focusing on promotion of positive health and well-being has been mentioned by *Charaka as naiṣṭhiki chikitsa*.[15]

INTEGRATION OF YOGA WITH BIOMEDICINE AND AYURVEDA

In the last two decades, rise in research in the domain of integration of yoga with modern medicine has led to enhanced acceptability of yoga as an adjunct to modern medicine, especially for noncommunicable lifestyle-related disorders including mental health disorders.[16] Scientific exploration has also been done to unravel the underlying mechanisms through which yoga may work. As yoga therapy evolved, for the therapists, the modern scientific mechanisms of yoga became the base for deciding the therapy. For example, the effect of certain practices on the autonomic nervous system (ANS) became the basis for indication or contraindication of a practice in a particular condition characterized by dominance of a particular limb of ANS. Though application of yoga using such scientific rationale is good and should be encouraged, the traditional holistic vision of seeing an individual should not be compromised.

Sankhya school of philosophy says that whole creation is made up of two components: (1) matter (prakriti) and (2) consciousness (purusha).[4] If we look at the roots, both Yoga and Ayurveda emerge from the *vedas*. Ancient texts of yoga actually use prakriti classification of Ayurveda (*doshas*) to describe the therapeutic effects of the yogic practices on the body. For example, Hatha Yoga Pradipika (HYP) describes *surya bhedana* as vata reducing practice (*vataghna*) (HYP 2.53), similarly, both HYP[17] and Gheranda Samhita (GS)[18] describe *kapalabhati* as "*kapha-dosha-vinashini*" means the destroyer of kapha (phlegm) dosha. **Table 2** provides several other such references from ancient yoga texts where Ayurveda-based prakriti classification has been used for therapeutic applications of yoga and suggesting various lifestyle corrections. In a research study, which aimed to understand guna-based clinical correlates of various psychiatric disorders, we applied vedic personality inventory (VPI, vedicpersonality.org) on 113 patients (73 males, 40 females) suffering from various psychiatric disorders and 113 age- and gender-matched healthy controls. This study showed that in comparison to healthy subjects, patients with psychiatric disorders had lower sattva scores. Patients with psychotic disorders had lowest sattva scores and highest tamas scores among all psychiatric disorders and those with anxiety disorders had highest "rajas" scores. This redefining of mental health disorders in terms of *doshas* and *gunas* is particularly important because

TABLE 2: Yoga practices for different Ayurveda-based prakriti types as per ancient yoga texts.

Type of dosha	Vata	Pitta	Kapha	Kapha-pitta	Vata-kapha	Tridosha
Helpful practices	Surya bhedana (HYP 2.50)	Śītalī (HYP 2.58)	Dhauti karma (HYP 2.25)	Daṇḍadhauti (GS 1.38)	Ujjjāyīkumbhakaṃ (GS 5.71-72)	Mayurasana (HYP 1.32)
	Jalabasti (GS:1.46-47)		Kapalabhati (HYP 2.35)	Vamanadhauti (GS 1.39)		Vastikarma (HYP 2.27)
			Ujjāyī (HYP 2.51-52)	Vastradhauti (GS 1.40-41)		Nauli (HYP 2.34)
			Jihvāmūladhauti (GS 1.30)	Śītalīkumbhakaṃ (GS 1.73-74)		Bhastrikā (HYP 2.62-65)
			Kapālarandhra (GS 1.34)			
			Netiyogaḥ (GS 1.50-51)			
			Kapālabhāti (GS 1.55)			

TABLE 3: Dietary recommendations to be followed by a yoga practitioner (sadhaka) as per traditional yoga texts.

S. No.	Dietary aspect	Word-to-word english translation of the recommendations in ancient texts with relevant example	Reference
1.	Diet for different gunas	*Sattvic diet:* Foods which increase life, purity, strength, health, joy and cheerfulness, which are juicy and oleaginous, substantial and agreeable, are dear to sattvic people (e.g., fresh ripened fruits as per the season, vegetables and salads, cows milk, grains, and nuts)	BG 17.8
		Rajasic diet: Foods that are bitter, sour, saline, excessively hot, dry, pungent and burning, are liked by the rajasic people and are productive of pain, grief, and disease (e.g., excessive use of salt, tamarind, chilly, garlic, onion; excessive consumption of tea, coffee, etc.)	BG 17.9
		Tamasic diet: That which is stale, tasteless, putrid, rotten and impure refuse (leftover foods), causing dullness of the mind, is the food liked by tamasic people (e.g., food left for more than 3–4 hours after cooking, dried and devoid of freshness—fermented foods and drinks, refined, canned and processed food. Many junk food items such as pizza, burger, cheese, etc., may fall under this category)	BG 17.10
2.	Value of moderation in eating	*Mitāhāraḥ* is defined as consumption of agreeable and sattvic food leaving one-fourth of the stomach free, and eaten (as an offering to God)	HYP 1.38
		He who practices yoga without moderation of diet, incurs various diseases, and obtains no success	GS 5.16
3.	Conducive food for yogi	The most conducive foods for the yogis are: good grains, wheat, Shashtika rice (variety of rice that needs 60 days to be harvested) barley, milk, ghee, butter, rock sugar, honey, dry ginger, patola (ridge guard), five vegetables [Balasaka (*Tinospora cordifolia*), Kalasaka (*Chenopodium album*), Patolapatraka (*Alternanthera sessilis*), Vastaka (*Amaranthus Polygonoides*), Himalochika (*Bacopa monnieri*)], mung and such pulses and pure water	HYP 1.62 & GS 5.20
		A yogi should eat rice, barley (roti) or wheat roti. He may eat mudga (green gram), masa beans (black gram), gram, etc. These should be clean, white and free from chaff	GS 5.17
		A yogi may eat patola (ridge guard), jackfruit, manakachu (*Alocasia macrorrhizos*), kakkola (*Piper cubeba*), the bonduc nut, cucumber, plantain, the unripe plantain, the small plantain, the plantain stem, the roots, brinjal, and medicinal roots and fruits	GS 5.18-19
		Easily digestible, agreeable and cooling foods which nourish the humors of the body, a yogi may eat according to his desire	GS 5.29
		Cardamomum, jaiphal, cloves, aphrodisiacs or stimulants, the rose-apple, haritaki (*Terminalia chebula*), and date palms, a yogi may eat while practicing yoga	GS 5.28
4.	Prohibited food for yogi	The foods which are prohibited for the yogi are: those which are bitter, sour, pungent, salty, heating, green vegetables (other those prescribed), sour gruel, oil, sesame and mustard, alcohol, fish, flesh foods, curds, buttermilk, horse gram, fruit of jujube (ber fruit), oil cakes, asafetida and garlic	HYP 1.59
		Unhealthy diet should not be taken, that is reheated after becoming cold, which is dry (devoid of natural oil), which is excessively salty or acidic, stale or has too many (mixed) vegetables	HYP 1.60
		A yogi should avoid hard (not easily digestible), sinful food (food that is obtained by hurting more evolved living beings), or putrid foods (fermented foods), or very hot, or stale food (kept for many hours after cooking), as well as very cooling (e.g., ice-creams, cold drinks, etc., after food) or very much exciting food (e.g., excess of chilly, garlic, onion, tea, coffee, etc.)	GS 5.30

ancient texts also provide specific lifestyle guidelines on correcting the imbalances in them.[17] For example, texts such as Bhagavad Gita (BG)[19] do mention about the diet that may be conducive for enhancing specific *gunas* and dietary advices for purity of the mind **(Table 3)**. Thus, it is important that even for diagnosis and management of disorders an integrative approach is followed for Yoga therapy, where modern scientific assessments are combined with *dosha*- and *guna*-based assessments to determine the appropriate therapy plan for the patients.

CONCLUSION

Approach to mental health has evolved over years from multifactorial causation to monocausal theories and back to a multifactorial model. With the increasing popularity of traditional systems of medicine, the emphasis has shifted back toward personalized holistic aspects in diagnosis and treatment of mental health disorders. Integration of biomedicine and traditional systems of medicine looks like the way forward in which mental healthcare would evolve in the years to come. It is important that traditional systems of medicine explore their full potential, and the vision provided in classical texts is tested in future research, with the aim to explore and amalgamate the best possible treatment approaches from different systems of medicine.

REFERENCES

1. Federoff HJ, Gostin LO. Evolving from reductionism to holism: is there a future for systems medicine? JAMA. 2009;302(9):994-6.
2. Kendler KS. From many to one to many—the search for causes of psychiatric illness. JAMA Psychiatry. 2019;76(10):1085-91.
3. Patwardhan B. Ayurveda and integrative medicine: riding a tiger. J Ayurveda Integr Med. 2010;1(1):13-5.
4. Sedlmeier P, Srinivas K. How do theories of cognition and consciousness in ancient Indian thought systems relate to current western theorizing and research. Front Psychol. 2016;7:343.
5. Acharya YT (Ed). Agniveśa, Charaka Samhita, redacted by Charaka and Dridhabala with Ayurveda Dipika commentary by Chakrapāṇi, 4th edition. Chapter no. 1: Sarira sthana; Sloka no.: 67-69. Varanasi, India: Chaukhamba Surbharati Prakashan; 2001.
6. Bhishagacharya HP. Aśhtaṅga Hṛdaya of Vāgbhaṭa with commentaries Sarvāṅga Sundari of Aruṇadatta and Āyurveda Rasāyana of Hemadri, 9th edition. Chapter no. 12: Sutra sthana; Sloka no.: 67. Varanasi, India: Chaukhamba Orientalia Publication; 2005.
7. Acharya YT (Ed). Agniveṣa, Charaka Samhita, redacted by Charaka and Dridhabala with Ayurveda Dipika commentary by Chakrapāṇi, 4th edition. Chapter no. 1: Nidana sthana; Sloka no.: 108. Varanasi, India: Chaukhamba Surbharati Prakashan; 2001.
8. Acharya YT (Ed). Agniveshạ, Charaka Samhita, redacted by Charaka and Dridhabala with Ayurveda Dipika commentary by Chakrapāṇi, 4th edition. Chapter no. 1: Sutra sthana; Sloka no.: 15, 16. Varanasi, India: Chaukhamba Surbharati Prakashan; 2001.
9. Acharya YT (Ed). Agnivesha, Charaka Samhita, redacted by Charaka and Dridhabala with Ayurveda Dipika commentary by Chakrapāṇi, 4th edition. Chapter no. 1: Sarira sthana; Sloka no.: 3. Varanasi, India: Chaukhamba Surbharati Prakashan; 2001.
10. Acharya YT (Ed). Agnivesha, Charaka Samhita, redacted by Charaka and Dridhabala with Ayurveda Dipika commentary by Chakrapāṇi, 4th edition. Chapter no. 11: Sutra sthana; Sloka no.: 27. Varanasi, India: Chaukhamba Surbharati Prakashan; 2001.
11. Acharya YT (Ed). Agnivesha, Charaka Samhita, redacted by Charaka and Dridhabala with Ayurveda Dipika commentary by Chakrapāṇi, 4th edition. Chapter no. 1: Sarira sthana; Sloka no.: 134. Varanasi, India: Chaukhamba Surbharati Prakashan; 2001.
12. Acharya YT (Ed). Agnivesha, Charaka Samhita, redacted by Charaka and Dridhabala with Ayurveda Dipika commentary by Chakrapāṇi, 4th edition. Chapter no. 1: Sarira sthana; Sloka no.: 95. Varanasi, India: Chaukhamba Surbharati Prakashan; 2001.
13. Acharya YT (Ed). Agnivesha, Charaka Samhita, redacted by Charaka and Dridhabala with Ayurveda Dipika commentary by Chakrapāṇi, 4th edition. Chapter no. 1: Sarira sthana; Sloka no.: 137. Varanasi, India: Chaukhambha Surabharathi Prakashana; 2001.

14. Acharya YT (Ed). Agniveśha, Charaka Samhita, redacted by Charaka and Dridhabala with Ayurveda Dipika commentary by Chakrapāṇi, 4th edition. Chapter no. 1: Sarira sthana; Sloka no.: 138, 139. Varanasi, India: Chaukhamba Surbharati Prakashan; 2001.
15. Acharya YT (Ed). Agniveśha, Charaka Samhita, redacted by Charaka and Dridhabala with Ayurveda Dipika commentary by Chakrapāṇi, 4th edition. Chapter no. 1: Sarira sthana; Sloka no.: 94. Varanasi, India: Chaukhamba Surbharati Prakashan; 2001.
16. Cramer H, Ward L, Saper R, Fishbein D, Dobos G, Lauche R. The safety of yoga: a systematic review and meta-analysis of randomized controlled trials. Am J Epidemiol. 2015;182(4):281-93.
17. Svatmarama YS. The Hatha Yoga Pradipika. Alexandria: Library of Alexandria; 1975. p. 97.
18. Digambarji S. Gheranda Samhita. Berlin, Germany: XinXii; 2017. p. 83.
19. Swarupananda S. Srimad Bhagavad Gita. Advaita Ashrama, Belur Math, Kolkata: Ramakrishna Math; 2016. p. 396.

SECTION 2

Neurobiological Dimensions

4. **Neurophysiology of Yoga**
   Kaviraja Udupa, Inbaraj G, Sathyaprabha TN

5. **Neurophysiology of Meditation**
   Ajay Kumar Nair, Bindu M Kutty

6. **Role of Neuroimaging in Understanding Mental Health Effects of Yoga**
   Vanteemar S Sreeraj, Venkataram Shivakumar, Vijay Kumar KG, Naren P Rao

7. **Role of Transcranial Magnetic Stimulation in Yoga Research**
   Ramajayam Govindaraj, Jitender Jakhar, Urvakhsh Meherwan Mehta

8. **Insights into Mode of Action of Yoga in Mental Disorders: A Summary of Biological Evidence**
   Monojit Debnath, Rima Dada, Michael Berk

CHAPTER 4

Neurophysiology of Yoga

Kaviraja Udupa, Inbaraj G, Sathyaprabha TN

INTRODUCTION

The exploration of the physiological benefits of yoga (which is one of the gems of Indian cultural heritage) has increased tremendously in the last few decades resulting in a plethora of scientific studies. These studies have looked into various physiological measures enhanced or improved by yoga through numerous well-structured research studies carried out globally. These physiological benefits of yoga have been extensively studied in healthy individuals who practiced short-term yoga, Siddhis (people who have mastered and attained extraordinary powers), and patients with various disorders. The cellular, molecular, and systemic effects of yoga have been well documented through studies that looked into electrical activities of the heart [electrocardiogram (ECG)], brain [electroencephalography (EEG)], and muscles [electromyography (EMG)], and assessment of the regulation of the autonomic nervous system (ANS), neuroendocrine axis, and radio imaging.

The human body tries to maintain homeostasis of various interconnected systems through several neurochemical, immunological, and molecular pathways. This homeostasis is altered in various disease conditions as a result of several cumulative factors, of which stress is of primary importance.

Yoga, an ancient Indian discipline known to bestow good health, is practiced widely across the globe. It has evolved over thousands of years as a way to control the mind and behavior. In its traditional context, yoga had its roots in the yoga sutras of Patanjali, from which many interpretations and translations have been made. Practicing yoga aims to develop a state of physical and mental well-being, inner harmony, and ultimately an experience involving the union of the self with the supreme. Yoga has become increasingly popular in the West, also because of its positive effects on health. These encouraging effects of yoga generated enhanced interest among the scientific community, resulting in growing numerous research studies exploring the positive impacts of yoga on multiple dimensions, including physiological parameters, emotional perceptions, and cognitive functionality.[1] In recent decades, publications on yoga-related research have exponentially increased. In general, physiological measures such as brain activity (electrophysiology and imaging measures), cardiorespiratory measures (pulse rate, respiratory rate, blood pressure, and variability of these measures over time), biochemical and immunological variables are the most commonly assessed parameters in both healthy volunteers and patients with various disorders to understand the physiology of yoga.

Yoga appears to be a perfect antidote for stress, effectively tackling the dreaded effects of stress acting via the modulation of sympathovagal, neuroendocrine and psycho-neuro-immunological balance, resulting in restoring good health. Although overall background ideas of yoga modulating the homeostasis are well established, there needs to be more long-term, in-depth and well-controlled studies to understand the complex interactions of yoga and stress coping mechanisms and provide scientific credibility to yoga research. These steps would hopefully enable mankind to adopt a disease-free and healthy lifestyle.

A neurophysiological overview suggests that control over respiration (breath, prana) seems to be a fundamental factor in controlling higher cortical functioning, leading to control over: lower medullary centers (seat of control of the visceral autonomic functions, cardiovascular and vagal regulation), emotional centers, and the hypothalamus.[2] The human body tries to achieve homeostasis by balancing neural, endocrine, and immunological functions in coherence with other systems. Further, these systems function as a coordinated orchestra at various molecular, cellular, and tissue levels to achieve homeostasis. However, in physical as well as mental disorders, the ability of these regulatory systems to achieve this balance is lost and this imbalance could be normalized with the practice of yoga. In this chapter, we will outline the major neurophysiological processes and neural circuits that are influenced by the practice of yoga.

■ THE BEGINNING OF YOGIC RESEARCH IN NEUROPHYSIOLOGY

Research on the psychophysiological correlates of yoga dates back to the 1920s with the work of Swami Kuvalyananda at Kaivalyadhama, Lonavala, Maharashtra. During that time, some yogis claimed that they could stop their heart from beating or survive without air. A study by Kothari et al. (1973) showed that yogis could control their heart rate by significantly reducing their metabolism and oxygen utilization.[3] Bagchi and Wenger (1957), in their studies on yoga practitioners, suggested that yogic meditation is a form of profound relaxation of the ANS without sleep or drowsiness.[4] Of course, these extreme practices require intense dedication, regular practice, and higher levels of consciousness. These practices and higher-level skills might not be relevant to most people who practice yoga as a means to improve health and reduce the risk of disease.

The possible mechanisms for the attainment of these skills could be neurophysiological [sympathovagal balance; fast (gamma and beta) and slow (theta and delta) frequencies of EEG; activation of default mode networks] and/or neurochemical [excitatory (glutamate and norepinephrine) and inhibitory (GABA) neurotransmitter balance] homeostasis. Once a constant periodic breathing control is established, there may be a reciprocal biochemical stability that helps to maintain that control. Further, autonomic control over the hypothalamus may also have a positive effect on endocrine functions. By willfully exercising the cortex, the individual can have complete control over the vital and emotional functions of the brain by creating a mutual link between the cortex, reticular system, and multiple centers of the brain. It is quite possible that in a yogi, both the reticular and the cerebral cortex are changed functionally and proliferated structurally.[2] In the 1970s, Elmer and Green from Menninger Foundation in Topeka, Kansas, conducted numerous biofeedback experiments on Swami Rama. They found Swami Rama could produce different brain waves at will, including theta and delta (sleep) waves while remaining aware of his environment. He was also able to create a temperature difference of 10°F between two points on the palm of his hand, evidently regulating blood flow through the radial and ulnar arteries. Thus, these "siddhis" (special powers) tend to have physiological bases, but we are still not clear about the cause/effect of these changes in the human body. In 1971, researchers proposed that transcendental meditation (TM) relaxes and stimulates physical as well as mental health by reducing stress, increasing creativity, and other intellectual skills.[5]

Initial work in the area of yoga and neurophysiology was carried out at National Institute of Mental Health and Neuro Sciences (NIMHANS) in the department of Neurophysiology, led by Professor Desiraju. He pioneered the move "Project Consciousness" and it involved studying the brain in different states of consciousness. Drs Telles and Desiraju conducted numerous research studies on pranayama and found that different pranayama breathing led to different types of alterations in brain oxygen consumption and metabolic rate. These physiological and psychological modifications are connected with both short-term and long-term yoga practices. The practice of yoga resulted in reduced metabolic and oxygen consumption, enhanced cognitive and cerebral neurophysiology effects, and improved neuromuscular and respiratory function.[6]

MODERN NEUROPHYSIOLOGICAL RESEARCH TOOLS USED IN STUDYING THE EFFECTS OF YOGA

There have been several advances in understanding the psycho-physio-neurobiology of yoga. The effects of yoga have been assessed using the following tools to understand the physiological basis of yoga: EEG, evoked potentials, ECG, heart rate and blood pressure variability. Research studies have attempted to understand the cortical excitability changes in patients with neurological and psychiatric disorders using transcranial magnetic stimulation (TMS), a non-invasive mode of brain stimulation technique. These studies observed that a single session of yoga practice resulted in a significant lengthening of the cortical silent period in the yoga group as compared to intermittent walking, thereby showing enhanced cortical GABA tone following yoga.[7] Thus yoga training enhances the inhibitory control or "braking" to bring about optimal control system to attain higher precision in both motor as well as cognitive functions.

Efficacy of Yoga Assessed using Cardiorespiratory and Autonomic Variables

The ANS regulates the functioning of visceral organs involuntarily through its sympathetic and parasympathetic limbs. These two limbs function in a complementary manner to maintain the balance and obtain the optimal functioning of the system. This sympathovagal balance is known to be altered in various psychosomatic disorders and the usual pattern observed has been increased sympathetic activity and reduced parasympathetic activity. The practice of yoga has shown beneficial effects in the modulation or normalization of the sympathovagal balance of the ANS evidenced in the form of reduced heart rate, blood pressure, respiratory rate, intraocular pressure, fasting blood sugar in diabetes, increased breath holding time, galvanic skin response, and better sympathovagal balance with normalization of baroreceptor sensitivity, and blood pressure variability. Heart rate variability (HRV), an effective technique to assess the regulation of the ANS, has been widely used to understand the intrinsic mechanisms underlying the potential effects of yoga. Several studies have shown the beneficial effects of yoga on HRV in short- and long-term practices. The majority of studies provide evidence that yoga enhances HRV and improves cardiovagal balance.[8]

A simple breathing practice (pranayama) ensures better use of oxygen and lung surface areas leading to the enhanced circulation of oxygenated blood throughout the body. Studies have shown that pranayama influences the ANS by exhibiting an increase in high-frequency (HF) power in HRV, reflecting increased vagal tone.[8] It also decreases the low-frequency power, denoting a reduction in sympathetic tone, thereby shifting the autonomic balance toward relative parasympathetic dominance.[9] Pranayama also inhibits the sympathetic tone of the skeletal muscle blood vessels leading to vasodilation, thereby reducing vascular resistance and diastolic blood pressure. The therapeutic benefits of breathing practice are mainly accomplished by the modulation of the ANS: by reducing the sympathetic tone and increasing the parasympathetic tone to normalize the altered sympathovagal balance.

Research from NIMHANS has found that yoga helps in modulating autonomic dysfunction, which is a known element in many ailments such as epilepsy, migraine, neurodegenerative disorders, depression, bipolar disorders, and schizophrenia. In one study, children with Duchenne muscular dystrophy were assessed for modulation in HRV measures following yoga therapy and it showed equal and beneficial effects compared to physiotherapy.[10] Similarly, it has been reported that individuals who practiced yoga had a significant reduction in seizure recurrence, needed lower doses of antiepileptic medications, and had fewer side effects of medications. Another study from NIMHANS found that the practice of yoga reduced seizure frequency and modulated the ANS by enhancing parasympathetic activity.[11] Meditation stimulates the vagus nerve and could reduce the seizure frequency by 28–38% by modulating the limbic system and ANS activity via the hypothalamus.[12] The conditioning of these brain regions by the practice of meditation is proposed to assist in maintaining normal homeostasis. Hence, stress reduction may play a pivotal role in the clinical improvement of these patients.

Effects of Yoga Assessed using Evoked Potentials and EEG

Evoked potentials indicate the response and the degree of attention of the subject to an individual stimulus. Studies on the peak latency and peak amplitude of the P300 auditory event-related potentials have shown that yoga reduces peak latencies, indicating better cortical inhibition and sensory discrimination. In cyclic meditation (CM) studies, participants showed a greater ability in the P300 auditory oddball test to distinguish hearing sounds from various pitches. These sustained latencies of evoked potentials, generated in the cerebral cortex following CM, support the concept of cortical inhibition following CM.[13] The mid-latency auditory evoked potential also showed a change in meditators suggesting that the neural generators in cortical regions are of longer latency.[14] This signifies greater cortical inhibition and effective subcortical neural modulation that leads to optimum autonomic neural functioning. EEG shows how the brain's coherent status is processed during cognitive and sensory inputs. The practice of Sudarshan Kriya Yoga (SKY) was shown to increase the beta activity of the brain in EEG studies. Similarly, TM practitioners showed an increase in alpha/delta power and a decrease in beta/alpha power.[15] Thus, neurophysiological evaluations of yoga using EEG studies have demonstrated the calming effects of yoga/meditation in terms of potentiation of slow waves, modulation of faster waves, and better discrimination abilities in cognitive processing tasks.

Effects of Yoga on Neuroplasticity

Yoga and its effect on neuroplasticity are evident from the fact that age-related gray matter volume (GMV) decline is reduced in individuals practicing meditation regularly. Brain-derived neurotrophic factor (BDNF), which is known to play a pivotal role and is positively correlated with enhanced neuroplasticity and neurogenesis, tends to increase with the practice of yoga. This enhancement has been seen at the level of morphometric, neural network, and molecular levels. As the key regulators of neuroplasticity, BDNF and its signaling cascades: receptor tyrosine kinase B (TrkB), and mechanistic target of rapamycin (mTOR) contribute to complex functions of the brain such as cognition and emotion. The practice of meditation reduces inflammation by reducing the levels of inflammatory marker interleukin-6 (IL-6) and down-regulation of the nuclear factor kappa B (NF-κB) pathway, an effect opposite to that of chronic stress on gene expression, leading to an increase in neuroplasticity. Yoga also helps achieve and maintain optimum cellular health by enhancing genomic stability, chromosomal integrity, and telomere length.[16]

YOGA AND STRESS

Yoga practice is especially effective in combating the negative effects of stress. Compared to other exercise modalities, practicing yoga has superior effects on certain stress tolerance and mood measures. Persistent activation of the "fight-or-flight" reaction is linked to the onset of psychiatric disorders such as anxiety and depression. A trial by Rocha[17] compared salivary cortisol concentrations in a 6-month-trained yoga and a periodic physical exercise group. The yoga group demonstrated considerably lower levels of cortisol than those of the physical exercise group following the program.[17] Another study with electroencephalographic recordings and measures of serum cortisol showed an increase in alpha rhythm frontally and a decrease in cortisol after a single yoga session.[18] In a study by Streeter,[19] an analysis of yoga practice on gamma-aminobutyric acid (GABA) levels suggested that yoga is effective in conditions with low-GABA such as depression, anxiety, and epilepsy. Further, the neurohemodynamic correlates of audible "OM" chanting were assessed using functional magnetic resonance imaging (fMRI) in right-handed healthy volunteers and the results showed significant deactivation of the limbic system, i.e., the bilateral orbitofrontal, anterior cingulate, parahippocampal gyri, thalami, and hippocampi.[20] Thus, yoga practice appears to balance emotional regulation in response to stress **(Flowchart 1)**.

YOGA AND CARDIOVASCULAR DISORDERS

Cardiovascular disorders (CVDs) are known to be associated with adverse changes in autonomic function, with elevated sympathetic

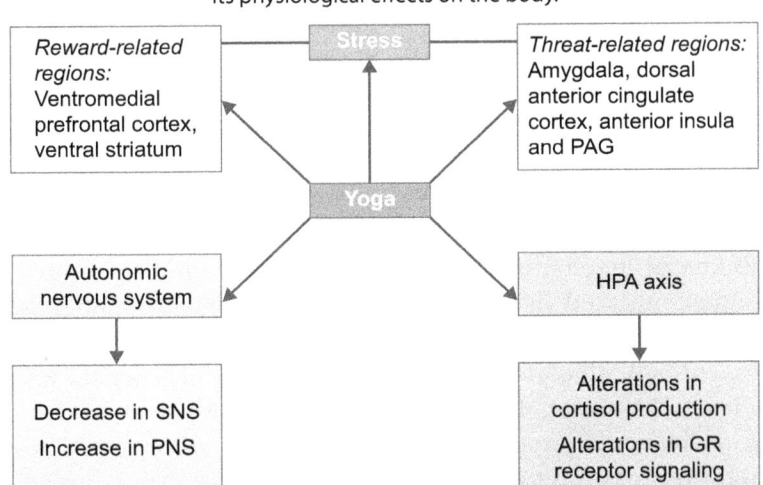

Flowchart 1: Diagrammatic representation of the effects of yoga in reducing stress and its physiological effects on the body.

(GR: glucocorticoid receptor; HPA: hypothalamic-pituitary-adrenal; PNS: parasympathetic nervous system; SNS: sympathetic nervous system)

activity for a prolonged period along with parasympathetic withdrawal. This rise in the sympathetic nervous system (SNS) activity mediates modification in the neuroendocrine system through the hypothalamic-pituitary-adrenal (HPA) axis. Bringing a change in the level of stress hormones (e.g., adrenaline, aldosterone, cortisol, and norepinephrine), leading to an increase in heart rate, blood pressure, and concentrations of blood glucose and lipids. This mechanism contributes to the advancement of atherosclerosis and CVDs, especially in people with chronic stress and a sedentary lifestyle. Various investigators have evaluated several cardiovascular indicators before and after a program/practice session of yoga and found decreased total peripheral resistance and enhanced arterial compliance, stroke volume, and cardiac output. Studies that looked at blood pressure and HRV have found that yoga significantly improves HRV and modulates the sympathovagal balance suggesting that yoga enhances the vagal tone and reduces sympathetic activity. Yoga is known to effectively tackle the dreaded impacts of stress on physiological systems mainly by achieving sympathovagal balance (short-term regulation) and helps to maintain homeostasis and restore health by modulating the long-term mediators (HPA axis, biochemical and inflammatory markers of stress). Thus yoga achieves homeostasis in various disorders by modulating the ANS, neuroendocrine, and psycho-neuro-immunological axis, and effectively integrating the functions of various systems of the body.

The neurohumoral mechanism which is found to be dysregulated in CVD can be favorably modulated through yoga, by reducing serum cortisol, aldosterone, and catecholamine levels. Moreover, the regular practice of yoga is known to improve nitric oxide bioavailability leading to reduced oxidative stress and enhanced endothelial function. Besides, yoga also reduces the rate pressure product (a measurable index of myocardial oxygen consumption and load on the heart), lipid profiles, and even enables atherosclerosis regression when combined with dietary and other lifestyle changes.[21] Systemic inflammation has been considered as a strong predictor of mortality in CVD. Yoga is found to reduce inflammation by reducing proinflammatory response genes and reverse the NF-κB-related transcription of proinflammatory cytokines. Thus yoga provides relief from the effect of stress and provides a sense of well-being.

A study by Huang et al., 2013 found that the practice of hatha yoga can reduce perceived stress and salivary cortisol, a major effector of SNS and HPA pathways, and enhance cardiometabolic health. Also, this study noted that even a single hatha yoga session (90 min) could significantly increase the HF power component of HRV.[22] In a 12-week yoga study by Hari Krishna et al., 2014, they showed that yoga in addition to standard medical treatment had significant improvement in parasympathetic activity and decreased sympathetic activity in patients with heart failure.[23] In another study by Muralikrishnan et al., 2012 Isha yoga practitioners had balanced positive vagal efferent activity and improved HRV while resting and breathing deeply compared to nonyoga practitioners.[24] A study by Patil et al., 2015 of elderly subjects with arterial stiffness found that yoga helped in reducing arterial stiffness along with a reduction in blood pressure when compared to brisk-walking. This study further showed that yoga helped to reduce sympathetic activity and enhance endothelial function with increased nitric oxide bioavailability.[25] Even in resting conditions, regular yoga practitioners have increased vagal tone as compared to nonyoga practitioners. These changes in autonomic balance coupled with positive changes in the HPA axis, endothelial functions, and oxidative stress mechanisms possibly

Flowchart 2: Diagrammatic representation of the effects of yoga in reducing cardiovascular disorders (CVD) and its pathophysiological steps.

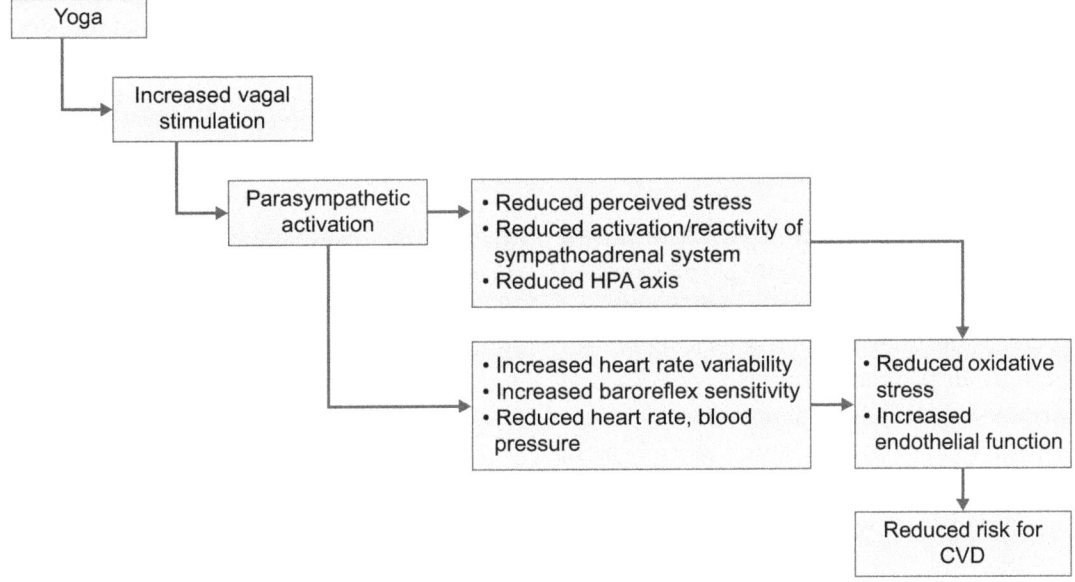

(HPA: hypothalamic-pituitary-adrenal)

protect an individual from cardiovascular morbidities. Thus, by improving cardiovagal activity and reducing sympathetic function, yoga modulates the neuro-cardiac regulation and reduces the risk of CVDs **(Flowchart 2)**.

NEUROPHYSIOLOGY OF PRANAYAMA

Pranayama or regulated breathing is an integral component of yoga, which is said to affect the physiological process. The voluntary control of the breath serves as a link between the brain and the body. Pranayama has shown beneficial effects on biochemical, psychophysiological, neurocognitive, and metabolic functions in healthy volunteers and subjects with various clinical conditions.[26] David S Shannahoff-Khalsa and his group unveiled the complexities of mind–body interactions and demonstrated how the nasal cycle is closely related to the ultradian rhythm of the cerebral hemispheric activity.[27] Using EEG they demonstrated that unilateral forced nostril breathing has a selective hemispheric activation, i.e., forced nostril breathing in one nostril generates a significant rise in EEG amplitude in the contralateral hemisphere.[28] Further, studies on yogic breathing evaluated the effect of Kapalabhati (15 min) on electroencephalogram activity.[29] The analysis revealed that there was enhanced alpha activity during the initial 5 minutes of Kapalabhati practice and in the later 15 minutes, theta activity was found to be enhanced in the occipital region. A study by Telles et al., 2013 on Bhastrika Pranayama, which was practiced for 18 minutes showed a reduction in anticipatory responses.[30] Mukha Bhastrika for nine rounds showed a significant reduction in visual reaction time and auditory reaction time in 22 healthy school children.[31] A study comparing the cumulative effect of slow and fast pranayama on cognitive functions in healthy volunteers has reported significant improvement in executive functions, perceived stress scale, and reaction time in both fast and slow pranayama groups, except reverse digit span, which showed improvement only in fast pranayama group.[32] Practicing Bhramari pranayama (female honeybee humming breath) has been shown to cause nonepileptic paroxysmal gamma waves in the EEG.[33] Also, the practice of Bhramari for 10 minutes improved inhibition and reaction time in the stop-signal task that involves cognitive inhibition.[34] A study by Telles et al., 2013 assessed the effect of alternate nostril yoga breathing (nadishuddhi pranayama) on P300 auditory evoked potentials compared to breath awareness. There was a significant increase in peak amplitudes of the P300 at various scalp locations, along with a decrease in peak latency in the frontal scalp region, which suggests a positive influence on the cognitive processes required for sustained attention.[35] Experienced yoga practitioners during consciously-controlled rhythmic breathing with breath-holding, showed an increase in Na-wave amplitude and decrease in latency, although no changes were observed in the Pa-wave.[36]

Hemodynamic observations were made on a yogic technique that claimed to help eliminate and prevent heart attacks. The technique is a breath per minute (BPM) respiratory exercise with slow inspiration for 20 seconds, breath retention for 20 seconds, and slow expiration for 20 seconds, for 31 consecutive minutes. Recordings were carried out at three time points: pre-exercise resting period, a 31-minute exercise period, and a postexercise resting period. Around fourteen beat-to-beat parameters were measured noninvasively along with the left stroke work index and stroke systemic vascular resistance index. This breathing technique induced a profound shift in all hemodynamic variables during the one BPM exercise and the postexercise resting period, seeming to have a particular effect on the cardiorespiratory center regulating the Mayer wave patterns (0.1–0.01 Hz) of the cardiovascular system.[37]

EFFECT OF PRANAYAMA ON PSYCHOPHYSIOLOGY

In humans, respiration is the only neurological system that is under both autonomic and voluntary nervous control. Yogic breathing techniques have a significant influence on the modulation of autonomic nervous system functioning (AFT). A three-arm randomized controlled trial (RCT) using HRV as the measure of autonomic activity showed sympathetic arousal in the right uninostril breathing (UNB) group, and vagal dominance in the left UNB group following 6-week nostril breathing.[38] An RCT found that 20 minutes of alternate nostril breathing for a week increased galvanic skin resistance (GSR), which denotes enhanced parasympathetic activity and reduced sympathetic tone.[39] Nadishuddhi pranayama at a rate of one BPM has been found to enhance sinus arrhythmia and reduce the low-frequency component of HRV.[40] Slow breathing at a rate of 6 BPM with or without Ujjayi Pranayama has demonstrated an increase in baroreflex sensitivity (BRS) and a decrease in blood pressure.[41]

EFFECT OF PRANAYAMA ON RESPIRATORY SYSTEM

Yogic breathing technique is an effective way of improving pulmonary functions. Slow breathing at a rate of 6 BPM showed an increase in vital capacity, forced vital capacity, forced inspiratory vital capacity, and peak inspiratory flow rate.[42] A 12-week training in slow and fast pranayama on pulmonary function testing revealed that in the slow pranayama group, peak expiratory flow rate and forced expiratory volume were significantly improved, whereas, in the fast pranayama group, ratio of forced expiratory volume in first second to forced vital capacity was improved significantly[43] indicating the differential effects of these practices. Further, studies linking the effects of pranayama on respiratory regulatory centers and thereby on to pulmonary functions have to be performed.

EFFECT OF PRANAYAMA ON METABOLISM

Oxygen consumption has been used as a means to understand the body's metabolic activity. Research investigating the effects of Ujjayi Pranayama along with short and prolonged Kumbhaka (breath-hold) has shown that oxygen consumption rose with short Kumbhaka and decreased with prolonged breath-holding.[6] The immediate effect of Kapalabhati (1 min) showed a decrease in blood urea, and an increase in creatinine and tyrosine levels, possibly due to decarboxylation and oxidation mechanisms.[44]

YOGA AND BODY AWARENESS

Fiori et al. (2014) evaluated proprioceptive and vestibular body signals, and the presence of self-transcendence (ST) in a group of advanced yoga practitioners and controls without any experience in yoga.[45] Body signals were processed using the rod and frame test (RFT) and ST was measured using the temperament character inventory (TCI) subscale. Overall, yoga professionals demonstrated greater precision in RFT and higher ST scores on the TCI. These results suggest that yoga professionals are more aware of their bodies and can relate to ST elements. Yoga practitioners tolerated pain better (as measured by the time they kept their hand in cold water) and they had more GMV in several regions such as the insula, cingulate cortex, medial prefrontal cortex, inferior and superior parietal lobule, and increased intrainsular white matter connectivity. Furthermore, insular GMV had a positive correlation with pain tolerance (left and right insula) and years of yoga practice (left insula only). Yoga also had a huge impact on attention, memory, and executive domains. Yoga practice also improved visual attention ability by enhancing the ability to detect flicker frequencies and visual color discrimination.[46]

CONCLUSION AND FUTURE DIRECTIONS

The practice of yoga has been shown to change several physiological functions in the human body and brain, including neurocognitive capacities, maintaining the homeostasis of neurotransmitters, and modulation of autonomic functions. Most of these changes seem to correspond to the traditional understanding of the flow of *Prana* (vital energy) controlling the physical functions of the body. Thus, several research studies have found beneficial effects of yoga in coordinating various physiological systems to face challenges and threats. This balance is achieved by strengthening the inhibitory control through GABA, vagal activities, and other molecular mediators to potentiate quality checks in the system. Further studies are needed to prove whether this is the cause or effect of yoga-mediated positive changes. This needs long-term studies with a multitude of parameters (including GABAergic inhibitory control and vagal modulation of autonomic balance), to understand the coordination of various systems in bringing homeostasis. Also, there needs to be more long-term, in-depth and well-controlled studies to help us understand these complex interactions of yoga and health: this will add scientific credibility to yoga.

ॐ सर्वे भवन्तु सुखिनः। सर्वे सन्तु निरामयाः।
सर्वे भद्राणि पश्यन्तु ।मा कश्चिद्दुःखभाग्भवेत् ।
ॐ शान्तिः शान्तिः शान्तिः॥

(Aum, May All be Happy, May All be Free from Illness. May All See what is Auspicious, May no one Suffer. Aum, Peace, Peace, Peace)

REFERENCES

1. Gard T, Noggle JJ, Park CL, Vago DR, Wilson A. Potential self-regulatory mechanisms of yoga for psychological health. Front Hum Neurosci. 2014;8:770.

2. Ramamurthi B. Some thoughts on neurophysiological basis of yoga. Anc Sci Life. 1981;1(1):20-4.
3. Kothari LK, Bardia A, Gupta OP. The yogic claim of voluntary control over the heart beat: an unusual demonstration. Am Heart J. 1973;86(2):282-4.
4. Bagchi BK, Wenger MA. Electrophysiological correlates of some yogi exercises. Electroencephalography and Clinical Neurophysiology. 1957;7:132-49.
5. Wallace RK. Physiological effects of transcendental meditation. Science. 1970;167(3926):1751-4.
6. Telles S, Desiraju T. Oxygen consumption during pranayamic type of very slow-rate breathing. Indian J Med Res. 1991;94:357-63.
7. Jakhar J, Mehta UM, Ektare A, Vidyasagar PD, Varambally S, Thirthalli J, et al. Cortical inhibition in major depression: investigating the acute effect of single-session yoga versus walking. Brain Stimulat. 2019;12(6):7-9.
8. Tyagi A, Cohen M. Yoga and heart rate variability: a comprehensive review of the literature. Int J Yoga. 2016;9(2):97-113.
9. Harinath K, Malhotra AS, Pal K, Prasad R, Kumar R, Kain TC, et al. Effects of Hatha yoga and Omkar meditation on cardiorespiratory performance, psychologic profile, and melatonin secretion. J Altern Complement Med N Y N. 2004;10(2):261-8.
10. Pradnya D, Nalini A, Nagarathna R, Raju TR, Sendhilkumar R, Meghana A, et al. Effect of yoga as an add-on therapy in the modulation of heart rate variability in children with Duchenne muscular dystrophy. Int J Yoga. 2019;12(1):55-61.
11. Sathyaprabha TN, Satishchandra P, Pradhan C, Sinha S, Kaveri B, Thennarasu K, et al. Modulation of cardiac autonomic balance with adjuvant yoga therapy in patients with refractory epilepsy. Epilepsy Behav EB. 2008;12(2):245-52.
12. Breit S, Kupferberg A, Rogler G, Hasler G. Vagus nerve as modulator of the brain-gut axis in psychiatric and inflammatory disorders. Front Psychiatry. 2018;9:44.
13. Subramanya P, Telles S. A review of the scientific studies on cyclic meditation. Int J Yoga. 2009;2(2):46-8.
14. Subramanya P, Telles S. Changes in midlatency auditory evoked potentials following two yoga-based relaxation techniques. Clin EEG Neurosci. 2009;40(3):190-5.
15. Lee DJ, Kulubya E, Goldin P, Goodarzi A, Girgis F. Review of the neural oscillations underlying meditation. Front Neurosci. 2018;12:178.
16. Szebeni A, Szebeni K, DiPeri T, Chandley MJ, Crawford JD, Stockmeier CA, et al. Shortened telomere length in white matter oligodendrocytes in major depression: potential role of oxidative stress. Int J Neuropsychopharmacol. 2014;17(10):1579-89.
17. Rocha KKF, Ribeiro AM, Rocha KCF, Sousa MBC, Albuquerque FS, Ribeiro S, et al. Improvement in physiological and psychological parameters after 6 months of yoga practice. Conscious Cogn. 2012;21(2):843-50.
18. Kamei T, Toriumi Y, Kimura H, Ohno S, Kumano H, Kimura K. Decrease in serum cortisol during yoga exercise is correlated with alpha wave activation. Percept Mot Skills. 2000;90(3 Pt 1):1027-32.
19. Streeter CC, Whitfield TH, Owen L, Rein T, Karri SK, Yakhkind A, et al. Effects of yoga versus walking on mood, anxiety, and brain GABA levels: a randomized controlled MRS study. J Altern Complement Med N Y N. 2010;16(11):1145-52.
20. Kalyani BG, Venkatasubramanian G, Arasappa R, Rao NP, Kalmady SV, Behere RV, et al. Neurohemodynamic correlates of "OM" chanting: a pilot functional magnetic resonance imaging study. Int J Yoga. 2011;4(1):3-6.
21. Ornish D, Scherwitz LW, Doody RS, Kesten D, McLanahan SM, Brown SE, et al. Effects of stress management training and dietary changes in treating ischemic heart disease. JAMA. 1983;249(1):54-9.
22. Huang FJ, Chien DK, Chung UL. Effects of Hatha yoga on stress in middle-aged women. J Nurs Res. 2013;21(1):59-66.
23. Krishna BH, Pal P, Pal G, Balachander J, Jayasettiaseelon E, Sreekanth Y, et al. A Randomized Controlled Trial to Study the Effect of Yoga Therapy on Cardiac Function and N Terminal Pro BNP in Heart Failure. Integr Med Insights. 2014;9:1-6.
24. Muralikrishnan K, Balakrishnan B, Balasubramanian K, Visnegarawla F. Measurement of the effect of Isha Yoga on cardiac autonomic nervous system using short-term heart rate variability. J Ayurveda Integr Med. 2012;3(2):91-6.
25. Patil SG, Aithala MR, Das KK. Effect of yoga on arterial stiffness in elderly subjects with increased pulse pressure: a randomized controlled study. Complement Ther Med. 2015;23(4):562-9.
26. Saoji AA, Raghavendra BR, Manjunath NK. Effects of yogic breath regulation: a narrative review of scientific evidence. J Ayurveda Integr Med. 2019;10(1):50-8.
27. Werntz DA, Bickford RG, Bloom FE, Shannahoff-Khalsa DS. Alternating cerebral hemispheric activity and the lateralization of autonomic nervous function. Hum Neurobiol. 1983;2(1):39-43.

28. Werntz DA, Bickford RG, Shannahoff-Khalsa D. Selective hemispheric stimulation by unilateral forced nostril breathing. Hum Neurobiol. 1987;6(3):165-71.
29. Stancák A, Kuna M, Srinivasan, Dostálek C, Vishnudevananda S. Kapalabhati—yogic cleansing exercise. II. EEG topography analysis. Homeost Health Dis Int J Devoted Integr Brain Funct Homeost Syst. 1991;33(4):182-9.
30. Telles S, Yadav A, Gupta RK, Balkrishna A. Reaction time following yoga bellows-type breathing and breath awareness. Percept Mot Skills. 2013;117(1):89-98.
31. Bhavanani AB, Madanmohan, Udupa K. Acute effect of Mukh bhastrika (a yogic bellows type breathing) on reaction time. Indian J Physiol Pharmacol. 2003;47(3):297-300.
32. Sharma VK, Rajajeyakumar M, Velkumary S, Subramanian SK, Bhavanani AB, Madanmohan, et al. Effect of fast and slow pranayama practice on cognitive functions in healthy volunteers. J Clin Diagn Res. 2014;8(1):10-3.
33. Vialatte FB, Bakardjian H, Prasad R, Cichocki A. EEG paroxysmal gamma waves during Bhramari Pranayama: a yoga breathing technique. Conscious Cogn. 2009;18(4):977-88.
34. Rajesh SK, Ilavarasu J V, Srinivasan TM. Effect of Bhramari Pranayama on response inhibition: Evidence from the stop signal task. Int J Yoga. 2014;7(2):138-41.
35. Telles S, Singh N, Puthige R. Changes in P300 following alternate nostril yoga breathing and breath awareness. Biopsychosoc Med. 2013;7(1):11.
36. Telles S, Joseph C, Venkatesh S, Desiraju T. Alterations of auditory middle latency evoked potentials during yogic consciously regulated breathing and attentive state of mind. Int J Psychophysiol. 1993;14(3):189-98.
37. Shannahoff-Khalsa DS, Sramek BB, Kennel MB, Jamieson SW. Hemodynamic observations on a yogic breathing technique claimed to help eliminate and prevent heart attacks: a pilot study. J Altern Complement Med. 2004;10(5):757-66.
38. Pal GK, Agarwal A, Karthik S, Pal P, Nanda N. Slow yogic breathing through right and left nostril influences sympathovagal balance, heart rate variability, and cardiovascular risks in young adults. North Am J Med Sci. 2014;6(3):145-51.
39. Turankar AV, Jain S, Patel SB, Sinha SR, Joshi AD, Vallish BN, et al. Effects of slow breathing exercise on cardiovascular functions, pulmonary functions and galvanic skin resistance in healthy human volunteers—a pilot study. Indian J Med Res. 2013;137(5):916-21.
40. Jovanov E. On spectral analysis of heart rate variability during very slow yogic breathing. Conf Proc IEEE Eng Med Biol Soc. 2005;2005:2467-70.
41. Mason H, Vandoni M, Debarbieri G, Codrons E, Ugargol V, Bernardi L. Cardiovascular and respiratory effect of yogic slow breathing in the yoga beginner: what is the best approach? Evid-Based Complement Altern Med. 2013;2013:743504.
42. Sivakumar G, Prabhu K, Baliga R, Kirtana Pai M, Manjunatha S. Acute effects of deep breathing for a short duration (2-10 minutes) on pulmonary functions in healthy young volunteers. Indian J Physiol Pharmacol. 2011;55(2):154-9.
43. Dinesh T, Gaur G, Sharma V, Madanmohan T, Harichandra Kumar Kt, Bhavanani A. Comparative effect of 12 weeks of slow and fast pranayama training on pulmonary function in young, healthy volunteers: a randomized controlled trial. Int J Yoga. 2015;8(1):22-6.
44. Desai BP, Gharote ML. Effect of Kapalbhati on blood urea, creatinine and tyrosine. Act Nerv Super (Praha). 1990;32(2):95-8.
45. Fiori F, David N, Aglioti SM. Processing of proprioceptive and vestibular body signals and self-transcendence in Ashtanga yoga practitioners. Front Hum Neurosci. 2014;8:734.
46. Telles S, Nagarathna R, Nagendra HR. Improvement in visual perception following yoga training. J Indian Psychol. 1995;(31):30-2.

CHAPTER 5

Neurophysiology of Meditation

Ajay Kumar Nair, Bindu M Kutty

■ INTRODUCTION

Spiritual practices are widely prevalent in India and around the world, and have been a source of solace for patients to cope with illness and stressors. As such, the importance of integrating spirituality into patient care has been highlighted.[1] Yoga and meditative practices have also become very popular over the last few decades. Meditation refers to a range of mind–body techniques that can elicit intense experiential states often leading to improvements in overall well-being. Meditative techniques may include concentration (on breath, a mantra, some object or idea, etc.), passive awareness of sensations and perceptions, guided visualizations, generating goodwill and compassion for oneself or for others, and so on. A common end result of a successful meditation session is temporary disengagement from day-to-day challenges and routine activities, and a sense of calm and tranquility. Meditative practices across a number of traditions have been associated with a range of psychological benefits, especially in terms of changes in emotional regulation and interpersonal issues.[2]

Since meditative techniques can be offered in a structured manner, they are increasingly being used in randomized clinical trials for improving mental health outcomes. Since there are clear differences in the techniques practiced, the impact on the physiology and psychology of the practitioner needs to be carefully considered before recommending a particular meditation practice to a patient. Further research into the neurophysiology of meditation is thus imperative.

■ HISTORICAL OVERVIEW

Yoga and meditation have been practiced for thousands of years and their benefits have been documented in traditional texts. Studies on the effects of meditation examine state effects (changes in neurophysiology while participants are meditating), trait effects (long-term persistent differences in anatomy or physiology seen in meditators, as compared to controls, even when they are not meditating) and finally state-trait interactions. The process of the brain's adaptation to experience is called neuroplasticity, and is manifested through trait effects and state-trait interactions.

The earliest electroencephalography (EEG) studies on the state effects of meditation were carried out in the 1950s and 1960s. BK Anand[3] and others reported predominant alpha waves during meditation that persisted even in the presence of distractors. A foundational set of studies on the neurophysiology of meditation was carried out by a group of researchers studying the effects of transcendental meditation (TM). These studies from RK Wallace and colleagues[4,5] starting in the 1970s showed that TM practice enhanced theta and alpha power as well as low frequency synchrony leading to greater integration of brain functions. Similar studies employing many different meditative traditions were carried out under the leadership of T Desiraju at National Institute of Mental Health and

Neuro Sciences (NIMHANS) from 1975 until the early 1990s.

A landmark study on the trait effects of meditation examined changes in cortical thickness. Insight meditation practitioners, as compared to age and gender matched controls, had greater thickness of the right anterior insula, and right middle and superior frontal sulci, areas that were *a priori* considered relevant for interoception and cognitive processing, respectively.[6] The overall cortical thickness in each group was comparable, suggesting that the changes were meditation specific. Overall, this study showed, for the first time, meditation linked changes in brain structure. A number of studies have subsequently reported structural changes in gray and white matter volume, attributed to meditation.

Over the last few decades, research into meditation has expanded considerably and has involved many modalities including EEG, polysomnography (PSG), event-related potentials (ERPs), and structural and functional magnetic resonance imaging (MRI and fMRI).

At NIMHANS, research in the department of neurophysiology over the past two decades has focused on cross-sectional studies of the neurophysiological and psychological effects of different meditative practices in expert as well as novice practitioners. The sections below provide examples from studies examining both state and trait effects. An overview of the traditions and specific meditation technique is given to provide context.

■ NEUROPHYSIOLOGY OF DIFFERENT MEDITATION STATES

Meditative practices have had a long history in a wide variety of cultures such as Buddhist, Hindu, Sufi, Kabbalistic, Christian Gnostic, Greco-Roman, Shamanic, and American-Indian.[7] Meditative practices when grounded in their traditions are said to have three phases in common—developing concentration, experiencing tranquility, and gaining insight. These practices help in improving spiritual well-being by reducing the turbulence in the outer and inner lives of practitioners by bringing harmony in their social and spiritual worlds.[7]

The sage Patanjali in his yoga aphorisms (*yoga sutras*) highlighted that a healthy body and a healthy mind have a close connection. He recommended several preliminary disciplines that would enable the practitioner to develop one-pointedness (*ekagrata*), concentration (*dharana*), spiritual mastery through meditation (*dhyana*), and reach a state of realization and equanimity (*samadhi*).[8] Patanjali's approach to meditation considers yoga to be the suppression of the fluctuations of the mind (*Yogas chitta vritti nirodhah*), in other words, to make the mind calm and silent.[8,9] The Bhagavad Gita also recommends meditations of different forms including the path of devotional meditation.

Meditation practices have been classified into open-monitoring (OM) and focused-attention (FA) categories.[10] A category for contemplative meditation (CM) has been suggested[11] and an additional category of "automatic self-transcending" has been proposed.[12] A more recent taxonomy suggests three meditation families "attentional, constructive, and deconstructive" on the basis of their primary cognitive mechanisms.[13]

In the Vipassana tradition as taught by SN Goenka, meditators go through a structured practice involving multiple techniques to stabilize in corresponding meditative states. Typically, they start with *Anapana-sati* which is based on attention to inhalation and exhalation without any regulation of the breath flow. This practice helps to stabilize the mental state and reduce mind wandering. Next, they practice *Vipassana-Bhavana*, during which a nonreactive state of awareness of body sensations is maintained. This step is meant to aid the development of insight into the nature of impermanence and thereby, improved mental balance. Finally, the practitioners engage in *Metta-Bhavana*, which involves generating a feeling of goodwill for all and indirectly enhancing the sense of personal well-being.

Changes in EEG for three groups of meditators (teachers, senior meditators, and novices) were examined as they went through the above timed and structured meditation sequence.[14] The group of teachers was the most proficient with over 10,000 hours of meditation practice, along with experience of instructing meditation courses for others. Senior meditators formed the next group, having similar duration of experience as teachers, but without any special training or teaching responsibilities. Novices were the least experienced group with about 1,000 hours of meditation experience on average. All meditators showed EEG power changes during the different states of meditation as compared to rest state. Specifically, EEG power was higher in the delta (0–4 Hz), theta (4–8 Hz), alpha (8–12 Hz), beta (12–30 Hz), and low-gamma (30–40 Hz) bands during meditation. Thus, the meditation sequence elicited a global increase in power. Additionally, there were clear group differences (seen in power spectra as well as complexity measures such as Higuchi fractal dimensions and permutation entropy) during practice of the three meditation techniques, indicating the effect of proficiency on changes in brain state.

Importantly, long-term meditators (i.e., both teachers and seniors) and novices had significant differences in the low-alpha and low-gamma power bands at rest when all participants were specifically instructed not to meditate. This demonstrates trait effects of meditation that contribute to the resting state physiology of the long-term meditators. This further implies that when the proficient practitioners start meditating, they are likely to easily or more effortlessly achieve a meditative state with reduced interference of mind-wandering. Sustained proficient practice facilitates progress toward higher states of consciousness as part of the spiritual journey that the meditation tradition espouses.[15]

The above findings underscore a crucial need for meditation studies to consider the specific meditation technique and the proficiency of the meditators while discussing any relevance to clinical applications.

■ NEUROPHYSIOLOGY OF MENTAL STATE SHIFTS

As discussed in the previous section, expert long-term meditators are likely to quickly and more effortlessly enter a meditative state. Indeed, true mastery of one's mental faculties would allow the person to efficiently and effectively achieve a desired mental state at will, on demand and under (almost) any condition. This ability was tested in a study involving Brahma Kumaris Rajayoga (BKRY) practitioners who include in their repertoire, techniques that involve quickly shifting between meditative states.

Brahma Kumaris Rajayoga employs meditation techniques that involve a conceptual foundation following a 7-day course on the nature of soul, God, karma, time, etc. (in stark contrast to the Vipassana meditation practice, for example, which explicitly discourages conceptual focus during meditation). BKRY uses many tools and techniques, including guided audio or visual commentaries, quiet contemplation, mentally traversing space and time, witness consciousness, soul consciousness, and communion with God. The first step in most of the techniques is soul consciousness—experiencing oneself as a soul or a point of light behind the center of the forehead. BKRY meditation is practiced with eyes open unlike most traditions that suggest keeping eyes closed during meditation. Pertinent to the study under discussion, BKRY practitioners use techniques such as "traffic control" and "spiritual drill". Traffic control involves suddenly disengaging from day-today activities for a short 2-minute meditation either in a timed manner or at random. The spiritual drill is a rapid sequence of several (usually five) distinct meditative states. The goal of these techniques is to help the practitioner be "ever-ready" in a state of well-being and spiritual outlook.

We recruited three groups of participants to undergo a protocol of quickly shifting in and out of a meditative state and examined evidence of any reliable EEG markers showing state shifts.[16] The long-term group had over 10,000 hours of BKRY practice, while the short-term group had about 1,000 hours of experience. The third group consisted of healthy nonmeditating controls. All groups were matched for age, gender, and socioeconomic background. The study protocol provided visual instructions and audio cues to shift between 16 different conditions—alternating between 1-minute long rest and soul-conscious meditation states, with eyes open and closed, before and after an engaging task. The soul-conscious state was chosen for meditation as it is the foundation for most of the techniques and thus practiced by all meditators. The instructions were also easy enough for the control participants to visualize so that all participants followed an identical protocol (this is not possible for many meditative states).

It was found that long-term meditators were able to achieve state shifts between rest and meditation (seen by changes in theta power) in all conditions, thus demonstrating mastery. Short-term meditators could not achieve state shifts reliably, but when all conditions were combined, they showed evidence of state shifts (indexed by lower alpha power) during eyes-closed condition. Control participants did not show any state shifts indicating that the protocol itself was not responsible for any differences in EEG power.

An important consideration is that both long-term and short-term meditators were highly proficient and, as compared to the controls, had significantly enhanced well-being as assessed by a number of measures.[17] Thus, proficient practice allows meditators to be able to reliably shift into and out of meditation states but in the initial stages it is effortful and takes time. However, with long-term practice, the neuroplastic changes facilitate the process and make state shifting faster and more effortless.

In order for the protocol to robustly assess state shifts, it was split across two sessions separated by a multilevel audiovisual cognitive task. The task [ANGEL (assessing neurocognition via gamified experimental logic)] is gamified such that participants perform well initially and make a number of mistakes toward the end. The fast pace and feedback-based approach keeps the task very engaging[18] and simulates practical day-to-day work life challenges that can be engaging and error-prone. The ability to quickly and reliably achieve meditative states under these conditions can be invaluable for those in high stress situations.

Although most control subjects reported feeling peaceful at the end of the short meditation protocol, it is important to bear in mind that they did not achieve any EEG-indexed state shifts, indicating that training and practice is needed for achieving a meditative state, and not merely compliance with instructions. From a clinical perspective, it is encouraging to note that given time, short-term meditators could reliably achieve meditative states and also benefit from enhanced well-being.

NEUROCOGNITIVE EFFECTS OF MEDITATION PRACTICE

How does meditation practice impact neurocognitive processing at a time when the practitioner is not meditating? This question was addressed[19] by examining ERPs and associated cognitive processing in the three groups of Vipassana meditators discussed earlier, using the ANGEL task.

Task instructions for the participants were very simple—press the left button on a response pad if a salient image appeared in the left half of a computer monitor, and press the right button if the image appeared on the right half. The cognitive processing challenge occurs due to a number of factors. The images could appear for less than a quarter of a second, were somewhat unpredictable, and were accompanied by audiovisual distractors. The EEG activity just before and after the stimulus presentation (considered to be an "event") was averaged to obtain an ERP. The task allows examination of many different types of events and therefore elicits many kinds of neurocognitive processing, i.e., changes taking place in the brain each time an event occurs.

For this study, the differential processing between rare and frequently occurring stimuli were examined. Typically, rarer events generate higher ERP amplitudes and the waveform is called P3, as it is a positive peak appearing about 300 ms after the event. The power spectral changes corresponding to P3 processing as well as intertrial coherence (i.e., frequency-linked similarities) were also examined. The P3 ERP is widely used as an example of cognitive processing in healthy and clinical populations.

The study found that the three groups showed proficiency-linked differences in event-related spectral perturbations. This is remarkable as participants were healthy meditators differing only in the extent of meditation proficiency. As can be expected, all participants performed the task well and could discriminate between the two conditions accurately when the task difficulty was low. The P3 ERP waveforms were reliably elicited and were similar for all three groups. An important consideration is that the ANGEL task was performed right after the meditators had completed their traditional meditation practice, providing state-trait interactions supporting the altered cognitive processing. Thus, a person who meditates right before a challenging situation is more likely to have a balanced perspective and be effective especially if the person is a long-term proficient meditator. Trait changes in neurocognitive processing might also contribute to enhanced well-being reported by meditation practitioners from a variety of traditions.

SLEEP NEUROPHYSIOLOGY IN MEDITATORS

One important confounder in any meditation study is the demand characteristic, which means that the participants in the study are aware of the purpose of the study and this might influence their meditation or task performance favorably or adversely. As discussed in the previous section, long-term meditation practice brings trait changes, i.e., experience-dependent neuroplastic changes. These changes persist even when the individual is not practicing meditation. Studying the sleeping brain is an ideal situation to avoid the demand characteristics and observe trait differences in their natural form. In this section, we summarize a few studies examining the alterations in the neurophysiology of sleep in Vipassana meditators.

During sleep, the brain undergoes a structured pattern of cyclical changes through the night. This sleep architecture can be studied using PSG, a method of recording brain activity by EEG and other sensors during sleep. Soon after sleep onset, brain waves become progressively slower with larger amplitudes and muscle activity reduces until the large slow waves become predominant. Then comes a state of minimal muscle activity but faster low amplitude EEG activity along with rapid eye movement (called REM, the eyes remain closed). This pattern of nonrapid eye movement (NREM) and REM sleep stages reappears in a predictable manner, multiple times during the night. Slow wave sleep is longer during the initial part of the night whereas toward the end, REM sleep tends to be more prolonged. Slow wave sleep, which is the deepest part of NREM sleep, is a form of restorative sleep involved in tissue repair and growth, as well as consolidation or refreshing of memory of facts and experiences. REM sleep is important for consolidating memories of skills that are more implicit in nature. Overall, sleep is very important for our immune system and healthy functioning. Sleep problems are associated with a number of mental health conditions as well as with age. Conversely, those with higher well-being might be able to sleep better, although the direction of causation is unclear.

Sulekha et al.[20] and Pattanashetty et al.[21] compared male Vipassana meditators and controls, and found that overall sleep duration was similar in both groups but meditators had increased slow wave sleep and REM sleep percentages as compared to controls. Sleep epochs containing REM activity are called phasic REM while those without explicit eye activity are called tonic REM. Maruthai et al.[22] found that senior meditators had more phasic REM activity than controls.

The consistent finding of enhanced REM, specifically phasic REM, in these meditators needs to be considered in the light of autonomic nervous system activity. The autonomic nervous system consists of two counteracting systems—sympathetic activity generates an aroused state with higher heart rate and systolic blood pressure whereas parasympathetic activity reduces both the heart rate and blood pressure to reach a more restful and restorative state. The enhanced phasic REM is associated with higher sympathetic surge activity and is considered to be a risk factor for adverse cardiac events. An evaluation of the cardiac autonomic function activity in Vipassana meditators is thus important to understand implications for clinical populations.

Nagendra et al.[23] examined heart rate variability (HRV) in senior Vipassana meditators and matched non-meditating controls, during different stages of sleep. Interestingly, sympathetic activity during REM did not differ across groups but meditators had significantly higher parasympathetic activity during slow wave sleep and REM. Overall, for each sleep stage, meditators showed higher parasympathetic predominance (reduced sympathetic to parasympathetic ratio). Thus, the increased sympathetic activity in meditators during the longer REM sleep is buffered by further increases in parasympathetic activity. Overall, there is considerable evidence for the trait effects of long-term Vipassana meditation seen through changes in sleep architecture and autonomic functions during sleep.

ADDITIONAL CONSIDERATIONS

The studies discussed in this chapter suggest that meditative practices from diverse traditions bring about neurophysiological changes during meditation as well as provide long-term changes in cognitive ability, cognitive flexibility, and even sleep physiology. While different meditation practices yield enhancements in well-being, they are not universally beneficial for all. Indeed, adverse effects are also possible and there have been case reports of psychoses following a variety of meditative practices.[24] Thus, suggestions have been made for personalized meditation practices that are guided by neurophysiological responses.[25]

CONCLUSION

This chapter presents a summary of the neurophysiological evidence for the state and trait effects of different forms of meditation. This evidence needs to be considered in the context of the meditation tradition, the type of meditation technique employed, and both proficiency and duration of meditation practice of participants. However, this field is still nascent and more work needs to be done before achieving the goal of personalized recommendations.

REFERENCES

1. Koenig HG. Religion, spirituality, and health: the research and clinical implications. ISRN Psychiatry; 2012. pp. 1-33.
2. Sedlmeier P, Eberth J, Schwarz M, Zimmermann D, Haarig F, Jaeger S, et al. The psychological effects of meditation: a meta-analysis. Psychol Bull. 2012;138(6):1139-71.
3. Anand B, Chhina GS, Singh B. Some aspects of electroencephalographic studies in yogis. Electroencephalogr Clin Neurophysiol. 1961; 13:452-6.
4. Wallace RK. Physiological effects of transcendental meditation. Science. 1970;167(3926): 1751-4.
5. Wallace R, Benson H, Wilson A. A wakeful hypometabolic physiologic state. Am J Physiol. 1971;221(3):795-9.
6. Lazar SW, Kerr CE, Wasserman RH, Gray JR, Greve DN, Treadway MT, et al. Meditation experience is associated with increased cortical thickness. Neuroreport. 2005;16(17):1893-7.
7. Fontana D. The Meditation Handbook: The Practical Guide to Eastern and Western Meditation Techniques. Duncan Baird Publishers; 2012.
8. Bryant EF. The Yoga Sutras of Patanjali: A New Edition, Translation, and Commentary. New York: North Point Press; 2015.
9. Bærentsen KB. Patanjali and neuroscientific research on meditation. Front Psychol. 2015; 6:1-4.
10. Lutz A, Slagter HA, Dunne JD, Davidson RJ. Attention regulation and monitoring in meditation. Trends Cogn Sci. 2008;12(4):163-9.
11. Shapiro SL, Schwartz GER, Santerre C. Meditation and positive psychology. In: Snyder CR, Lopez SJ (Eds). Handbook of Positive Psychology. Oxford University Press; 2002.
12. Travis F, Shear J. Focused attention, open monitoring and automatic self-transcending: categories to organize meditations from Vedic, Buddhist and Chinese traditions. Conscious Cogn. 2010;19(4):1110-8.
13. Dahl CJ, Lutz A, Davidson RJ. Reconstructing and deconstructing the self: cognitive mechanisms in meditation practice. Trends Cogn Sci; 2015. pp. 1-9.
14. Kakumanu RJ, Nair AK, Venugopal R, Sasidharan A, Ghosh PK, John JP, et al. Dissociating meditation proficiency and experience dependent EEG changes during traditional Vipassana meditation practice. Biol Psychol. 2018;135:65-75.
15. Nair AK, Kutty BM. Meditation, Cognitive Reserve and the Neural Basis of Consciousness. In: Menon S, Nagaraj N, Binoy VV (Eds). Self, Culture and Consciousness. Springer Nature: Singapore; 2017. pp. 51-8.
16. Nair AK, Sasidharan A, John JP, Mehrotra S, Kutty BM. Just a minute meditation: rapid voluntary conscious state shifts in long-term meditators. Conscious Cogn. 2017;53:176-84.
17. Nair AK, John PJ, Mehrotra S, Kutty BM. What contributes to wellbeing gains—proficiency or duration of meditation-related practices? Int J Wellbeing. 2018;8(2):68-88.
18. Nair AK, Sasidharan A, John JP, Mehrotra S, Kutty BM. Assessing Neurocognition via Gamified Experimental Logic: A Novel Approach to Simultaneous Acquisition of Multiple ERPs. Front Neurosci. 2016;10:1.
19. Kakumanu RJ, Nair AK, Sasidharan A, John JP, Mehrotra S, Panth R, et al. State-trait influences of Vipassana meditation practice on P3 EEG dynamics. Prog Brain Res. 2019;244:115-36.
20. Sulekha S, Thennarasu K, Vedamurthachar A, Raju TR, Kutty BM. Evaluation of sleep architecture in practitioners of Sudarshan Kriya yoga and Vipassana meditation. Sleep Biol Rhythms. 2006;4(3):207-14.
21. Pattanashetty R, Sathiamma S, Talakkad S, Nityananda P, Trichur R, Kutty BM. Practitioners of Vipassana meditation exhibit enhanced slow wave sleep and REM sleep states across different age groups. Sleep Biol Rhythms. 2010;8(1):34-41.
22. Maruthai N, Nagendra RP, Sasidharan A, Srikumar S, Datta K, Uchida S, et al. Senior Vipassana meditation practitioners exhibit distinct REM sleep organization from that of novice meditators and healthy controls. Int Rev Psychiatry. 2016;28(3):279-87.
23. Nagendra R, Sulekha S, Sasidharan A, Sathyaprabha T, Pradhan N, Raju TR, et al. Vipassana meditation practices enhance the parasympathetic activity during sleep: a case-control study of heart rate variability across sleep cycles. Int J Complement Altern Med. 2017;5(2):00145.
24. Sharma P, Mahapatra A, Gupta R. Meditation-induced psychosis: a narrative review and individual patient data analysis. Ir J Psychol Med; 2019. pp. 1-7.
25. Fingelkurts AA, Fingelkurts AA, Kallio-Tamminen T. EEG-guided meditation: a personalized approach. J Physiol Paris. 2015;109(4-6):180-90.

Role of Neuroimaging in Understanding Mental Health Effects of Yoga

CHAPTER 6

Vanteemar S Sreeraj, Venkataram Shivakumar, Vijay Kumar KG, Naren P Rao

INTRODUCTION TO YOGA AND ITS UTILITY IN MENTAL HEALTH

Mental illnesses are major causes of loss of productive lives and contribute to 32.4% of years lost due to disability (YLDs) and 13% of disability-adjusted life years (DALYs).[1] Understandably, mental illness is a major concern to the global community today. The global burden of mental illness has been on the rise for various reasons: Important among them are the stigma associated with mental illness and the lack of effective treatments. The predominant treatment modalities, so far, have been pharmacological and psychotherapeutic approaches. Although these treatment modalities have changed the course of illness and reduced the burden to some extent, their effects are limited mostly to the acute phases of illness. In addition, some of the side effects associated with many pharmacological agents add to the burden of patients and care givers.[2]

Amidst this conundrum of treatment resistance and rising burden of psychiatric disorders, biopsychosocial approaches have been revisited in the last 15 years. Of late, the biopsychosocial models often include the mind-body component in addition to the biological, psychological, and social factors. Yoga has been at the forefront of this renewed biopsychosocial model of treatment approach.[3] Yoga, an ancient Indian practice, has been revisited with a new vigor, given its comprehensive and holistic approach towards preventive and curative health and disease. There has been a blurring of lines between physical/mental/emotional/spiritual boundaries, thereby bringing biopsychosocial approaches such as mind-body medicine to the fore. Yoga, since the last decade, has been considered as one of the mainstream approaches in mind-body medicine. Yoga, derived from the word "Yuj", meaning "to bind", is believed to unite mind and body, thereby modulating bodily functions by enhancing the capacity of one's mind. Yoga, as per the traditional definition *"chitta vritti nirodaha"*, is therapeutic to mental illness and brings harmony.

Over the last few years, yoga has been shown to improve psychiatric conditions in addition to a number of physical illnesses. An increasing number of studies have documented the positive effects of yoga in mental well-being and psychiatric disorders. Several systematic studies have reported the efficacy of yoga as an add-on treatment in various psychiatric disorders including, depression, anxiety, post-traumatic stress disorder (PTSD), and psychotic disorders.

POTENTIAL BIOLOGICAL MECHANISMS OF YOGA IN MENTAL HEALTH

Mechanisms underlying the mental health benefits of yoga are less known as they are underexamined. Probably the most common biological mechanism examined is the effect of yoga on the hypothalamic-pituitary-adrenal axis and the sympathetic nervous system response; several studies have reported the downregulation of hypothalamic-pituitary-adrenal axis and the decreased tone of the sympathetic nervous system. Some studies have even quantified peripheral stress markers such as serum cortisol in disorders such as depression and anxiety. Only a few studies have examined the potential neuroplasticity effects of yoga by examining the peripheral BDNF (brain-derived neurotrophic factors) levels in disorders such as schizophrenia and depression. Despite its importance in treatment of psychiatric disorders, only a handful of studies have utilized neuroimaging modalities in understanding the neurobiological mechanisms underlying the beneficial effects of yoga in mental illness.

NEUROIMAGING IN ELUCIDATING THE MECHANISMS UNDERLYING PSYCHIATRIC DISORDERS

Brain is a complex organ system and each part of the brain is unique in its structure and function. It is a precious organ which is covered by the skull bone from all the sides which makes it difficult to approach directly using investigative modalities. Mapping the structure and functions of the brain requires specialized techniques to observe the tissue beyond the skin, soft tissue, and the skull. Ultrasound waves, which are commonly used in medical evaluations of other body systems, cannot pass through the skull. Hence, its utility in brain imaging is limited to infants and small children before the fusion of skull bones.

Electromagnetic radiations across different spectra can pass through the skull and hence are commonly used in neuroimaging. Electrical currents are produced naturally within the brain circuits and can be recorded using electroencephalography (EEG) as graphs. These electric currents also produce magnetic fields which are recorded by magnetoencephalography (MEG). However, neuroimaging typically refers to the techniques that create visual representations/images of the brain (and exclude EEG/MEG where time vs. activity is plotted graphically).

Electromagnetic waves in the X-ray spectrum are differentially absorbed by different body tissues. They can be sent across the brain and the ones that are unabsorbed by the body tissue are measured in different axes to create the sliced images in computed tomography (CT) scan. Similarly, electromagnetic waves in near-infrared spectrum pass through the skull and get reflected by hemoglobin (Hb). These reflected waves are measured as a proxy for blood flow in specific regions in near-infrared spectroscopy (NIRS). Alternatively, small quantities of radioactive substances are injected, and the concentration of these decaying molecules is measured through the emissions in positron emission tomography (PET) and single-photon emission computed tomography (SPECT). Hydrogen atoms in the omnipresent water molecules in the brain can be polarized using strong magnetic fields. These excited hydrogen atoms emit radiofrequency signals which are measured to create images in magnetic resonance imaging (MRI).

Brain changes in yoga are very subtle and CT scan is sensitive to investigate only gross structural changes. Hence, neuroimaging research in yoga mostly comprises of studies with MRI and functional NIRS (fNIRS). Although PET and SPECT studies provide valuable information on neurochemistry, they have been underutilized. Hence in this chapter, we will be reviewing two neuroimaging modalities, namely, MRI and fNIRS.

MAGNETIC RESONANCE IMAGING TECHNIQUES

Magnetic resonance imaging has become an integral part of studies trying to understand the neurobiological basis of psychiatric disorders. The search term "Neuroimaging and Psychiatry" in PubMed brings up more than 30,000 publications in the last 10 years that have used MRI, underscoring its important role in understanding the neurobiology of psychiatric disorders. This magnitude of research utilizing neuroimaging in psychiatry could be attributed to advanced MRI techniques elaborating the structure and functions of brain in vivo like never before. The availability of standardized protocols and sophisticated analyses techniques have further encouraged its application in psychiatry resulting in the emergence of "psychoradiology" as a new field within radiology.[4]

There are different MRI techniques measuring various parameters of the brain. For the sake of simplicity and in relevance to the current chapter, MRI techniques can be broadly classified into structural, functional, and chemical neuroimaging. These techniques are discussed below, in brief, along with current evidence in yoga and future applicability.

Structural Neuroimaging

Structural neuroimaging includes structural MRI (sMRI) and diffusion tensor imaging (DTI), which have been used predominantly in psychiatric research. Structural MRI includes several sequences, of which T1-weighted image is the most commonly used because of its ability to delineate the anatomy of the brain in greater detail, enabling quantification of the volume and related parameters such as shape, cortical thickness, sulcus depth, and gyrification indices of various brain regions. DTI is a neuroimaging technique that details the white matter structure and integrity in great detail, enabling one to understand the structural connectivity within the brain in vivo.

Functional Neuroimaging

Popularly called as functional MRI (fMRI), this is a neuroimaging technique that maps brain activity by recording changes in the brain's hemodynamic responses **(Figs. 1A and B)**. fMRI quantifies the blood-oxygen-level-dependent (BOLD) changes which is dependent on cerebral blood flow. This BOLD change which serves as a proxy for neural activity can measure the brain activity following a cognitive task or at rest, providing details on functional connectivity between various brain regions. These are termed as task-based fMRI and resting state fMRI (rs-fMRI), respectively.

Chemical Neuroimaging

Utilization of neuroimaging techniques to quantify neurotransmitter levels or brain

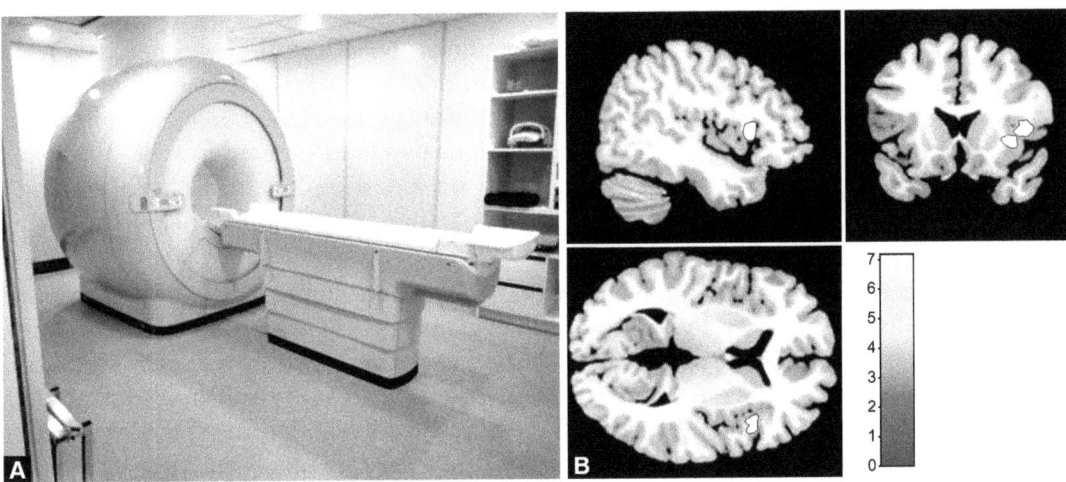

Figs. 1A and B: Photographs illustrating an MRI scanner (A) and sample functional magnetic resonance imaging (fMRI) activation map overlaid on a structural brain template (B).

metabolite levels in vivo in the brain is called neurochemical imaging. This technique involves predominantly two types imaging, magnetic resonance spectroscopy (MRS) and PET. PET although can be used as a functional imaging technique, its application in exploring neurotransmitters and their receptor functions are of more relevance today.

MRI Studies in Yoga

There is a dearth of studies examining the neurobiological correlates of yoga therapy in psychiatric disorders. So far, studies that have utilized neuroimaging techniques to evaluate the neurobiological effects of yoga therapy are primarily in nonpsychiatric populations. These studies have been carried out in healthy controls and long-term yoga practitioners or yoga gurus.[5] Majority of these studies are functional studies reporting a significant improvement in functional activation of several brain regions following different forms of yoga.[6,7] Further, several studies have also examined structural changes such as alterations in cortical thickness and gray matter volume of several regions following yoga.[8-10] Some studies have also examined the white matter tracts using DTI techniques reporting increase in fractional anisotropy (FA) values in several regions.[10,11] In addition, some studies have also examined the effects of yoga on gamma-aminobutyric acid (GABA) levels in healthy subjects.[12]

To summarize, MRI studies in healthy people have utilized various yoga techniques such as *Kundalini yoga*, mindfulness meditation, *Zen*, *Vipassana*, *Kriya yoga*, and so on and results of these studies are wide-ranging and inconsistent. This can mostly be attributed to the use of different yoga techniques and MRI methodology. However, despite these shortcomings, some brain regions such as dorsolateral prefrontal cortex, orbitofrontal cortex, fusiform gyrus, supramarginal gyrus, and middle and inferior temporal gyrus have been consistently implicated in yoga-related changes.[5]

Potential Utility of MRI for Yoga in Psychiatric Disorders

Recent research has indicated cognitive dysfunction as one of the key features associated with socio-occupational dysfunction in psychiatric disorders. Such cognitive dysfunction is seen in several cognitive domains such as attention, perception, working memory, learning, memory, emotion, and social cognition. These domains of cognition can be examined using task-based fMRI by measuring the brain activation patterns in response to various cognitive tasks with yoga as an intervention. Further, the rs-fMRI seems to be a worthy investigative tool to look into the psychophysiological effects of yoga, given the difficulty in administering task-based fMRI in patients with psychiatric disorders.

Resting state fMRI detects the spontaneous BOLD fluctuations at rest in the absence of any goal-oriented task/stimuli. The coactivation patterns between regions can be mapped as resting state functional connectivity (rs-FC) which can be further used to construct functional brain networks called resting state networks (RSNs). Several recent studies have also examined rs-FC and RSNs in healthy controls practicing yoga and have found a significant increase in connectivity within the default mode networks (DMN) and the functional connectivity between other regions.[13] RSNs and their connectivity with other parts of the brain have been associated with the cognitive and clinical symptoms in various psychiatric disorders. These changes can be examined before and after yoga intervention to get objective measures of yoga-induced neurobiological changes.

Given that neuroplasticity deficits and resultant brain structural changes are frequently observed in various psychiatric disorders, the same can be examined by quantifying the change in gray matter volumes of brain regions following long-term yoga therapy in psychiatric patients. This would provide more evidence for the neuroprotective role of yoga. In addition to this, MRS studies could be used to map the changes in GABA and glutamate levels in specific brain regions which are deranged in psychiatric disorders.

FUNCTIONAL NEAR-INFRARED SPECTROSCOPY

Functional near-infrared spectroscopy is a noninvasive neuroimaging technique using electromagnetic waves in the near-infrared spectrum (750–1,400 nm) **(Figs. 2A to C)**. A small window of wavelength between 700 and 900 nm can pass through the skin, bone, and soft tissue above the brain but gets absorbed by Hb. The light emitted by optodes placed on the scalp, thus pass through the tissue gets absorbed partially by the Hb, few scattered by neuronal tissue and rest follow a ballistic path. A detector placed at around 3–5 cm distance from optode on the scalp will measure the attenuated light which has taken an elliptical path (Banana-shaped curve).

Hemoglobin is the chromophore (molecule giving distinct color) in the blood. Hb supplying oxygen to brain can be in two forms: oxyhemoglobin (HbO) and deoxyhemoglobin/reduced Hb (HbR). HbO carries oxygen from lungs to brain tissue and once brain utilizes the oxygen, Hb is left without oxygen as HbR. Relative changes in the HbO and HbR are measured by differences in their absorption spectra. An isosbestic point is seen at 810 nm where both HbO and HbR have an identical absorption coefficient. Two continuous waves of wavelengths one above and one below the isosbestic point are generally used to calculate the relative concentrations of the HbO and HbR, respectively, using modified Beer–Lambert law.

Commonly used fNIRS devices employ the above principle using light with distinct intensity which is continuously emitted from one source and detected from a detector called continuous wave NIRS (CW-NIRS), and provides data on relative changes in concentrations of HbO/HbR. Three other types of devises are also available: (1) spatially resolved NIRS (SRS-NIRS), (2) frequency domain NIRS (FD-NIRS), and (3) time domain NIRS (TD-NIRS). SRS-NIRS is similar to

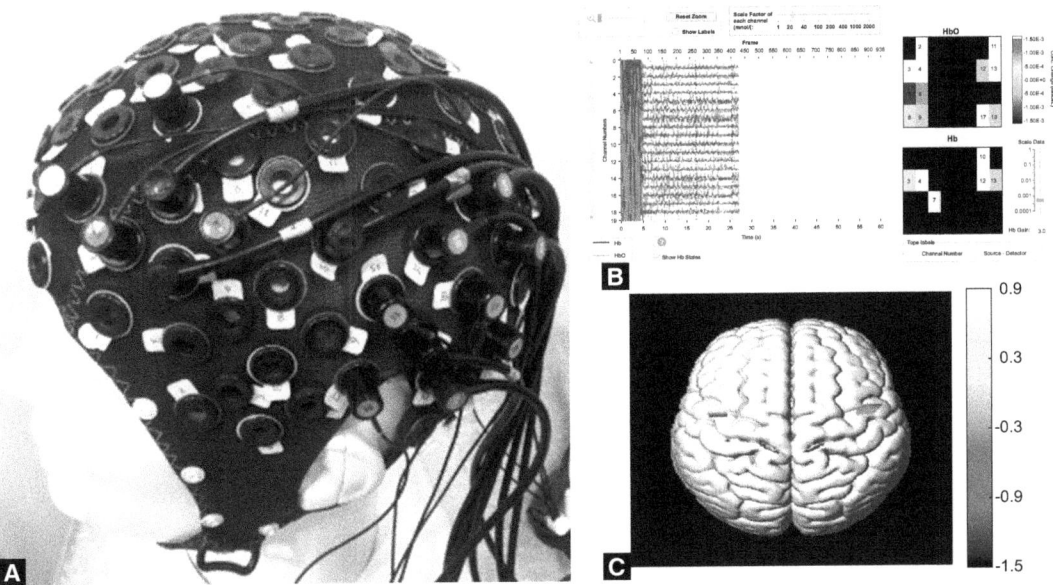

Figs. 2A to C: Photographs illustrating a portable functional near-infrared spectroscopy (fNIRS) set-up (A), raw data during acquisition (B) and fNIRS activation maps overlaid on a brain template (C).

FW-NIRS but uses two detectors and can calculate absolute changes in concentrations of chromophores (HbO/ HbR). FD-NIRS modulates the amplitude of waves of distinct intensity, whereas TD-NIRS sends waves in pulses. These two devices calculate absolute concentration of chromophores but are more time-consuming and less sensitive to changes in concentration.

Comparison of fNIRS with fMRI

Functional MRI is currently considered as the gold standard method of investigating functioning of the brain through hemodynamic activity. Functional NIRS has an advantage over MRI in being less expensive, portable, and more robust to motion artifacts. This last feature comes handy in yoga-related research where fNIRS can provide real time changes in brain activity during yoga asanas compared to MRI where only post-yoga changes can be measured. A comparative profile of fMRI and fNIRS is given in **Table 1**, which can be used to choose the modality for investigation.

Functional NIRS in Yoga and Mental Health Research

Functional NIRS, being a relatively novel modality, is still in its infancy with respect to optimal method of acquiring and analyzing the signals. Functional NIRS is used in psychiatric conditions with relative ease.[14] However, only a handful of studies have evaluated cerebral effects of yoga using fNIRS. Published studies on its applicability in mental health settings are even fewer. Studies have mostly looked at the hemodynamic activity at prefrontal cortex during or after one or two sessions of

TABLE 1: Comparison of functional magnetic resonance imaging (fMRI) and functional near-infrared spectroscopy (fNIRS).

	fMRI	fNIRS
Measuring parameter	BOLD (blood oxygen level dependent) signal changes from HbR (deoxyhemoglobin) concentrations	Scatter optic waves based on attenuation coefficient of specific optic waves of HbO (oxyhemoglobin) and HbR
Physical properties operated	Paramagnetic properties	Optical absorption
Safety	Safe with adequate precautions (cannot be done in subjects with metallic implants, claustrophobia)	Safe
Imaging	Three-dimensional	Two-dimensional
Deeper structure	Good	Poor (only cortical surface up to a depth of around 1.5 cm can be measured)
Spatial resolution	Good	Poor
Temporal correspondence	Poorer	Better
Robustness to motion	Poor	Good
Combining with other modalities (e.g., EEG, TMS, tDCS, eye tracking, etc.) and BCI applications	Hard	Simple
Price	Costlier	Cheaper
Portable	No	Yes
Adaptable to realistic environment/real-life experiments	No	Yes
Signal-to-noise ratio	Higher	Lower

(BCI: brain-computer interface; EEG: electroencephalography; TMS: transcranial magnetic stimulation; tDCS: transcranial direct current stimulation)

yogic postural exercise, breathing exercise, and mediation.

Changes in bilateral prefrontal activation during a fluid cognition task were evaluated with a single session of yoga, moderate intensity exercise, severe intensity exercise, and sedentary control in a cross-over design. Moderate intensity aerobic exercise increased oxygenation during the task much higher than other three interventions. More importantly, on combined analyses all the three exercise groups showed an improved hemodynamic efficiency of cognitive processing. Increase in efficiency of the neural activity with a lesser hemodynamic activity was apparent with improved processing speed after acute exercises.[15]

Kapalbhati, a high frequency yogic breathing exercise at 2 Hz, was performed by patients with schizophrenia and healthy controls. Functional NIRS showed an increase in bilateral prefrontal hemodynamic activity (increased HbO and total Hb) in the healthy but a reduction in right prefrontal HbR in patients with schizophrenia. On comparing the two groups during high frequency breathing, the prefrontal hemodynamic activation was significantly higher in healthy people as compared to those with schizophrenia, showing hyporesponsiveness of prefrontal hemodynamics to kapalbhati in schizophrenia.[16] This increase in prefrontal hemodynamic activity in healthy yoga practitioners with 2 Hz breathing is in contrast to the two other studies in healthy controls which evaluated prefrontal activity after 1 Hz breathing. After 1 Hz frequency breathing, a reduction of HbO activity was noted which lasted around 10 minutes postactivity.[17,18] Thus, with kapalbhati, the rate at which the breathing exercise is practiced may have a differential effect on the brain. Another study looked at the effects of uninostril breathing on prefrontal activity and found that right nostril breathing increased oxygenation and blood volume in left prefrontal cortex.[19] Breath awareness has been found to reduce HbR levels in different studies.[18,19]

Prefrontal activation during Stroop task was compared between "om" chanting and "ss" chanting. Performance in Stroop task improved with lesser prefrontal hemodynamic activation after "om" chanting in comparison to "ss" chanting. This again suggests an increased neural efficiency with "om" chanting, specifically in right prefrontal cortex.[20]

A cross-sectional evaluation of a mindfulness task in long-term meditation experts was compared with controls. A wide spread increase in activity with more localization in higher auditory areas (BA 1, 6, and 40) was noted in meditation experts but a decrease in activity was noted in these areas in controls during an auditory mindfulness task. The higher activation in the brain areas (BA 39, 40, 44, and 45) beyond the meditative task in the experts could possibly be an indication of long-term positive effects on empathy, metacognitive skills, and subjective well-being.[21]

A 6-week meditation intervention was provided to patients with open-angle glaucoma. Improved HbO in prefrontal cortex was noted in patients who underwent meditation but not the control group using fNIRS. This was noted in parallel to improvement in ocular pressure, quality of life, and BDNF levels.[22]

Potential Application of fNIRS

Functional NIRS is increasingly used in sports medicine research. It is considered as a state-of-the-art neuroimaging tool to investigate the effects of mind–body medicine activities such as yoga on cerebral oxygenation and hemodynamic activity due to its noninvasiveness and ability to quantify HbO and HbR even during motion. It can thus be used even in children and subjects who have conditions which are contraindications for fMRI.

Real-time measurement of changes in hemodynamic activity can provide newer insights into the mechanisms through which yoga brings about effects on mental health and well-being. It can be used to determine the cerebral effects of different forms and limbs/domains of yoga. Apart from immediate and short-term effects, fNIRS can also be used in understanding the long-term effects and differential activations in long-term practitioners and yoga-naïve subjects. Knowledge on the neurobiological effect of yoga in psychiatric patients is sparse. fNIRS could provide a necessary tool to understand the differential effects of yoga in health and disease that could guide in customizing yoga as a specific therapeutic modality. The clinical utility and mechanism of clinical benefits can be determined by evaluating the long-term rather than very short-term effects. A comparison of different durations and types of yogic exercises, and comparing with other types of physical and mental exercises would provide better understanding of the specific effects of yoga as a therapeutic modality.

CONCLUSION

Preliminary evidence suggests a potential role for neuroimaging techniques including fNIRS in elucidating the mechanistic basis of yoga as a treatment for psychiatric disorders. The neuroimaging evidence available so far is only in healthy controls and similar studies have to be conducted in various psychiatric disorders in a systematic fashion before arriving at any definitive conclusion. fNIRS although examined by few in psychiatric disorders, requires further rigorous systematic research in larger numbers.

Evidence from healthy control studies have major inconsistencies in results probably due to differences in the yoga protocols used. Hence, adopting a uniform yoga protocol would ascertain the reliability of results. In addition to this, studies must incorporate long-term yoga therapy approaches with a longitudinal design for better understanding of the effects of yoga. Establishing a dose-response effect for yoga is essential, as single session yoga-related effects could be affected by chance findings in neuroimaging examination. Further, studies should concentrate on an apriori region of interest (ROI)-based approach rather than fishing through the whole brain. Results from such studies would give more insights into the potential neurobiology of yoga. Given the difficulties associated with blinding of yoga therapy, the outcome measures being examined like clinical assessments and neuroimaging parameters have to be assessed in a blinded manner. Demonstration of brain connectivity changes using neuroimaging would provide the much-required objective evidence as a complement to clinical studies which have reported improvement using clinical measures.

Each neuroimaging modality and technique has its own pros and cons, and they can also complement each other. Future studies have to focus on utilizing multimodal neuroimaging techniques in a randomized controlled fashion incorporating a rigorous blinding at the level of image analysis. Adopting study-specific uniform yoga protocols in various psychiatric conditions would elucidate the neurobiological effects of yoga and encourage its wider application in mental health.

REFERENCES

1. Vigo D, Thornicroft G, Atun R. Estimating the true global burden of mental illness. Lancet Psychiatry. 2016;3(2):171-8.
2. Abosi O, Lopes S, Schmitz S, Fiedorowicz JG. Cardiometabolic effects of psychotropic medications. Horm Mol Biol Clin Investig. 2018;36(1).
3. Taylor M. Creating a biopsychosocial bridge of care: linking yoga therapy and medical rehabilitation. Int J Yoga Ther. 2012(22):93-4.
4. Huang X, Gong Q, Sweeney JA, Biswal BB. Progress in psychoradiology, the clinical application of psychiatric neuroimaging. Br J Radiol. 2019;92(1101):20181000.
5. Hazari N, Sarkar S. A review of yoga and meditation neuroimaging studies in healthy subjects. J Altern Complement Ther. 2014; 20(1):16-26.

6. Gothe NP, Hayes JM, Temali C, Damoiseaux JS. Differences in brain structure and function among yoga practitioners and controls. Front Integr Neurosci. 2018;12:26.
7. Kalyani BG, Venkatasubramanian G, Arasappa R, Rao NP, Kalmady SV, Behere RV, et al. Neurohemodynamic correlates of 'OM' chanting: A pilot functional magnetic resonance imaging study. Int J Yoga. 2011;4(1):3-6.
8. Hariprasad VR, Varambally S, Shivakumar V, Kalmady SV, Venkatasubramanian G, Gangadhar BN. Yoga increases the volume of the hippocampus in elderly subjects. Indian J Psychiatry. 2013;55(Suppl 3):S394-S6.
9. Lazar SW, Kerr CE, Wasserman RH, Gray JR, Greve DN, Treadway MT, et al. Meditation experience is associated with increased cortical thickness. Neuroreport. 2005;16(17):1893-7.
10. Luders E, Toga AW, Lepore N, Gaser C. The underlying anatomical correlates of long-term meditation: larger hippocampal and frontal volumes of gray matter. Neuroimage. 2009;45(3):672-8.
11. Tang YY, Lu Q, Geng X, Stein EA, Yang Y, Posner MI. Short-term meditation induces white matter changes in the anterior cingulate. Proc Natl Acad Sci USA. 2010;107(35):15649-52.
12. Streeter CC, Whitfield TH, Owen L, Rein T, Karri SK, Yakhkind A, et al. Effects of yoga versus walking on mood, anxiety, and brain GABA levels: a randomized controlled MRS study. J Altern Complement Med. 2010;16(11):1145-52.
13. Santaella DF, Balardin JB, Afonso RF, Giorjiani GM, Sato JR, Lacerda SS, et al. Greater anteroposterior default mode network functional connectivity in long-term elderly yoga practitioners. Front Aging Neurosci. 2019;11:158.
14. Kumar V, Shivakumar V, Chhabra H, Bose A, Venkatasubramanian G, Gangadhar BN. Functional near infra-red spectroscopy (fNIRS) in schizophrenia: a review. Asian J Psychiatr. 2017;27:18-31.
15. Moriarty T, Bourbeau K, Bellovary B, Zuhl MN. Exercise intensity influences prefrontal cortex oxygenation during cognitive testing. Behav Sci (Basel). 2019;9(8):83.
16. Bhargav H, Nagendra HR, Gangadhar BN, Nagarathna R. Frontal hemodynamic responses to high frequency yoga breathing in schizophrenia: a functional near-infrared spectroscopy study. Front Psychiatr. 2014;5:29.
17. Telles S, Gupta RK, Singh N, Balkrishna A. A functional near-infrared spectroscopy study of high-frequency yoga breathing compared to breath awareness. Med Sci Monit Basic Res. 2016;22:58-66.
18. Telles S, Singh N, Gupta RK, Balkrishna A. Optical topography recording of cortical activity during high frequency yoga breathing and breath awareness. Comment to: Non-invasive assessment of hemispheric language dominance by optical topography during a brief passive listening test: a pilot study. Stefano Bembich, Sergio Demarini, Andrea Clarici, Stefano Massaccesi, Domenico Grasso. Med Sci Monit. 2011;17(12):CR692-697. Med Sci Monit. 2012;18(1):LE3-4.
19. Singh K, Bhargav H, Srinivasan TM. Effect of uninostril yoga breathing on brain hemodynamics: a functional near-infrared spectroscopy study. Int J Yoga. 2016;9(1):12-9.
20. Bhargav H, Manjunath NK, Varambally S, Mooventhan A, Bista S, Singh D, et al. Acute effects of 3G mobile phone radiations on frontal haemodynamics during a cognitive task in teenagers and possible protective value of Om chanting. Int Rev Psychiatry. 2016;28(3):288-98.
21. Gundel F, von Spee J, Schneider S, Haeussinger FB, Hautzinger M, Erb M, et al. Meditation and the brain—Neuronal correlates of mindfulness as assessed with near-infrared spectroscopy. Psychiatry Res Neuroimaging. 2018;271:24-33.
22. Gagrani M, Faiq MA, Sidhu T, Dada R, Yadav RK, Sihota R, et al. Meditation enhances brain oxygenation, upregulates BDNF and improves quality of life in patients with primary open angle glaucoma: a randomized controlled trial. Restor Neurol Neurosci. 2018;36(6):741-53.

CHAPTER 7

Role of Transcranial Magnetic Stimulation in Yoga Research

Ramajayam Govindaraj, Jitender Jakhar, Urvakhsh Meherwan Mehta

INTRODUCTION

The brain is a complex network of neurons with electrical signals as its essential tool of communication. Ideas of electricity within nerve cells started in the 1780s when Galvani discovered that muscles of a dead frog's leg twitched when struck with an electrical spark.[1] Since then, numerous studies on animals and humans have tried modulating the endogenous electrical signals within the brain, spinal cord, or neuromuscular system with exogenous electrical signals.[2,3] Meanwhile, in the late 1800s and early 1900s, it was also discovered that alternating magnetic fields could also stimulate the central and peripheral nervous system just as the electrical signals could.[4]

With growing interest in the effects of electrical and magnetic signals on the nervous system, in 1985, Anthony Barker and his colleagues at the University of Sheffield came up for the first time with a transcranial magnetic stimulator that could stimulate the human brain.[5] Earlier in 1980, Merton and Morton[6] had demonstrated the feasibility of stimulating the human motor cortex transcranially with direct electrical current over the scalp, which was painful, unlike transcranial magnetic stimulation (TMS), which is painless. In the last two decades, TMS has gained popularity both in therapeutic and investigational aspects in the field of medicine, especially in neuroscience. With a growing body of research in the field of yoga and neuroscience, TMS, as a noninvasive brain probing tool, has many promising roles in understanding the neuroscience of yoga.

OVERVIEW OF THE TMS MACHINE AND ITS PRINCIPLE

The two essential components of a TMS machine are magnetic stimulator and magnetic coil (**Fig. 1**). The magnetic stimulator has multiple components (charging system, energy storage capacitors, energy recovery circuitry, thyristor switch, and pulse-shape circuitry) to generate a high-intensity magnetic field (~2.5 Tesla) from high voltage electricity. The magnetic coil consists of one or more well-insulated copper wires. As current passes through these copper wires, it generates a varied pattern of a magnetic field, and it induces an electric current in a conductor (in this case, brain, i.e., the head of the subject)

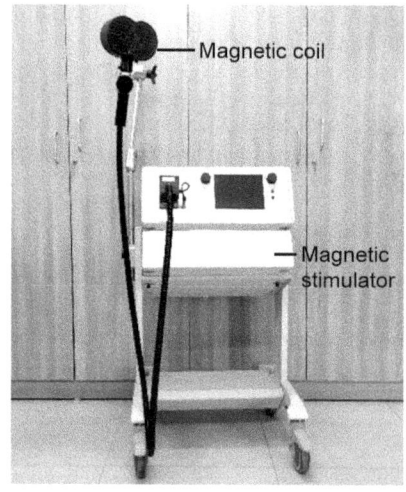

Fig. 1: Transcranial magnetic stimulation machine.

placed in this varying magnetic field as per Faraday's law of electromagnetic induction.[7] Thus there is a painless stimulation of the brain with the induced electrical field through a magnetic coil. Different types of coils are available based on the research or therapeutic need, and the most commonly used coil is a figure of eight coil **(Fig. 1)**.

UNDERSTANDING THE TMS TECHNIQUE

When a pulse is delivered through TMS coil on the scalp surface, as shown in **Figure 2**, the magnetic field (B) generated in the coil induces an electric field (E) in the opposite direction in the brain.

This electrical field probably stimulates the nerves at the bend[8] of neuronal axons (if they are vertically placed in the cortex like the pyramidal neurons) as shown in **Figure 2**, or it stimulates the neurons which are placed parallelly (horizontally) in the cortex (e.g., the interneurons). Based on the stimulation site on the scalp and the underlying cortical region, varied responses could be obtained, which can be measured objectively. For example, delivering a TMS pulse on the scalp overlying the hand region of the motor cortex elicits a visible twitch in the corresponding hand muscle, and an electromyography (EMG) electrode attached to the hand muscle can capture the twitch. Depending on the stimulation site, different kinds of behavioral responses could be studied. Based on the type of delivered stimulus and corresponding responses, one could infer information regarding the neurotransmission in the cerebral cortex.

DIFFERENT RESEARCH PARADIGMS WITH TMS

Different kinds of TMS research paradigms are available based on: (A) the number of pulses delivered (single pulse, paired-pulse, triple pulse, quadri pulse, repetitive pulses, patterned pulses), (B) the interval between the delivered pulses, strength of the pulse(s), and (C) the site where the pulses are delivered. More details on various research paradigms are described elsewhere by other researchers.[9]

With all these available TMS research paradigms, one could study about cortical reactivity (inhibition/facilitation) within and between cortical hemispheres, cortical plasticity [with high- or low-frequency repetitive TMS (rTMS); continuous or intermittent theta-burst stimulation; paired associative stimulation techniques], cortical connectivity [combining TMS with electroencephalogram (EEG) and functional magnetic resonance imaging (fMRI)], cortical mapping (through virtual lesion effects), and mirror neuron system (MNS) activity.

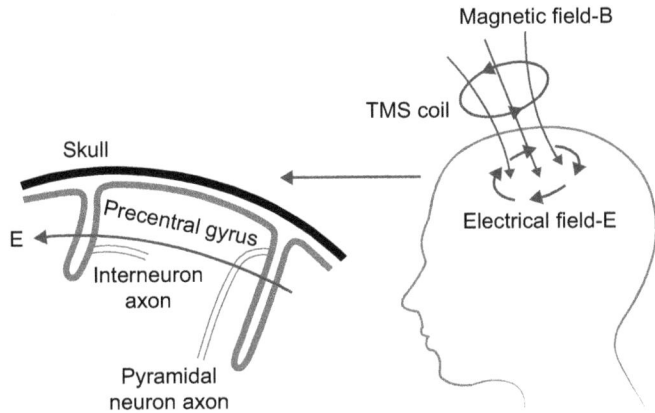

Fig. 2: Magnetic stimulation of cerebral cortex with transcranial magnetic stimulation (TMS) coil.

APPLICATIONS OF THE TMS IN YOGA RESEARCH

Global Cortical Excitability[10,11]

Global cortical excitability is a function of the overall effect of various excitatory and inhibitory neurotransmitters in the brain. It depends on multiple factors such as age, sleep/sleep disturbances, drugs (especially benzodiazepines), and neuropsychiatric disorders such as Alzheimer's disease, multiple sclerosis, amyotrophic lateral sclerosis, schizophrenia, and cocaine dependence. Yoga as a mind–body technique is commonly used in most of the disorders described above. TMS could be one of the tools to study global cortical excitability in yoga research involving the disorders mentioned above as well as other related conditions. TMS could also be used in healthy long-term yoga practitioners to examine if their cortical excitability is different from that of healthy controls not practicing yoga.

Global cortical excitability can be measured with TMS using motor-evoked potential (MEP) input-output (IO) curves evoked with varying strength of magnetic pulse delivered at the motor cortex. The MEP IO curve is obtained by plotting different strengths of magnetic pulses delivered against the corresponding MEP amplitude in microvolts recorded from the EMG electrode connected to specific muscle group stimulated from the cortex with TMS coil. Greater the slope of the MEP IO curve, the higher the cortical excitability. It is speculated that a calm mind might need greater strength of magnetic stimulation than a distracted mind, and the slope of the MEP IO curve in long-term yoga practitioners might be lesser compared to non-yoga practitioners.

Gamma-aminobutyric Acid and Glutamate Neurotransmission

Gamma-aminobutyric acid (GABA) and glutamate are the major inhibitory and excitatory neurotransmitters in the brain, respectively. Most of the brain functions: cognitive, emotional, and behavioral—are dependent on the optimal functioning of the GABA and glutamate neurotransmission. Stress models in animal studies have shown that the GABA-glutamate ratio influences specific behavioral responses with changes in the prefrontal cortex and amygdala.[12,13] Many of the behavioral deficits observed in psychiatric disorders such as autism and schizophrenia are hypothesized to be due to an imbalance in excitatory-inhibitory function mediated by GABA and glutamate. Thus GABA-glutamate balance is crucial for normal functioning, and its imbalance due to various causes, especially stress,[14] has important implications in many of the neuropsychiatric disorders such as depression, anxiety, epilepsy, and schizophrenia. Most of the neuropsychiatric disorders are reported to have less GABAergic tone leading to a tilt toward glutamate in the excitatory-inhibitory (E-I) balance, i.e., increased E-I balance.

Yoga is one of the common antidotes for stress used by people alike from different walks of life. Enhanced inhibitory tone mediated by GABA in the brain could be one of the possible mechanisms for the relaxing effect of yoga. Recent evidence with TMS and magnetic resonance spectroscopy (MRS) studies had shown that yoga enhances GABAergic inhibitory tone in the cortex and thalamus.[15-17] Thus, it is reasonable to believe that yoga could be one of the potential tools to revert the increased E-I balance in stress and related disorders by increasing the GABAergic inhibitory tone.[18]

In the context of stress, with yoga and neuropsychiatric disorders converging at a common pathway through GABA and glutamate neurotransmission, TMS as a cost-effective, noninvasive brain stimulation technique has practical relevance in enhancing the knowledge related to the neuroscience of yoga.

Given below are the different TMS paradigms[19] for studying cortical GABA or glutamate neurotransmission, which are relevant for yoga research.

Short-interval Intracortical Inhibition

Short-interval intracortical inhibition (SICI) is a paired-pulse paradigm in which the effect of a subthreshold conditioning stimulus diminishes the MEP amplitude (measured from the EMG electrode attached to corresponding muscle group in hand stimulated through the cortex) of a suprathreshold test stimulus when the two stimuli are delivered from a single coil with an interstimulus interval of 3–6 milliseconds. SICI is a marker of cortical GABAergic neurotransmission at the $GABA_A$ receptor.

Long-interval Intracortical Inhibition

Long-interval intracortical inhibition (LICI) is a paired-pulse paradigm in which the effect of a suprathreshold conditioning stimulus diminishes the MEP amplitude of another suprathreshold test stimulus when the two stimuli are delivered from a single coil with an interstimulus interval of 100 milliseconds. LICI is a marker of cortical GABAergic neurotransmission at $GABA_B$ receptor.

Intracortical Facilitation

Intracortical facilitation (ICF) is a paired-pulse paradigm in which the effect of a subthreshold conditioning stimulus enhances the MEP amplitude of a suprathreshold test stimulus when the two stimuli are delivered from a single coil with an interstimulus interval of 6–10 milliseconds. ICF is a marker of cortical glutamatergic neurotransmission at the NMDA receptor.

Cortical Silent Period

Cortical silent period (CSP) is a single pulse paradigm, in which a suprathreshold magnetic pulse is delivered at the motor cortex when the corresponding muscle is in sustained contraction. When the pulse is delivered, while the muscle is contracting, the EMG amplitude due to contraction of the muscle becomes flat for few milliseconds (25–300 ms) before it regains the EMG amplitude once again. The duration for which the EMG amplitude becomes flat is CSP. CSP is a marker of GABAergic neurotransmission at the $GABA_B$ receptor. Unlike LICI, which is a marker of *cortical* GABAergic neurotransmission at the $GABA_B$ receptor, the initial few seconds (20–30 ms) of the silent period is due to *spinal* GABAergic neurotransmission at $GABA_B$ receptor.

All the paradigms mentioned above could be used alone or in combination to study the GABA and glutamate neurotransmission at the level of the cortex in relevant yoga research.

Complexity Measure of Consciousness

Consciousness is a complex term that neuroscience finds challenging to assess objectively. Although most of the effects of yoga are directly related to change at the level of consciousness, they are never measured due to the absence of a valid tool. At present, consciousness is assessed through neural correlates in most of the studies. Very commonly, fMRI is used in the study of neural correlates of consciousness (NCC). With the advent of TMS-EEG, NCC could be assessed as a function of complexity measures in the TMS-evoked EEG signal on the scalp. One such correlate for the complexity measure of consciousness is the perturbation complexity index (PCI).[20] In simple terms, PCI is a measure based on difficulty in compressing EEG signals generated by a TMS stimulus. The compression algorithm used is similar to the one used for compressing folders on the computer. Similar kinds of files inside the folder make it easier to compress against a variety of files that are relatively difficult to compress. In similar terms, EEG signals which are more synchronized as in sleep or meditation are easier to compress and hence have a lesser PCI value than during a cognitive task in wakefulness.

Perturbation complexity index is assessed using a single-pulse TMS (at the subject's motor threshold) delivered at the motor cortex, and the TMS-evoked EEG waves are recorded from the scalp EEG electrodes from multiple sites. Based on the spread and synchrony of the evoked EEG waves, PCI varies from zero to one. Though consciousness, as perceived in yoga, is not measurable with available tools in science, objective measures such as PCI, derived from activities in neural substrates related to consciousness, would guide yoga research in expanding the mechanistic evidence base.

A recent study by Bodart et al.[21] used a new measure called divergence index (DI) obtained by TMS-EEG with meditation as an intervention. This measure (DI) was initially developed by Casarotto et al. in 2010.[22] As the name suggests, DI is the percentage of TMS-evoked EEG signals that differ significantly across all channels compared to a cut-off value determined by a normative data tested by test-retest variability. DI, along with other EEG parameters, could be used to explore and differentiate states of mind attained by meditation. Unlike PCI, which deals with the compressibility of EEG signals, DI deals with the variability of EEG signals across channels against a known cut-off value.

Note: Both PCI and DI are based on information integration theory (IIT) proposed by Tononi.[23] For a comprehensive understanding of PCI and DI, readers are requested to refer to articles published elsewhere.[20,22]

Mirror Neuron System

Mirror neurons are a specialized network of neurons (frontal and parietal cortex) that get activated when a person acts or observes someone performing an action. For example, when a cricket match is being viewed on television, one might feel an urge to move (or even a twitch in one's body) in the direction one's favorite player is moving in order to complete a run or take a catch. This urge to move is likely to be mirror neuron driven. Activation of mirror neurons is relevant for understanding others' emotions, the intentions underlying their actions, and expressing meaningful behavior in social interactions.

Mirror neuron activity has been demonstrated by various means[24]—direct method, single-cell electrode recordings, and indirect methods such as fMRI, EEG, magnetoencephalography (MEG) as well as TMS.

Transcranial magnetic stimulation is a noninvasive method to transiently excite the cerebral cortex. When applied to the primary motor cortex, it produces peripheral MEPs, which are recorded using EMG from hand muscles. Observation of actions using specific muscle enhances the amplitude of MEPs recorded from those muscles—this enhancement has been purported to be indirectly reflective of the premotor MNS activity.

Mirror neuron system could be studied in a variety of neuropsychiatric disorders. For example, compared to healthy individuals, patients with autism and schizophrenia have reduced mirror neuron activity, and this is speculated as one of the reasons for impaired social functioning in these patients. It is hypothesized that yoga would enhance mirror neuron activity through the process of imitation while one learns yoga from the yoga instructor, as well as the experience of being imitated.[25] The method of learning yoga asana and pranayama by imitating the yoga instructor should help train the patients to activate the mirror neurons, potentially leading to better social functioning.

RESEARCH STUDIES ON YOGA WITH TMS
Research on Healthy Volunteers

Four published studies are available on TMS with yoga-based interventions. Three studies assessed the CSP and one study assessed DI.

In a single group prepost design study, Govindaraj et al.[26] found an increase in CSP following 20 sessions (60 min a day) of yoga, which included asana, pranayama, and yoga-based relaxation and om chanting. The subjects were 15 healthy volunteers who enrolled in a 1-month yoga appreciation course. Earlier in a pilot observation, Mehta et al. reported longer CSP in experienced yoga practitioners ($n = 6$) compared to an age and gender-matched nonyoga practitioners ($n = 10$).[18] Another study by Gugleiti et al.[27] found an increase in CSP following a single 60 minutes meditation session. The subjects were 35 meditators (practicing at least 3 hours per week regularly) and 35 nonmeditators who were engaged in a nonmeditative activity that approximated the levels of sedentariness associated with meditation.

Results of these studies suggest that yoga-based intervention could enhance GABAergic (in particular $GABA_B$) neurotransmission in the cortex.

Bodart et al.[21] in a single case study (69-year-old expert meditation practitioner with 60,000 hours of meditation practice) used DI along with power and phase-locking factor and demonstrated that different states of meditation could be assessed locally (at a particular stimulation site on the scalp) and globally with combined TMS-EEG study.

Research on Patients with Depression

Two studies are available related to depression. One study used TMS as an investigative tool to assess CSP following yoga, and the other research (case report) had used TMS as a therapeutic tool along with yoga-based intervention in refractory depression.

Patients with depression have deficits in GABAergic neurotransmission, and yoga is found to improve symptoms of depression as a monotherapy or as an add-on treatment. A recent study by Jakhar et al.[28] demonstrated a single session of yoga increased CSP significantly compared to walking in patients with depression, suggesting increased cortical GABAergic (GABA-B) neurotransmission. These findings are corroborated by increased cortical and thalamic GABAergic neurotransmission demonstrated in magnetic resonance spectroscopy studies by Streeter et al.[16,17] In another interesting case report by Pradhan et al.,[29] rTMS was combined with mindfulness-based cognitive therapy (MBCT) in a patient with refractory depression. MBCT was clubbed with rTMS sessions. In the first 30 minutes of each rTMS, the patient was trained to do focused attention meditation guided by real-time EEG feedback to attain a state of mental calmness. In the last 10–15 minutes of each rTMS session, MBCT was delivered simultaneously. Combined rTMS with MBCT reduced the number of rTMS sessions required from 36 (usual number of sessions for refractory depression) to 30 and the patient's refractory depression (for more than 30 years) not only remitted but also remained in remission (HAM-D17 depression scale score of 6) at 8 months follow-up.

SAFETY OF TRANSCRANIAL MAGNETIC STIMULATION

The general understanding of single-pulse stimulation is that they are safe. The high frequency of rTMS provides a much stronger effect on the brain and, albeit unlikely, can induce seizures. Other common side effects include nausea, arms jerking, transient headache, and facial pain caused by the activation of scalp and neck muscles, and safe intensity limits using rTMS are suggested to help reduce the risk of discomfort. The consensus is that TMS is safe. However, one should remain mindful of minimizing the risks.

CONCLUSION

Transcranial magnetic stimulation as a tool of investigation and therapy is gaining popularity as it is noninvasive and can modulate the cortical reactivity in real-time in a reversible manner. Applications of TMS in neuroscience are enormous, although we have discussed only a few of the relevant ones here. Understanding these basic applications of TMS in neuroscience would enable the yoga researcher to explore a vast majority of hypotheses ranging from cortical connectivity and plasticity, cortical and spinal motor conduction time, consciousness and its correlates, and neurochemical substrates underlying cortical reactivity in the context of yoga. TMS applications are safe, and it could be combined with different modalities such as EEG, fMRI, peripheral nerve stimulation techniques, and other neuromodulation techniques such as tDCS (transcranial direct current stimulation) and tACS (transcranial alternating current stimulation) for better understanding of the mechanisms underlying yoga.

REFERENCES

1. Gallone P. Galvani's frog: Harbinger of a new era. Electrochimica Acta. 1986;31(12):1485-90.
2. Ferrier D (Ed). The Functions of the Brain. Smith: Elder; 1886.
3. Ferrier D. The Croonian lectures on cerebral localisation. Br Med J. 1890;2(1541):68.
4. Geddes L. History of magnetic stimulation of the nervous system. J Clin Neurophysiol Off Publ Am Electroencephalogr Soc. 1991;8(1):3-9.
5. Barker AT, Jalinous R, Freeston IL. Non-invasive magnetic stimulation of human motor cortex. The Lancet. 1985;325(8437):1106-7.
6. Merton P, Morton H. Stimulation of the cerebral cortex in the intact human subject. Nature. 1980;285(5762):227-7.
7. Barker AT. An introduction to the basic principles of magnetic nerve stimulation. J Clin Neurophysiol Off Publ Am Electroencephalogr Soc. 1991;8(1):26-37.
8. Amassian VE, Eberle L, Maccabee PJ, Cracco RQ. Modelling magnetic coil excitation of human cerebral cortex with a peripheral nerve immersed in a brain-shaped volume conductor: the significance of fiber bending in excitation. Electroencephalogr Clin Neurophysiol Potentials Sect. 1992;85(5):291-301.
9. Hallett M. Transcranial magnetic stimulation: a primer. Neuron. 2007;55(2):187-99.
10. Ridding M, Rothwell J. Stimulus/response curves as a method of measuring motor cortical excitability in man. Electroencephalogr Clin Neurophysiol Mot Control. 1997;105(5):340-4.
11. Van der Kamp W, Zwinderman AH, Ferrari MD, van Dijk JG. Cortical excitability and response variability of transcranial magnetic stimulation. J Clin Neurophysiol. 1996;13(2):164-71.
12. Drouet JB, Fauvelle F, Maunoir-Regimbal S, Fidier N, Maury R, Peinnequin A, et al. Differences in prefrontal cortex GABA/glutamate ratio after acute restraint stress in rats are associated with specific behavioral and neurobiological patterns. Neuroscience. 2015;285:155-65.
13. Page CE, Coutellier L. Prefrontal excitatory/inhibitory balance in stress and emotional disorders: evidence for over-inhibition. Neurosci Biobehav Rev. 2019;105:39-51.
14. Gao J, Wang H, Liu Y, Li Y, Chen C, Liu L, et al. Glutamate and GABA imbalance promotes neuronal apoptosis in hippocampus after stress. Med Sci Monit. 2014;20:499-512.
15. Streeter CC, Jensen JE, Perlmutter RM, Cabral HJ, Tian H, Terhune DB, et al. Yoga Asana sessions increase brain GABA levels: a pilot study. J Altern Complement Med. 2007;13(4):419-26.
16. Streeter CC, Whitfield TH, Owen L, Rein T, Karri SK, Yakhkind A, et al. Effects of yoga versus walking on mood, anxiety, and brain GABA levels: a randomized controlled MRS study. J Altern Complement Med. 2010;16(11):1145-52.
17. Streeter CC, Gerbarg PL, Brown RP, Scott TM, Nielsen GH, Owen L, et al. Thalamic gamma aminobutyric acid level changes in major depressive disorder after a 12-week iyengar yoga and coherent breathing intervention. J Altern Complement Med. 2020;26(3):190-7.
18. Mehta UM, Gangadhar B. Yoga: balancing the excitation-inhibition equilibrium in psychiatric disorders. In: Progress in Brain Research. Elsevier; 2019. pp. 387-413.
19. Hallett M, Chokroverty S. Magnetic stimulation in clinical neurophysiology. Elsevier Health Sciences; 2005.
20. Casali AG, Gosseries O, Rosanova M, Boly M, Sarasso S, Casali KR, et al. A theoretically based index of consciousness independent of sensory processing and behavior. Sci Transl Med. 2013;5(198):198ra105.
21. Bodart O, Fecchio M, Massimini M, Wannez S, Virgillito A, Casarotto S, et al. Meditation-induced modulation of brain response to transcranial magnetic stimulation. Brain Stimul Basic Transl Clin Res Neuromodulation. 2018;11(6):1397-400.
22. Casarotto S, Lauro LJR, Bellina V, Casali AG, Rosanova M, Pigorini A, et al. EEG responses to

TMS are sensitive to changes in the perturbation parameters and repeatable over time. PloS One. 2010;5(4):e10281.
23. Tononi G. An information integration theory of consciousness. BMC Neurosci. 2004;5(1):1-22.
24. Rizzolatti G, Craighero L. The mirror-neuron system. Annu Rev Neurosci. 2004;27:169-92.
25. Mehta UM, Keshavan MS, Gangadhar BN. Bridging the schism of schizophrenia through yoga—Review of putative mechanisms. Int Rev Psychiatry. 2016;28(3):254-64.
26. Govindaraj R, Mehta UM, Kumar V, Varambally S, Thirthalli J, Gangadhar BN. Effect of yoga on cortical inhibition in healthy individuals: a pilot study using Transcranial Magnetic Stimulation. Brain Stimul Basic Transl Clin Res Neuromodulation. 2018;11(6):1401-3.
27. Guglietti CL, Daskalakis ZJ, Radhu N, Fitzgerald PB, Ritvo P. Meditation-related increases in GABAB modulated cortical inhibition. Brain Stimulation. 2013;6(3):397-402.
28. Jakhar J, Mehta UM, Ektare A, Vidyasagar PD, Varambally S, Thirthalli J, et al. Cortical inhibition in major depression: investigating the acute effect of single-session yoga versus walking. Brain Stimul Basic Transl Clin Res Neuromodulation. 2019;12(6):1597-9.
29. Pradhan B, Makani R, Chatterjee M. Combining mindfulness based cognitive therapy (MBCT) with brain stimulation using concurrent repetitive transcranial magnetic stimulation (rTMS) and focused attention meditation during the rTMS session for refractory depression: a case report. EC Neurol. 2018;10(4):241-51.

CHAPTER 8

Insights into Mode of Action of Yoga in Mental Disorders: A Summary of Biological Evidence

Monojit Debnath, Rima Dada, Michael Berk

INTRODUCTION

Mental illnesses constitute a major public health burden, both in developed and developing countries, due to disability, direct and indirect costs, elevated rates of morbidity and mortality. Smoking, poor dietary habits, obesity, and sedentary lifestyle are more common among people with mental disorders. These variables might further drive underlying common pathophysiological pathways for mental and physical disorders, promoting neuroprogression and somatoprogression, respectively,[1] thereby aggravating poor health outcomes in this population. Notably, side effects associated with some psychotropic medications like second-generation antipsychotic drugs such as weight gain and metabolic alterations increase medical comorbidity and depression.

Over the past few years, lifestyle interventions that combine exercise, smoking cessation, dietary counseling, and health promotion have shown promising results in preventing obesity as well as reducing cardiometabolic risk factors, thus impacting mental disorders and their somatic comorbidities. It has also become apparent that lifestyle intervention therapies, particularly yoga, seem to be efficacious in improving quality of life and reducing symptoms in patients with serious mental illnesses. However, the present state of knowledge on the beneficial effects of yoga on mental disorders remains limited to symptomatic changes. It would be useful to establish whether such beneficial effects are driven by cellular and/or molecular processes of an individual; this will help to scientifically validate yoga as a safe and effective therapeutic intervention. Attempts have been made to identify cellular/molecular mechanisms that may help to demonstrate the underlying biological basis of yoga's mode of action. Preliminary understanding suggests that yoga therapy might have effects on multiple biological systems/pathways such as immune, neuroendocrine, autonomic and stress-regulatory, to name a few. Contextually, many of these pathways have pathobiological relevance in major mental disorders. Although the precise mechanisms through which yoga brings changes in the above biological pathways are inadequately known, it is assumed that regulatory changes in genetic and epigenetic processes might at least, in part, be involved in driving these changes.

MODE OF ACTION OF YOGA: BIOLOGICAL PERSPECTIVES

To facilitate the understanding of the biological bases of yoga, we have tried to integrate findings from multiple candidate pathways that essentially highlight the underlying cellular, molecular as well as physiological mechanisms.

Cellular Mechanisms/Pathways

Cellular Aging

Yoga practice in healthy individuals has significant effect on markers of cellular aging. Yoga is shown to reduce the rate of cellular aging and subsequently our biological age. The underlying mechanisms through which yoga might improve cellular longevity are now beginning to be understood. Many mechanisms/factors, such as genomic stability, deoxyribonucleic acid (DNA) repair mechanisms, telomere metabolism, stress-regulatory system, apoptotic machinery, and so on, are central in maintaining cellular homeostasis including longevity. Importantly, yoga practice has been shown to have enduring effects on all these cellular processes within a cell. The levels of antiapoptotic *Bcl2* and *Cox2* genes in lymphocytes are upregulated in healthy yoga practitioners, implying that this could lead to better immunoregulation by prolonging the life span of lymphocytes. In various disease conditions, the percentage of apoptosis, the extent of DNA damage, the rate of shortening of telomere, and production of oxidative stress-related markers were found to be influenced by yoga therapy.

Immune Pathways

Aberrant immune system functioning has been proposed as one of the most predominant pathobiological mechanisms in patients with a range of mental disorders and their medical comorbidities. Diverse lines of evidence support the immune dysfunction hypothesis, which include (1) altered counts of various immune cells such as T-lymphocytes, B-lymphocytes, dendritic cells, and natural killer (NK) cells; (2) production of proinflammatory cytokines in the peripheral blood; and (3) aberrant expression of genes regulating immune functions, both in the peripheral blood and brain of patients with mental illnesses. Large-scale genomic studies also provided evidence of a genetic link between immune system and mental illnesses. Stress with raised cortisol levels causes persistent activation of the hypothalamic-pituitary-adrenal (HPA) axis and dysregulation of the immune system and may lead to autoimmune diseases and even cancer if left untreated. Raised cortisol levels are also neurotoxic and chronic stress is associated with reduced hippocampal volume, lowered antioxidant defenses and diminished levels of brain-derived neurotrophic factor (BDNF), a key determinant of neuroplasticity.

Yoga practice also has an impact on the immune system. Several immune components which are involved in initiating and mediating immuno-inflammatory responses such as C-reactive protein (CRP), inflammatory cytokines such as interleukin-12 (IL-12) and interferon-gamma (IFN-γ) are downregulated by yoga practice in healthy people and industrial workers, as well as in individuals suffering from various systemic and nervous system disorders.[2] Besides, yoga therapy is found to result significant improvement in the count of NK cells in patients with metastatic breast cancer.[3] The mechanism(s) through which yoga brings about changes in the blood levels of various immune mediators as well as percentage of immune cells are incompletely understood. Data obtained from preliminary studies demonstrated the impact of yoga not only on the expression levels of genes coding inflammatory mediators but also on key factors that are crucially involved in driving inflammatory cascade, such as nuclear factor-kappa B (NF-κB).[4] It is likely that yoga modulates the nongenetic processes involved in transcriptional regulation of the expression of immune function-related genes and subsequently, the production of proteins. The immune-dampening capacity of yoga might form a part of the mechanistic basis through which yoga offers clinical benefits in patients with mental disorders.

Neurochemicals and Neural Pathways

Stress can lead to imbalance of the autonomic nervous system, with decreased parasympathetic nervous system activity and increased sympathetic nervous system (SNS) activity, and may blunt activity of the gamma-aminobutyric acid (GABA) system.

Magnetic resonance spectroscopy studies have demonstrated reduced or abnormal GABA concentrations in various neuropsychiatric disorders such as anxiety disorders and depression.[5] Recent understanding suggests that yoga has a direct influence on the parasympathetic and sympathetic activity in the autonomic nervous system. Yoga, through pressure on the baroreceptors results in enhanced parasympathetic system activity and can modulate heart rate variability, blood pressure, and oxygen metabolism. Furthermore, different components of yoga such as breathing, calming effects of pranayama and physical movement due to asanas can reduce sympathetic activation and increase levels of GABA. A 12-week yoga intervention was associated with improved mood and decreased anxiety, thought to be due, at least in part, to increased thalamic GABA levels.[6]

Neurotrophic factors such as BDNF and vascular endothelial growth factor (VEGF) play a crucial role in development and plasticity of the brain. Altered BDNF production and signaling are implicated in the pathophysiology of many neuropsychiatric disorders including bipolar disorder and schizophrenia. Yoga practices led to increased blood BDNF levels in healthy subjects, premenopausal women with chronic low back pain, as well as in patients with major depression.[7,8] Another study demonstrated an increase in levels of BDNF, dehydroepiandrosterone-sulfate (DHEA-S), serotonin, and melatonin in patients with depression.[8]

Molecular Processes/Events

Telomere and Telomerase Activities

Telomeres are DNA sequences at the ends of chromosomes that protect the genome from nucleolytic degradation and interchromosomal fusion during cellular replication. Telomeres undergo shortening with each cell division. Telomerase enzyme activity influences telomere length by adding DNA sequences onto telomeres during cell division. Progressive shortening of telomeres is associated with senescence, apoptosis, and oncogenic transformation of somatic cells. Importantly, shortened telomere length and reduced telomerase are linked to a host of health risks and increased incidence of diseases. Telomere length and telomerase activity may be regulated by psychological stress and stress appraisals. Oxidative stress targets telomeres and causes their accelerated shortening and thus premature aging. About 40 base pairs (bp) are lost from telomere ends each year; however, psychological stress and associated oxidative stress due to reduced total antioxidant capacity causes 120 bp loss each year. Importantly, telomere length has been explored as a useful "psychobiomarker" linking stress and disease.[9] There is a documented association between significant telomere loss and neuropsychiatric disorders including schizophrenia and bipolar disorder. Increased telomerase activity and reduced levels of oxidative stress aid in maintenance of telomere length and thus reduce our biological age.[10] Yoga also upregulates the levels of sirtuins (SIRTs), the longevity genes, independent of caloric restriction, and intake of resveratrol.[10] SIRTs act as antiapoptotic regulators which aid cell survival in stress conditions and inhibit p53 and NF-κB signaling. SIRTs promote growth of neurons and protect cortical neurons against hydrogen peroxide (H_2O_2) stimulated oxidative stress by regulating mitochondrial Ca^{2+} homeostasis and mitochondrial dysfunction. SIRTs are also known to inhibit the death of neurons and inflammatory responses in central nervous system (CNS) through mammalian target of rapamycin (mTOR) signaling and by controlling excessive activation of microglia through NF-κB deacetylation, respectively.

Lifestyle factors can negatively influence health and life span of an individual, at least in part, by altering telomere length. The leukocyte telomere length is found to be better preserved in healthy individuals practicing yoga. Long-term yoga practice improves mental and cognitive functioning, lowers depressive symptoms and is associated with increased telomerase activity. This raises the possibility that the clinical benefits of yoga therapy in mental disorders could also be influenced by telomere length and the activity of telomerase.

Conserved Transcriptional Response to Adversity and Transcriptional Regulation

Stress is an important risk factor for mental disorders. Various biological pathways that are relevant to the pathophysiology of mental disorders undergo rapid changes during psychological stress. The HPA axis and SNS are the predominant pathways that mediate biological responses to stress. These stress axes further influence a number of adaptive behavioral and physiological processes. For example, acute/chronic psychological stress can result in immediate immunomodulation, which in turn is associated with endocrine and autonomic functions. It is important to note that chronic stress, by modulating neuroimmunoendocrine functions, can lead to increased risk for multiple noncommunicable diseases and chronic medical diseases that share an immune diathesis and plays a part in both neuroprogression and somatoprogression of mental and physical disorders, respectively. Although yoga appears to reduce endocrine, immune, and behavioral responses to psychological stress, the exact mechanisms remain unclear. Chronic stress by immune dysregulation can lead to autoimmune diseases and yoga aids in re-establishment of immunological tolerance and thus establishes molecular remission.[11] Yoga also resulted in elevated levels of human leukocyte antigen-G (HLA-G) and immunosuppressive cytokines and reduced expression levels of proinflammatory genes such as *IL-2, IL-6, IL-17, tumor necrosis factor-*α *(TNF-*α*)*, and NF-κB in cases with rheumatoid arthritis and comorbid depression.

Transcription factors play a crucial role in the inflammation biology. NF-κB is a key transcription factor, produced when stress activates the SNS, which then translates stress into inflammation by influencing the expression of inflammatory genes. It is hypothesized that the effect of stress might be translated through a host of immune function relates genes, especially the ones which are part of conserved transcriptional response to adversity (CTRA). The CTRA is considered as a molecular signature of chronic stress. CTRA is proposed to serve as a common molecular pattern in people exposed to various adversities such as bereavement, trauma, and socioeconomic impoverishment. Many such adverse conditions act as early risk determinants for psychiatric conditions. Altered CTRA reflects upregulation of proinflammatory genes that subsequently lead to major inflammation at the cellular level. Given the influence of yoga on inflammation, it seems that yoga most likely alters CTRA and neutralizes the stress-induced inflammatory responses in various mental illnesses.

Epigenetic Modulation

Epigenetics is the study of heritable changes in gene expression that are not due to changes in nucleotide sequences. Epigenetic processes operate at the interface of gene and environment in many diseases. Since almost all mental illnesses are complex and multifactorial, a significant role of epigenetic processes has been suggested in these disorders. Epigenetic changes are recognized signatures of adverse events in early life and are relevant biomarkers for mental illnesses. Epigenetic processes involve DNA methylation, histone acetylation and microRNA expression, of which DNA methylation has been widely studied in various mental disorders. It is now becoming evident that yoga therapy might influence epigenetic processes. Although data pertaining to the significant modulatory effects of various mind-body therapies such as meditation and Tai chi on various epigenetic events such as global modifications of histone, expression of histone deacetylase and DNA methylation are available, attempts to test the effect of yoga on epigenetics are indeed very few. However, preliminary findings have shown that even brief yoga interventions can induce DNA methylation changes in genes, particularly those involved in inflammation.

Physiological Processes/Pathways

Modulation of Biological Rhythms

Melatonin, a pineal hormone, is a critical mediator of biological rhythms. Apart from protecting the body's biological clock, melatonin regulates many biological and physiological processes including cell renewal, strengthening of the immune system, sleep and body temperature regulation. Melatonin is also an antioxidant that easily passes the blood-brain barrier. An altered secretory pattern of melatonin has been reported in various psychiatric disorders such as bipolar disorder, schizophrenia, anorexia, and panic disorder.[12] Yoga practice increases plasma melatonin levels, even at night-time. This implies that yoga practices in the form of psychophysiological stimuli can increase endogenous secretion of melatonin which might be associated with an improved sense of well-being and better sleep.

Modulation of HPA Axis and Stress-regulatory System

Dysfunctional HPA axis and SNS are reported in a range of mental disorders. Hypercortisolemia is observed in several psychiatric disorders such as schizophrenia, bipolar disorder, and major depression. Over the past few years, yoga has been found to be effective in reducing stress and biomarkers of stress such as blood/salivary cortisol levels. Yoga practice in young healthy people led to reduced plasma levels of adrenaline and increased plasma levels of serotonin.[2] In depression, treatment with yoga significantly reduced cortisol levels.[13] Further, 6 months of yoga practice was reported to be associated with reduced salivary cortisol levels, as well as parameters related to stress, depression and anxiety, and improved cognition scores in healthy male volunteers.[14]

Oxidative and nitrosative stress pathways along with immunoinflammation are implicated in the pathophysiology of many mental disorders.[15,16] The ameliorative effect of yoga on oxidative stress due to a reduction in lipid peroxidation has been demonstrated in multiple studies. Regular yoga practice led to significantly decreased serum levels of nitric oxide, F2-isoprostane, and lipid peroxide, while increasing serum total glutathione (GSH), activities of GSH-peroxidase and GSH-s-transferase, as well as total antioxidant status, suggesting an improved antioxidant defense system.[2,17] Healthy individuals practicing yoga had significantly lower levels of blood lactate, and higher levels of superoxide dismutase (SOD), GSH, and catalase, indicative of altered mitochondrial biogenesis and redox effects, respectively.[18] In addition, elevated gene expressions of glutathione S-transferase, Cu-Zn SOD, Mn-SOD, glutathione peroxidase, and catalase were reported in yoga practitioners.[19] Yoga practices were also seen to reduce seminal oxidative stress and oxidative damage and the levels of mutagenic base 8-hydroxy-2′-deoxyguanosine (8-OHdG). Accumulation of this base additionally causes epimutations. Increased levels of this base and high levels of DNA damage are associated with *de novo* germline mutations and dysregulated sperm transcripts. These are associated with increased incidence of genetic and epigenetic disorders in the offspring, autosomal dominant disorders, schizophrenia, depression and bipolar disorders in the offspring. Yoga reduces levels of 8-OHdG and oxidative DNA damage and thus may play a significant role in reducing incidence of these complex disorders.[20] Based on the above findings, it can be hypothesized that yoga benefits patients with mental disorders by modulating stress-regulatory and mitochondrial biogenesis pathways.

Regulation of Energy Metabolism and Metabolic Pathways

Stress has been linked to heightened sympathetic activity, increased energy expenditure and changes in the inflammasome, and thus places metabolic burden on homeostasis. Psychological stress can cause chronic mitochondrial dysfunction, oxidative stress, and subsequently risk the development of metabolic syndrome such as hypertension, obesity, and insulin-resistant diabetes mellitus. Compelling evidence suggests that there is a higher prevalence of metabolic syndrome in patients with severe mental illnesses such as schizophrenia and chronic mood disorders.[21,22] A recent genome-wide association study (GWAS) data on patients with depressive disorders in comparison to controls provided evidence of genetic links between genes involved in bioenergetics.[23] It is important to note that long-term yoga practice has been linked to lower metabolic rates and greater metabolic efficiency. This is becoming increasingly important given recent evidence that other therapies that boost mitochondrial biogenesis might reduce depression.[24] In another study, the practice of relaxation response was associated with rapid changes in gene expression that are linked to pathways responsible for energy metabolism, electron transport chain, biological oxidation and insulin secretion.[25]

Oxytocin and Social Cognition

Yoga-based interventions have produced improvements in psychopathology as well as social cognition parameters in patients with psychosis. A possible mediator is the "cuddling hormone" oxytocin, which is associated with the feeling of well-being. Changes in oxytocin levels during the practice of yoga have been evaluated. Those patients who participated demonstrated significant benefits in emotion recognition following yoga. However, no such benefit was demonstrated in waitlisted subjects. Oxytocin levels increased threefold in the yoga group after 1 month, with no such change evident in the waitlisted group.[26]

■ PROMISES AND CHALLENGES

Multiple studies have shown that yoga offers potential therapeutic benefits in several neuropsychiatric disorders. For example, patients with schizophrenia who practice yoga show more improvement in their positive and negative symptom scores, social functioning scores, and aspects of cognition. Results of some meta-analyses are also encouraging. In a recent meta-analysis of 29 studies comprising 1,109 patients, yoga therapy was found to offer better results on several key features such as reduction in depressive symptoms and global functioning than exercise in people diagnosed with schizophrenia spectrum disorders.[27] People practicing integrated yoga also experienced a significant decrease in anxiety-related symptoms. Some of the mechanisms of action of yoga include changes in multiple biological components such as levels of cortisol, immune mediators, expression of BDNF, immune function-related genes, neurotransmitters, and activity of HPA axis.

However, there are multiple limitations in current randomized control trials, as many of them consisted of small and heterogeneous groups of subjects. Furthermore, the duration of interventions has also not been uniform; some studies used shorter duration, which may not be adequate to detect changes in markers of various pathways. Another important question in yoga research studies is the "dose" of yoga, i.e., the duration of the yoga practices and the length of time for which the intervention is continued. Traditional yoga schools require daily training followed by similar practice at home for optimal benefits, both for learning and therapy. Most research trials from India require at least 2–4 weeks of supervised training followed by daily practice at home for the next 8–12 weeks. Also, the "spiritual" aspects of yoga practice need to be explored in terms of its contribution to therapeutic effects. There could also be several other benefits of practicing yoga that clinical rating scales may fail to demonstrate, such as boosting self-efficacy, control, social networks, and perceived support (and may even be seen as "side effects"). Future research needs to find a way to overcome these limitations. The possible adverse effects of yoga practices also need to be documented and studied if yoga as an intervention is to be held to the same standards as other scientific methods of treatments.

CONCLUSION

In this chapter, we have highlighted the biological candidate pathways/mechanisms related to yoga and have provided a perspective for future biological research on yoga in mental disorders. Despite limitations, current evidence suggests that yoga has salutary effects on the brain and behavior, and has been recommended as a safe therapy in a recent meta-analysis.[28] The positive effects of yoga on neural networks and neural plasticity have received recent attention. The neuroprotective effects of yoga may provide crucial clues about the neural bases of its potential clinical effects. Yoga therapy may also potentially help to preserve the cognitive domains of patients with severe mental disorders. The most salient finding from the current literature is the effect of yoga in inducing changes in molecules involved in energy metabolism. A correlation between yoga and the immune system is supported by functional genomic studies. In summary, yoga may offer beneficial effects on candidate components/pathways that are relevant in the pathogenesis of mental and comorbid physical disorders, and may offer benefits over and above current treatment approaches.

REFERENCES

1. Morris G, Puri BK, Walker AJ, Maes M, Carvalho AF, Walder K, et al. Shared pathways for neuroprogression and somatoprogression in neuropsychiatric disorders. Neurosci Biobehav Rev. 2019;107:862-82.
2. Lim SA, Cheong KJ. Regular yoga practice improves antioxidant status, immune function, and stress hormone releases in young healthy people: a randomized, double-blind, controlled pilot study. J Altern Complement Med. 2015;21(9):530-8.
3. Rao RM, Vadiraja HS, Nagaratna R, Gopinath KS, Patil S, Diwakar RB, et al. Effect of yoga on sleep quality and neuroendocrine immune response in metastatic breast cancer patients. Indian J Palliat Care. 2017;23(3):253-60.
4. Black DS, Cole SW, Irwin MR, Breen E, St Cyr NM, Nazarian N, et al. Yogic meditation reverses NF-κB and IRF-related transcriptome dynamics in leukocytes of family dementia caregivers in a randomized controlled trial. Psychoneuroendocrinology. 2013;38(3):348-55.
5. Chang L, Cloak CC, Ernst T. Magnetic resonance spectroscopy studies of GABA in neuropsychiatric disorders. J Clin Psychiatry. 2003;64(Suppl 3):7-14.
6. Streeter CC, Whitfield TH, Owen L, Rein T, Karri SK, Yakhkind A, et al. Effects of yoga versus walking on mood, anxiety, and brain GABA levels: a randomized controlled MRS study. J Altern Complement Med. 2010;16(11):1145-52.
7. Naveen GH, Thirthalli J, Rao MG, Varambally S, Christopher R, Gangadhar BN. Positive therapeutic and neurotropic effects of yoga in depression: a comparative study. Indian J Psychiatry. 2013;55(Suppl 3):S400-4.
8. Tolahunase MR, Sagar R, Faiq M, Dada R. Yoga- and meditation-based lifestyle intervention increases neuroplasticity and reduces severity of major depressive disorder: a randomized controlled trial. Restor Neurol Neurosci. 2018;36(3):423-42.
9. Epel ES. Psychological and metabolic stress: a recipe for accelerated cellular aging? Hormones (Athens). 2009;8(1):7-22.
10. Tolahunase M, Sagar R, Dada R. Impact of yoga and meditation on cellular aging in apparently healthy individuals: a prospective, open-label single-arm exploratory study. Oxid Med Cell Longev. 2017;2017:7928981.
11. Gautam S, Tolahunase M, Kumar U, Dada R. Impact of yoga based mind-body intervention on systemic inflammatory markers and comorbid depression in active rheumatoid arthritis patients: a randomized controlled trial. Restor Neurol Neurosci. 2019;37(1):41-59.

12. Pacchierotti C, Iapichino S, Bossini L, Pieraccini F, Castrogiovanni P. Melatonin in psychiatric disorders: a review on the melatonin involvement in psychiatry. Front Neuroendocrinol. 2001;22(1):18-32.
13. Thirthalli J, Naveen GH, Rao MG, Varambally S, Christopher R, Gangadhar BN. Cortisol and antidepressant effects of yoga. Indian J Psychiatry. 2013;55(Suppl 3):S405-8.
14. Rocha KK, Ribeiro AM, Rocha KC, Sousa MB, Albuquerque FS, Ribeiro S, et al. Improvement in physiological and psychological parameters after 6 months of yoga practice. Conscious Cogn. 2012;21(2):843-50.
15. Anderson G, Berk M, Dodd S, Bechter K, Altamura AC, Dell'osso B, et al. Immuno-inflammatory, oxidative and nitrosative stress, and neuroprogressive pathways in the etiology, course and treatment of schizophrenia. Prog Neuropsychopharmacol Biol Psychiatry. 2013;42:1-4.
16. Anderson G, Berk M, Dean O, Moylan S, Maes M. Role of immune-inflammatory and oxidative and nitrosative stress pathways in the etiology of depression: therapeutic implications. CNS Drugs. 2014;28(1):1-10.
17. Sinha S, Singh SN, Monga YP, Ray US. Improvement of glutathione and total anti-oxidant status with yoga. J Altern Complement Med. 2007;13(10):1085-90.
18. Sharma H, Sen S, Singh A, Bhardwaj NK, Kochupillai V, Singh N. Sudarshan Kriya practitioners exhibit better antioxidant status and lower blood lactate levels. Biol Psychol. 2003;63(3):281-91.
19. Sharma H, Datta P, Singh A, Sen S, Bhardwaj NK, Kochupillai V, et al. Gene expression profiling in practitioners of Sudarshan Kriya. J Psychosom Res. 2008;64(2):213-8.
20. Kumar SB, Chawla B, Bisht S, Yadav RK, Dada R. Tobacco use increases oxidative DNA damage in sperm—possible etiology of childhood cancer. Asian Pac J Cancer Prev. 2015;16(16):6967-72.
21. Falissard B, Mauri M, Shaw K, Wetterling T, Doble A, Giudicelli A, et al. The METEOR study: frequency of metabolic disorders in patients with schizophrenia. Focus on first and second generation and level of risk of antipsychotic drugs. Int Clin Psychopharmacol. 2011;26(6):291-302.
22. Toalson P, Ahmed S, Hardy T, Kabinoff G. The metabolic syndrome in patients with severe mental illnesses. Prim Care Companion J Clin Psychiatry. 2004;6(4):152-8.
23. CONVERGE consortium. Sparse whole-genome sequencing identifies two loci for major depressive disorder. Nature. 2015;523(7562):588-91.
24. Berk M, Tye S, Walder K, McGee S. Hyperthermia for major depressive disorder? JAMA Psychiatry. 2016;73(10):1095-6.
25. Bhasin MK, Dusek JA, Chang BH, Joseph MG, Denninger JW, Fricchione GL, et al. Relaxation response induces temporal transcriptome changes in energy metabolism, insulin secretion and inflammatory pathways. PLoS One. 2013;8(5):e62817.
26. Jayaram N, Varambally S, Behere RV, Venkatasubramanian G, Arasappa R, Christopher R, et al. Effect of yoga therapy on plasma oxytocin and facial emotion recognition deficits in patients of schizophrenia. Indian J Psychiatry. 2013;55(Suppl 3):S409-13.
27. Dauwan M, Begemann MJ, Heringa SM, Sommer IE. Exercise improves clinical symptoms, quality of life, global functioning, and depression in schizophrenia: a systematic review and meta-analysis. Schizophr Bull. 2016;42(3):588-99.
28. Cramer H, Ward L, Saper R, Fishbein D, Dobos G, Lauche R. The safety of yoga: a systematic review and meta-analysis of randomized controlled trials. Am J Epidemiol. 2015;182(4):281-93.

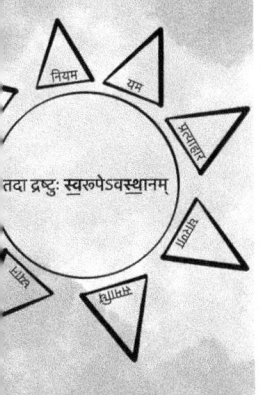

SECTION 3

Yoga for Clinical Conditions

9. **General Guidelines for Yoga Therapy**
   Hemant Bhargav, Shivarama Varambally

10. **Yoga Therapy for Depression**
    Praerna H Bhargav, Sneha J Karmani, Muralidharan Kesavan

11. **Yoga for Anxiety Disorders**
    Pooja More, Rakesh Chander, Narayana Manjunatha, Daniel Mintie

12. **Yoga in Obsessive Compulsive Disorder**
    Sanchari Mukhopadhyay, Nishitha Jasti, Shubha Bhat, Shubham Sharma

13. **Yoga Therapy for Schizophrenia**
    Elizabeth Visceglia, Rashmi Arasappa, Ramajayam Govindaraj

14. **Evidence for Efficacy of Yoga in Geriatric Psychiatry**
    Palanimuthu T Sivakumar, Shiva Shanker Reddy Mukku, Hariprasad VR, BV Kathyayani

15. **Yoga for Childhood and Adolescent Psychiatric Disorders**
    Shalu Abraham, Rashmi Arasappa, Kankan Gulati, Umesh Chikkanna

16. **Yoga for Substance Use Disorders**
    Venkata Lakshmi Narasimha, Sumana Venugopal, Bharath Holla, Hemant Bhargav

17. **Yoga in Chronic Pain Syndromes**
    Sowjanya Dumbala, Kankan Gulati, Sundarnag Ganjekar, Geetha Desai

18. **Yoga for Low Back Pain**
    Ameya Patwardhan, Vinod Kumar, Tarachand Joshi, Suman Bista

19. **Yoga for Migraine**
    Usha Rani MR, Sujan MU, Kaviraja Udupa, Sathyaprabha TN

20. **Yoga in Parkinson's Disease**
    Diya Chatterjee, Shantala Hegde, Arun Thejaus KP, Pooja Mailankody

21. **Yoga for Epilepsy**
    Praveen Angadi, Nivedha Mohan Raj, Malla Bhaskara Rao

CHAPTER 9

General Guidelines for Yoga Therapy

Hemant Bhargav, Shivarama Varambally

INTRODUCTION

The discipline of yoga arose as a systematic method of achieving mastery of the self and spiritual union with universal consciousness (*Samyoga yoga ityukto jivatma paramatmanah;* "yoga is the union of the individual soul with the universal soul"—*Ahirbudhnya Samhita*).[1] However, the understanding and practice of yoga has progressively become more practical in keeping with the times. In the last few decades, yoga has been increasingly seen as a health care practice and there is now convincing evidence of the benefits of regular yoga practice in several physical and mental disorders.[2] Yoga therapy is a recognized therapeutic intervention worldwide and charges for yoga sessions are reimbursed by health insurance companies in several countries. These developments have led to a significant increase in research studies evaluating the effects of yoga-based interventions in various disorders, and also the development of yoga regimens or modules designed for specific physical and mental conditions.

While some of these developments are likely to be very helpful for people suffering from these problems, they also mean that yoga trainers and therapists are seen as healthcare service providers. This may be encouraging to these therapists professionally and socially as evidenced by the exponential increase in the number of recognized courses and training facilities for yoga therapy all around the world; however, this status comes with several attendant responsibilities applicable to doctors, nurses, physiotherapists, and other healthcare professionals. The foremost among these is the expectation to take responsibility for both salutary effects as well as potential adverse effects of the practices which may be recommended. This highlights the urgent need for some standardization and guidelines to ensure that the primary principle of bioethics in healthcare practice is not violated (*Primum non nocere;* "first do no harm"). The field of yoga therapy, particularly in mental health disorders, is still in a nascent stage and would benefit from systematic research to provide such guidelines. This manual is a humble attempt in this direction, and we wish to start the section dealing with yoga as a therapy in clinical conditions with a set of simple guidelines which may be beneficial for therapists to incorporate when dealing with mental health disorders.

YOGA AS THERAPY FOR PSYCHIATRIC AND NEUROLOGICAL DISORDERS

Given the significant burden of mental health disorders that the world carries today as well as the huge treatment gap[3] [National Mental Health Survey (NMHS) report 2016], healthcare providers including yoga professionals have a responsibility to help people deal with their physical and mental health problems. In the new millennium, several yoga-based intervention modules have been designed for specific physical and mental health conditions. Some of these have been validated by consultation with experts, and a proportion of these have also been evaluated for feasibility and efficacy in randomized controlled trials (RCTs). Among mental health and neurological conditions, there are yoga-based modules published for depression, schizophrenia, obsessive compulsive disorder, substance use disorder, mild cognitive impairment of the elderly, and Parkinson's disorder, to name a few.[4-9]

In this regard, yoga therapists dealing with mental and neurological disorders have to be aware of certain precautions and relative contraindications for particular yoga practices in specific disorders. Ideally, the yoga "package" or module for each patient should be individualized; however, this is difficult in group therapy and tele-yoga settings which are likely to reach larger numbers of people. This chapter aims to highlight some of these precautions so that the risk of adverse effects of yoga is minimized.

Potential Adverse Effects of Yoga Practices

There have been several case reports of injuries sustained during yoga practices and some reports of precipitation of psychotic episodes with intense meditation practices. However, a majority of the earlier studies on yoga have not reported adverse effects in a systematic manner, and this is a very important credibility gap in yoga research which current researchers should consciously attend to. A recent review included 94 RCTs published from 1975–2014 with a total of 8,430 participants that had reported adverse effects due to yoga. The authors concluded that although there were several minor adverse effects, yoga was as safe as usual care and exercise.[10] Another review that focused on adverse effects of yoga in patients with psychiatric disorders included 19 studies with descriptions of 28 cases. This review described the types of meditative practices involved, including Transcendental, Mindfulness, Vipassana, Qigong, Zen, Theraveda, Bikram yoga, Pranic healing, and Hindustan type meditation. However, the review opined that it was difficult to attribute a causal relationship between the meditative practice and the adverse effect with current evidence.[11,12] Some yogic practices such as *kapalabhati* and *bhastrika* which involve voluntary hyperventilation may induce panic attacks and seizures, although hyperventilation can be a cause, a correlate and a consequence of panic attacks. An article published in 2010 suggested that the practice of *kumbhaka* (holding of the breath) reverses the hyperventilation process and may help in panic attacks.[13]

DURATION, FREQUENCY AND ASSESSMENT OF YOGA TRAINING FOR PATIENTS

A review by Cramer et al.[14] which compared results of yoga trials in India and other countries suggested that the Indian trials had better results, possibly because of higher intensity and frequency of the yoga sessions. Some recent studies have shown that the effects of a single yoga session do not last for more than a week, and that at least three sessions of yoga per week were required for clinical effects in patients with psychiatric disorders.[15] Although some trials have reported very early results (within a week) with yoga practices, based on our clinical experience, we suggest that at least 10 sessions over 2–3 weeks may be required to adequately learn the practices and start deriving benefits from the practice. We also suggest a minimum of three sessions a week (45 minutes to 1-hour sessions each) to obtain and sustain clinical benefits. Sessions can be practiced either in the morning before breakfast or in the evening before dinner. Ideally, it is recommended that modules which require dynamic physical and breathing practices should be performed at least 3 hours after full meal or 2 hours after light snacks.

Another lacuna in yoga research is that most studies have not assessed whether the patient has learnt the practice properly, as this could be a major factor in response. Therefore, we recommend that therapists should attempt to assess whether the patient has learnt the practice properly including the sequence of practices, the ability to regulate breathing, and to relax during the practice itself, which are critical in yoga for neuropsychiatric disorders. As an example, some recent studies have used a Yoga Performance Assessment (YPA) scale where the therapist assesses each of these on a scale of 1–4 for this purpose.[6] Once the patient has learnt the practices properly, future sessions may focus on slowing down the practices and enabling her/him to relax and enjoy the practices rather than worry if they are doing it properly. Another suggestion is to ask the patient to record his/her own session of supervised yoga therapy so that it can be used later for home practice.

SUGGESTIONS AND PRECAUTIONS FOR YOGA THERAPY IN COMMON PSYCHIATRIC DISORDERS

In **Table 1**, we have attempted to summarize some practices which may be useful in specific disorders which may be emphasized and some others which may be avoided unless the therapist is very confident of the same.

PATIENT-THERAPIST INTERACTIONS

Rapport building is a crucial aspect of any intervention that aims at improving mental health. Mental health disorders are conditions which demand more empathy and care from the Yoga therapist, but at the same time, the therapist should remain aware of the professional boundaries and learn the art of observing the stance of "empathy with detachment" while dealing with such patients.

Conducting the first session with the patient on a one-on-one basis is always a good idea. This will prepare the patient for a common group session and allow the therapist to understand the specific needs of each and every individual to modulate the sessions accordingly. What should the therapist do in the first one-on-one session with the patient? There are three important goals of the first session: (1) Understand the physical and mental constitution of the patient, her/his major illness and comorbidities; (2) Provide the patient an overview about what kind of yoga practices will be taught to her/him and how these practices may help improve his/her condition; and (3) Correct the patient as he/she performs the indicated practices and demonstrate the practices that he/she should avoid.

In the section below, we provide a tentative simplistic first yoga session format for the yoga therapists to give them an idea as to how the first yoga session with a patient should be planned. Therapists may modify the same as per the need.

A general format to be followed by the Yoga therapist in the first yoga therapy session with a patient is given below:

1. Every new patient must get at least a 45-minute one-to-one first session.
2. The 45-minute session should include first 15 minutes of theoretical introduction to yoga therapy and 30 minutes of practice of the specific yoga module.
3. In the first 15-minute introductory session, the following points need to be conveyed to the patient:
   - Greetings and welcome
   - *Introduce yourself*: Name and designation
   - *Ask whether the patient has any other health issue, injury or surgery in the past* and note it down.
   - *Introduce yoga*: Yoga is a holistic therapy which utilizes various mind-body practices to enhance overall health. Yoga emphasizes on bringing balance at different levels: 1st physical

TABLE 1: Details of the yoga practices to be emphasized in different psychiatric disorders.

Diagnosis	Yoga practices to be emphasized	Yoga practices to be avoided
Moderate-to-severe depression	Energizing and activating practices such as sun salutations, asanas involving backbends and chest opening, *bhastrika, kapalabhati*, right nostril breathing and loud mantra chanting	Advanced meditative practices, very slow practices and maintenance of the same posture for a long time
Anxiety disorders	Gentle relaxing practices with mild-to-moderate intensity. Practices such as: slow and deep breathing with prolonged exhalations, e.g., moon pose breathing, left nostril breathing, cooling breath, humming breath, *shavasana* with deep abdominal breathing	Fast breathing practices such as *kapalabhati* and *bhastrika* exceeding speed of 30 breaths/min. High-intensity practices
Schizophrenia and other psychotic disorders	Practices which are easy to learn but to be performed more intensely with rapid change of postures synchronized with dynamic breathing after sufficient warm-up. Some useful practices are: jogging, twisting poses, dynamic sun salutations, fast yoga breathing practices, loud mantra chanting with brief periods of relaxations (with eyes open) in between	Meditation which involves sense organ withdrawal and internalization of awareness (e.g., *vipassana* meditation) or those involving guided imageries (such as *Yoga nidra*). Maintenance of a yoga posture for a longer duration (more than a minute), and closure of the eyes for a longer duration
Bipolar affective disorder—manic/hypomanic episode	A balance has to be achieved by avoiding slow practices and preventing overdoing of fast practices. This can be achieved by keeping the patient engaged with dynamic change of practices from one to another interspersed with brief periods of relaxation in *shavasana* (corpse pose). Practices may also alternate between high-intensity and mild-to-moderate intensity	Patients may have the tendency of overdoing yogic practices which may be harmful, on the other hand slow-paced instructions and longer meditative practices may make patient more agitated
Obsessive compulsive disorder	Regulated breathing and mental relaxation should be emphasized. Left nostril breathing should be emphasized. Practices which are mild-to-moderate in intensity interspersed with deep relaxation and mantra chants should be emphasized	Emphasis on performing a particular practice for a specific number of times or for an exact duration or naming of body parts in a certain sequence should be avoided (instructions can be more general)
Mild cognitive impairment and dementia	Short modules of easy-to-do practices which have been proven useful in enhancing cognition such as humming breath, loud mantra chanting, right nostril breathing followed by left nostril breathing, slow gentle *kapalabhati* breathing (20 breaths/min or less), loosening of the joints with breath synchronization and *trataka* should be emphasized	Complicated practices, too many practices, frequent change of sequence should be avoided. For elderly, standing poses should always be performed besides a wall for support. Fast breathing practices should not exceed the speed of 30 breaths/min. Postures with increased risk of fall such as *trikonasana* (triangle pose), *vrikshasana* (tree pose), forward-backward bending should be avoided. Closure of the eyes while performing any standing posture should be avoided
Somatoform pain disorders, chronic pain syndromes, low back pain, and neck pain	Stretching should be emphasized more in the poses. Mild backward bending poses such as serpent pose (*bhujangasana*) or half-camel pose (*ardha ustrasana*) or half-wheel pose (*ardha chakrasana*) are useful in low	Extreme forward and backward bends should be avoided, especially patients with low back pain should avoid practices which involve bending forward, e.g., *padahastasana* (hand-to-feet pose), *paschimottanasana* (seated

Contd...

Contd...

Diagnosis	Yoga practices to be emphasized	Yoga practices to be avoided
	back pain and neck pain. Slow and deep breathing, alternate nostril breathing and deeply relaxing practices such as *Yoga nidra* or deep relaxation technique to enhance equal distribution of body awareness should be emphasized	forward bend pose), *Surya Namaskar* (sun salutations) or *shashankasana* (moon pose). In patients with neck pain, neck rotation and movements should be avoided, raising of the hands above the head should be avoided. Fast breathing practice such as *kapalabhati* and *bhastrika* should be performed very gently with caution
Migraine and other headaches	Slow deep breathing practices such as alternate nostril breathing, sectional breathing and humming should be emphasized. Deep relaxation of body parts should be delivered in the direction from head to toes	Fast breathing practices (*kapalabhati* and *bhastrika*) which involve hyperventilation should be avoided. Loud of chanting of mantras and rapid forward and backward bending should be avoided
Substance use disorders and other behavioral addictions	During acute withdrawal phase only mild intensity practices, e.g., left nostril breathing, joint loosening, deep relaxation technique and mantra chants should be taught. In the maintenance phase, more challenging poses and breathing practices with retention of breath (*kumbhaka*) could be added. Sleep special techniques (deep breathing, left nostril breathing, humming breath, OM chanting and reverse deep relaxation technique) should be advised at bedtime just before sleep	Fast breathing practices and intense yoga postures should be avoided when patients are experiencing acute withdrawal symptoms. Practices which are too slow and those requiring maintenance of posture for a longer duration or highly contemplative practices (e.g., *Yoga nidra*) should be avoided in the beginning
Seizure disorders	Practices with moderate intensity such as sun salutations, whole body joint loosening, alternate nostril breathing, humming breath with closure of the eyes (*Bhramari in shanmukhi mudra*), gentle chanting of mantras (such as OM) should be emphasized	Practices such as *kapalabhati* and *bhastrika* are contraindicated. "*Jyoti trataka*" which involves intense focusing of the gaze on candle flame without blinking of the eyes should be avoided
Autism and attention deficit hyperactivity disorder (ADHD)	Practices which can be performed together in groups, e.g., *Mandalam yoga* where children come together and form a combined pose, e.g., a lotus where each child contributes as a petal. Chanting mantras in chorus. Interesting breathing practices which children can relate to different animals such dog breathing, rabbit breathing, lion's breath, etc. Encourage imitation of postures	Sequence of postures and sitting arrangements should not change often. Complex practices which are difficult to learn, very slow-paced practices or meditations should be avoided

level by asanas, 2nd energy level by pranayama, and 3rd mental level by relaxation techniques, chanting, and meditation.
- *Asanas* work by enhancing blood circulation and removing congestion from different body parts, they allow fresh oxygenated blood to circulate to different body parts which are not exercised generally during our routine.
- *Pranayama* works by balancing the stimulating and relaxing parts of our nervous system. *Pranayama* also enhances proper channelization of subtle energy to different body parts. It improves lung functions and brings stability to the mind.

- *Relaxation techniques*: Part by part relaxation of the body leads to rejuvenation of each and every cell in the body **(Appendix 1.17)**. Chanting mantra sounds generates vibrations which allow body cells to resonate and relax. This also has an internal massaging effect on the organs. Patient may use mantras or sounds as per his/her sociocultural values, but feeling resonance in the body is the important component.
- How yoga will help you?
  - Stress is considered a major contributor toward aggravation of various physical and mental illnesses and hence addressing stress is very important.
  - The three aims of Yoga therapy are: (1) relax the body, (2) slow down the breath, and (3) calm down the mind.
  - Yoga practice has been proven to reduce stress and improve quality of life.
  - After this, add a section on how Yoga practices may help address the problem of the patient for which he/she has sought clinical consultation.
- Important key points that should be advised to patients:
  - *Keep your awareness on the body part that is being moved during asanas*: When I ask you to lift your hand up during an asana, kindly see to it that your awareness also moves to the hand that is being moved. Similarly, keep shifting your awareness to the body part that is moved or stretched during the asana practice. This enhances subtle energy flow to that part, increases efficacy of the asana, improves body awareness, and keeps your mind in the present moment.
  - *Keep your awareness on the touch of the air in your nostril during pranayama*: It is important that you remain aware of the touch of the air in your nostrils when you do pranayama. This stimulates necessary nerves at the root of your nose which are connected to various centers in the brain.
  - *Feel the vibrations when you chant during relaxation*: It is important that you feel the vibrations of the sound in your body when you chant mantra sounds (e.g., AA, UU, and MM). You may be able to feel the vibration of AA in your abdomen and chest, UU in your neck area, and MM in the head region.
  - *Avoid forceful and jerky exhalations during pranayama*: Pranayama practices should be gentle and smooth, done with a calm mind without unnecessary body movements.
  - *Avoid straining beyond your limits*: Kindly do not compare your practice with others in the group who may have been doing yoga for a longer duration and who may be more flexible than you. Kindly do not over strain, do what you can within your comfort limits.
  - *Avoid food immediately before and after the yoga practice*: You can practice yoga 3 hours after a meal and 1.5 hours after breakfast. You should avoid food for 30 minutes after yoga practice.
  - *Wear loose clothes*: Kindly avoid wearing a tight dress or saree during yoga practice. You may wear track pants and loose T-shirts.
  - *Make yoga a part of your lifestyle*: As bathing is necessary to keep the body clean, yoga is necessary for

cleaning the mind every day. Kindly do not stop the practice once you feel alright.

- *About the yoga module that is being taught*: The yoga module which we have decided to teach you is a ---- minute practice specifically designed for your problem(s). Your yoga module contains the following types of practices: (1) Preparatory loosening practices such as ---- (name them), (2) Asanas in standing (two asanas name them), sitting (number and names), prone (number and name), and supine (number and names) positions. Then, relaxation in lying down position. This is followed by pranayama practice which involves ---- practices ---- (number and names) and then, finally relaxation with chanting sounds of ---- .
- *Depending on the problem that you suffer from, you should avoid these practices from the module*: Write the name of the practice on a piece of paper and give it to the patient. For your other problem (say, e.g., back pain), I will teach you one extra practice which is not there in the module but you may continue practicing it at home.

4. *Teaching the yoga module*: Now I will teach you one round of each practice that you are going to do in a group tomorrow in detail [Kindly teach 1 or 2 rounds of all the practices that are there in the module and correct the patient (if he performs any practice incorrectly): 30 minutes].
   - Teach any additional practice if he needs, which he can continue at home for any specific problem other than the problem for which module is prescribed.
   - Explain clearly and show the practices that need to be avoided (If you are unclear, kindly discuss with the Doctor).

5. *End the session*: Thank the patient and encourage him to come for all the sessions for better results.

CONCLUSION

Overall, like any other system of medicine, yoga therapy also needs to be delivered by someone with clinical expertise and experience in the field. The therapist should not only develop necessary skills of imparting suitable yoga techniques as per the major illness and comorbidities of the patient, but he/she should also have a good understanding of the underlying pathology of disorders and awareness of natural course of these disorders. Finally, therapist should also understand the scope of the yoga therapy, set realistic goals, and always work in liaison with clinical consultants, psychotherapists, and physiotherapists.

REFERENCES

1. Matsubara M. Pancaratra Samhitas and Early Vaisnava Theology, with a Translation and Critical Notes from Chapters on Theology in the Ahirbudhnya Samhita. New Delhi, India: Motilal Banarsidass; 1994.
2. Varambally S, George S, Gangadhar BN. Yoga for psychiatric disorders: from fad to evidence-based intervention? Br J Psychiatry. 2020;216:291-3.
3. National Mental Health Survey of India, 2015–16. [online] Available from http://indianmhs.nimhans.ac.in/Docs/Report2.pdf [Last accessed September, 2020].
4. Bhat S, Varambally S, Karmani S, Govindaraj R, Gangadhar BN. Designing and validation of a yoga-based intervention for obsessive compulsive disorder. Int Rev Psychiatry. 2016;28(3):327-33.
5. Naveen GH, Rao MG, Vishal V, Thirthalli J, Varambally S, Gangadhar BN. Development and feasibility of yoga therapy module for out-patients with depression in India. Indian J Psychiatry. 2013;55(Suppl 3):S350-6.
6. Hariprasad VR, Varambally S, Varambally PT, Thirthalli J, Basavaraddi IV, Gangadhar BN. Designing, validation and feasibility of a yoga-based intervention for elderly. Indian J Psychiatry. 2013;55(Suppl 3):S344-9.

7. Govindaraj R, Varambally S, Sharma M, Gangadhar BN. Designing and validation of a yoga-based intervention for schizophrenia. Int Rev Psychiatry. 2016;28(3):323-6.
8. Kakde N, Metri K, Varambally S, Nagaratna R, Nagendra HR. Development and validation of a yoga module for Parkinson disease. J Complement Integr Med. 2017;14(3).
9. Bhargav H, Pilli Devi V, Sumana V. Development, validation and feasibility testing of a yoga module for opioid use disorder. Adv Mind Body Med. 2020;20(1):20-5.
10. Cramer H, Ward L, Saper R, Fishbein D, Dobos G, Lauche R. The safety of yoga: a systematic review and meta-analysis of randomized controlled trials. Am J Epidemiol. 2015;182(4):281-93.
11. Sharma P, Mahapatra A, Gupta R. Meditation-induced psychosis: a narrative review and individual patient data analysis. Ir J Psychol Med; 2019. pp. 1-7. doi: 10.1017/ipm.2019.47.
12. Schlosser M, Sparby T, Vörös S, Jones R, Marchant NL. Unpleasant meditation-related experiences in regular meditators: prevalence, predictors, and conceptual considerations. PLoS One. 2019;14(5):e0216643.
13. Meuret AE, Ritz T. Hyperventilation in panic disorder and asthma: empirical evidence and clinical strategies. Int J Psychophysiol. 2010;78(1):68-79.
14. Cramer H, Lauche R, Langhorst J, Dobos G. Are Indian yoga trials more likely to be positive than those from other countries? A systematic review of randomized controlled trials. Contemp Clin Trials. 2015;41:269-72.
15. Streeter CC, Gerbarg PL, Brown RP, Scott TM, Nielsen GH, Owen L, et al. Thalamic gamma-aminobutyric acid level changes in major depressive disorder after a 12-week Iyengar Yoga and Coherent Breathing Intervention. J Altern Complement Med. 2020;26(3):190-7.

CHAPTER 10

Yoga Therapy for Depression

Praerna H Bhargav, Sneha J Karmani, Muralidharan Kesavan

■ INTRODUCTION

Depression is the most common mental health disorder affecting 2–6% of the population.[1] According to the recent Indian National Mental Health Survey (2015–2016), one person in 20 suffers from depression, with higher incidence in urban areas and women.[2] A person with depression is 20 times more likely to commit suicide than someone who is not.[3] All these factors make depression a significant contributor to the global burden of disease and disability.

Depression is a ubiquitous syndrome often starting in mid-adult life, characterized mainly by pervasive sadness, loss of interest or pleasure in activities enjoyed earlier and feelings of tiredness at rest, with an inability to carry out day-to-day activities. These symptoms may be accompanied by various other physiological and psychological symptoms such as disturbances in appetite (excess appetite or low appetite), sleep (excess sleep or reduced sleep), change in weight (weight loss or weight gain), anxiety, reduced concentration and attention, indecisiveness, restlessness, feelings of guilt or low self-worth or hopelessness and thoughts of self-harm or suicide. Based on the severity of these symptoms, a depressive episode can be categorized as mild, moderate or severe. In mild depression, one is able to function with minimal impairment whereas severe depression is disabling, rendering him/her almost nonfunctional. Mild depression, if prolonged for 2 years or more, is termed as "dysthymia" whereas a depressive episode of varying severity appearing either as isolated or recurrent episodes, lasting for 2 weeks is called as "major depressive disorder (MDD)". Dysthymia and major depression can co-occur, with the latter being superimposed on the former.

No single cause can be implicated in the etiology of depression. Faulty mood regulation by the brain, genetic vulnerability, major life changes, trauma or stress, physical illnesses, and medications have all been implicated in its etiology.

■ YOGIC UNDERSTANDING OF DEPRESSION

Scriptures such as *Upanishads*, *Ramayana*, *Bhagavad Gita* (also known as BG), *Patanjali's Yoga Sutras*, and Ayurvedic texts provide ancient perspectives of depression. The symptomatology described under the term "*Vishada*" is found to be very similar to that of depression. Bhagavad Gita, a popular yoga text, starts with the chapter—"*Arjuna Vishada Yoga*" ("the despondency of *Arjuna*") which narrates the expression of *Arjuna's* anxiety, disappointment, despondence, fear, sadness, guilt, and dejection which leads to a state of inaction after being caught up in the battlefield against his own kinsmen in the enemy camp. Gita contains dialogues between *Krishna* and *Arjuna* where *Krishna* clarifies doubts raised by *Arjuna and helps* restore his functioning as a warrior.[4] *Bhagavad Gita* describes three attributes of the human mind called as "*Gunas*".

The three gunas are: (1) *Sattva*, (2) *Rajas*, and (3) *Tamas* (BG 4.5).[4] *Sattva guna* consists of qualities such as flexibility, balance, selfless service, and surrender to a higher principle in life. *Rajas guna* is characterized by activities done with selfish motive, ambitiousness, restlessness, and strong desire for pleasure. *Tamas guna* consists of qualities of dullness, lack of sensitivity, inertia, procrastination, and destructive tendencies.[4] As per the *Bhagavad Gita*, depression is found to be associated with dominance of *Tamas guna* with hypofunctional *Rajas* and *Sattva guna*.[5] *Charaka*, the editor of the Ayurvedic classical text "*Charaka Samhita*" has defined *vishada* as:

> *sarvadā manaù khedaù (ca sü20/11)* and *väkkäyacittävasädoviñäd (ca ci 33/6)*
> "*Vishada is a condition characterized by persistent sadness and global reduction in activities of speech, body, and mind.*"[6]

This above definition is in line with the current understanding of depression. *Patanjali's Yoga Sutras* (PYS) describe *Chittavikshepa* as a distracted state of the mind. This is an outcome of one's identification with *klishta chitta vrittis* (disturbing thought waves of mind). *Chittavikshepa*s are the obstacles to stable mental health and may manifest in one or more of the following forms: disease, mental laziness, doubt, carelessness, sloth, craving for sense pleasure, delusion, despair caused by failure to concentrate and instability (PYS I.30). Further, the text describes four symptoms which accompany these *chittavikshepa*s: (1) grief, (2) despondency, (3) bodily tremors, and (4) breathing disorders (PYS I.31).[7] A similar cluster of symptoms can also be seen in the ICD-10 criteria for diagnosis of depression.

■ FIVE LAYERS OF EXISTENCE—PANCHAKOSHA MODEL: PATHOGENESIS OF DEPRESSION

A holistic concept of human existence was given in *Taittiriya Upanishad* called the "*Panchakosha* model". According to this concept, human beings exist at five layers of consciousness. The grossest layer comprises of the physical body called *Annamaya kosha* followed by subtler layers of *Pranamaya kosha* (comprised of *prana* or life force), *Manomaya kosha* (a layer of emotions with forces of likes and dislikes without clear insight), *Vijnanamaya kosha* (a deeper layer of the mind responsible for insight, wisdom, and power of discrimination) and finally the very core of existence *Aanandamaya kosha* (consisting of pure bliss and unconditional happiness characterized by a perfect state of balance and harmony).

According to the yogic concept of disease, *Yoga Vashishtha* classifies disease into two types based on the mode of occurrence, i.e., (1) *Adhija vyadhi* (internal cause)—stress-borne diseases originating at the *Manomaya kosha* level and (2) *Anadhij avyadhi* (external cause) resulting out of injuries or infections at the *Annamaya kosha* level. According to the yogic understanding of disease, depression is categorized under "*Adhija vyadhi*"—a mental illness caused by clouding of the *Vijnanamaya* and *Aanandamaya kosha* respectively due to higher density and imbalance at the level of *Manomaya kosha*. This has been depicted in the **Figure 1**. This clouding is a result of imbalance at the level of emotions caused by strong likes and dislikes, leading to accumulation of stress (*Klesha*) in the system. This stress manifests in depression as the momentum of thoughts (*rajas*) in initial stages and leads to a blockage of thought process (*tamas*) after a certain threshold is crossed. Just as in a piece of rock, enormous amount of energy is stored in the mind but is not visible. Similarly, in depression, poor mastery over emotions such as fear, anxiety, anger, frustration, and so on generates uncontrolled momentum of thoughts which later on stagnates. It has disturbing implications over the life force or subtle energy (*prana*) balance which manifests as disturbances in breathing pattern.

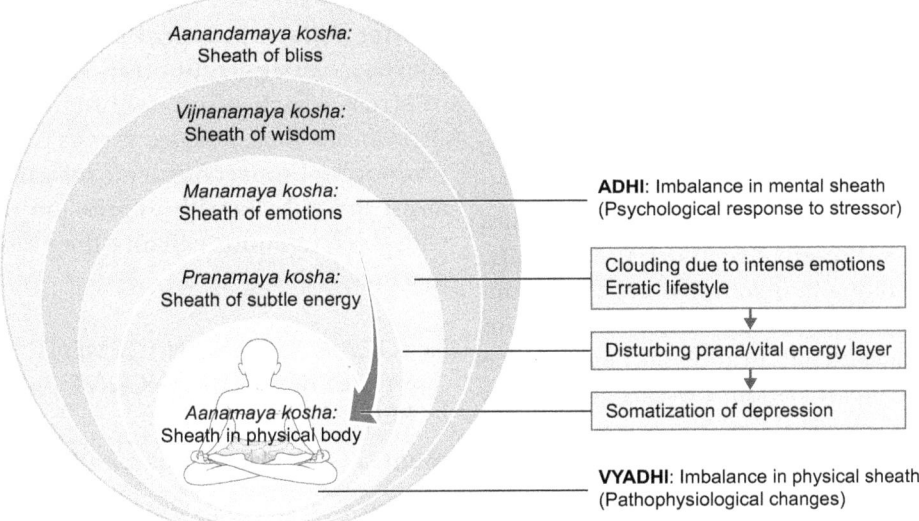

Fig. 1: Pathological conception of depression based on *Panchakosha* model.

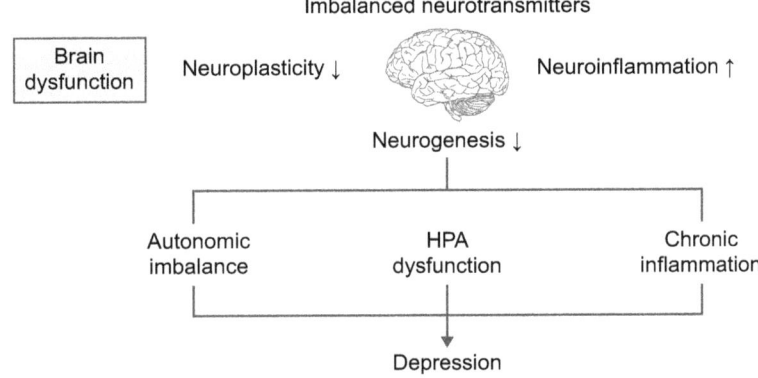

Fig. 2: Pathophysiology of depression (HPA: hypothalamic-pituitary-adrenal).

Further, prompted by chronic suppressed stresses and erratic lifestyle this may percolate down into physical layer as somatic symptoms including headache, body pain, and digestive disturbances.[8]

STRESS AND DEPRESSION

Stress is defined as "a phylogenetic response pattern to a demanding situation", i.e., the response of an individual to demanding situations either through "fight" or "flight" mode. This response initiates several adaptive changes in the body-mind complex mediated through brain via neurotransmission, endocrine regulation at the center, and autonomic nervous system via sympathetic and parasympathetic system at the periphery.[9] Studies have noted that chronic stress is an important trigger and precipitating factor for depression, and that depressed subjects have significantly higher autonomic imbalance than healthy subjects.[10] Also growing number of literature has shown that stress primes neuroinflammatory pathways and predisposes one to psychiatric disorders such as depression.[11] **Figure 2** shows how stress triggers pathophysiological changes and results in psychiatric disorder—depression.

CONVENTIONAL MANAGEMENT OF DEPRESSION

Conventional treatment options for management of depression usually involve antidepressants, electroconvulsive therapy (ECT) and psychosocial interventions. Current strategies for treating depression are not sufficient for many individuals, often resulting in incomplete recovery from depressive symptoms which continue to impair functionality. In addition, patients have several concerns about existing treatments and Uebelacker et al. (2010) in their systematic review suggested that yoga may be an attractive alternative to, or a good way to augment current treatment strategies. This review also detailed plausible biological, psychological, and behavioral mechanisms by which yoga may have an impact on depression. Among the traditional therapies, yoga is one of the most popular and sought-after therapies for depression.[12]

RATIONALE FOR USE OF YOGA IN DEPRESSION

Yoga is an evidence-based, cost-effective, safe and easy-to-implement technique for balancing the mind. *Bhagavad Gita* defines *"yoga as a state of mental equanimity"* (*samatvam yoga ucyate;* BG 2.28). Sage *Vasishtha* (Vashishtha) in his *Yoga* text defined yoga "as a strategy to calm down the mind" (*manah prashamanopayah yoga ityabhidhiyate*). Yoga therapy not only treats the patient's symptoms but brings deeper corrections at all the five layers of existence described earlier. Yoga techniques bridge psychosocial and somatic aspects of care and also address the subject's spiritual needs. When the yoga practice is done with active involvement and a sense of self-control, awareness and attention combined with relaxation, it helps in altering the perceptions and mental responses to both external and internal stimuli. This reduces hyper-reactive responses to such stimuli and instills a greater sense of control over situations, thereby causing reduction in the levels of stress which ultimately helps combat depression. Thus, practice of yoga as a health promoting biopsychosocial resource may assist individuals with depression to cope with stress and thus enhance their resilience and mood.[8]

YOGA-BASED MANAGEMENT OF DEPRESSION: ANCIENT PERSPECTIVES

Mantra Chanting, Asanas, and Relaxation

Patanjali, in his Yoga Sutras, stated various ways which can help in removing the *chittavikshepa* mentioned earlier. One of them was the repeated chanting of the *vedic mantra "Om"* with meditation upon its meaning (PYS I.27-28).[7] Thus, techniques like *"Om"* chanting and *"Om"* meditation may be effective in treating depression. Interestingly, a functional neuroimaging study done at the National Institute of Mental Health and Neuro Sciences (NIMHANS) demonstrated that *"Om"* chanting produced deactivation of the limbic cortex in healthy volunteers.[13] Limbic cortex is the area of the brain associated with memories related to negative emotions. The authors hypothesized that this effect of *"Om"* chanting may be due to stimulation of the auricular branch of the vagus nerve. Vagus nerve stimulation is a recognized treatment modality for depression, and *"Om"* chanting may be considered as an autogenous method of vagal stimulation.

Other yogic techniques such as *Shavasana* (HYP: I.32) and *Trataka* (HYP: II.32) have also been described in ancient texts as being helpful in removing tiredness and fatigue, which are symptoms of depression.[14]

Diet from Yoga Perspective

From the perspective of yoga, diet is very important. Diet, according to yoga, is classified as *Tamasic*, *Rajasic*, and *Sattvic* depending on the kind of effect it produces on the body-mind complex to promote respective *guna* in the mind. Diet can have an important role in alleviating depression. *Sattvic* foods boost strength, stamina and purity and increase the lifespan (BG 17.8). They also promote health, happiness, and satisfaction. Such nourishing foods are sweet, oleaginous, enduring, and palatable—for example, fresh seasonal fruits, green vegetables, wholesome grains, cow's milk and ghee. Foods that taste bitter, sour, and salty and are very hot, or pungent and dry in nature cause burning and lead to distress, misery, and diseases termed as *Rajasic* (BG 17.9). Examples of *Rajasic* foods are: green chilli, pepper, spicy food items, etc. Stale, tasteless, stinking, left over and impure foods are *tamasic* in nature (BG 17.10). These include fermented, refrigerated, stale, reheated food items, tinned food, etc. Patients with depression should avoid *tamasic* food as they lack vitality and energy whereas they may require more of *rajasic* and *sattvic* food. Although *Rajasic* foods are energizing and boost the metabolism but they do not lead to clear balanced energy; *sattvic* foods not only nourish but also add vitality to the system and bring a state of calm alertness and lightness without deranging the overall energy state.[4]

Recreation and Activities

The state of mind during performance of action/activities (*karma*) has been classified into three types based on the *guna* system as mentioned in *Bhagavad Gita*. All the activities performed with enthusiasm and in accordance with duty, not motivated by false ego and without attachment to the result are *Sattvic* in nature (BG 18.23). In contrast, *Rajasic* activities involve great effort and are enacted from a sense of false ego with a longing to gratify one's desires (BG 18.24). *Tamasic* activities are performed in ignorance without considering the consequences which are impractical and result in distress to oneself as well as others (BG 18.25). Yogic behavioral advice in depression includes bringing awareness and insight to the subject regarding *tamasic* activities and promoting *rajasic* and *sattvic* activities.[4]

Sleep

Sleep disturbance is an important symptom of depression. Yoga texts also describe various techniques to promote quality of sleep. *Mandukya Upanishad* divides consciousness into three states: (1) Wakefulness (*Jagrata*), (2) Dream (*Swapna*), and (3) Sleep (*Sushupti*) (MU I.2-5).[15] It advocates use of three sounds AAA, UUU, and MMM (humming sound) to promote each of the three states, respectively. Thus, a patient with depression should try to stay more in the *Jagrata* state by chanting the sound AAA during the day. This will help in reducing tiredness, fatigue, and ruminations. Patients should spend more time in *Sushupti* during night by making use of the humming sound (MMM), i.e., *Bhramari pranayama*. This will help improve quality of sleep.[15]

■ YOGA FOR DEPRESSION: CURRENT SCIENTIFIC EVIDENCE

In the last few decades, various yoga-based practices have been used extensively for treatment of depression in clinical settings, with several studies reporting decreases in psychological and physical symptoms of depression and stress in individuals practicing yoga.[12] *Sudarshan Kriya Yoga* (SKY), a breathing-based yoga practice propounded by the Art of Living foundation has been reported to produce a sense of well-being and relief from dysphoria, and studies have found neurobiological effects such as increased parasympathetic drive, calming of stress response systems, and neuroendocrine release of hormones and thalamic generators.[16] A study assessing the effect of *Sahaja Yoga* (meditation-based yoga practice) as an add-on to antidepressants in patients with MDD, found it to be more effective than antidepressants alone. Significant improvements in memory and various other cognitive domains were also found, possibly because of the neuroplastic effects of yoga.[17] Another study showed that practice of yoga (emphasizing more on postures that involve chest openings which included backbends and inversions) results in increase in positive mood and reduction in negative mood possibly by helping an individual to cope with depressed affect.[18] An ongoing study from NIMHANS examining the effect of add-on yoga to standard antidepressant therapy has shown that although the Hamilton Depression Rating Scale (HDRS; also known as HAM-D) scores decreased in both the yoga and waitlist groups over time, time to remission was faster in the yoga group as compared to the waitlist group.[19] A summary of controlled yoga trials in depression is presented in **Table 1**.

Yoga as Monotherapy for Depression

According to the current scientific evidence, yoga may be prescribed as monotherapy for mild-to-moderate cases of depression.[27] In a recent randomized controlled trial (RCT) by Prathikanti et al., Hatha yoga given as

TABLE 1: Summary of controlled trials of yoga in depression.

Author/Year	Sample	Yoga technique	Control	Duration of yoga	Results
Khumar et al., 1993[20]	Major depressive disorder (MDD) (n = 50) RCT	Shavasana Yoga (n = 25)	No treatment (n = 25)	4 weeks	Yoga significantly superior
Rohini et al., 2000[21]	DSM-IV MDD (n = 30)	Sudarshan Kriya Yoga (SKY) (n = 15)	Partial SKY (without cyclical breathing) (n = 15)	4 weeks	Reduced the Beck Depression Inventory (BDI) scores in both groups; no difference at 4 weeks Remission: 12 SKY subjects and 7 partial SKY subjects
Janakiramaiah et al., 2000[22]	DSM-IV MDD (n = 45) RCT: Three groups	SKY (n = 15)	Electroconvulsive therapy (ECT) (3/week) and adequate dose of imipramine (n = 15 each)	4 days/week for 4 weeks	Significant reductions in HDRS and BDI scores in all three groups; ECT superior, improvement similar in IMN and SKY groups
Sharma et al., 2006[17]	DSM-IV MDD (n = 30) RCT: Two groups	Sahaja Yoga meditation + antidepressants (n = 15)	Antidepressant (n = 15)	8 weeks	Found lower HDRS scores after 8 weeks in Sahaja Yoga group
Prathikanti et al., 2017[23]	MDD (BDI—14–28) n = 38 RCT: Two groups	Yoga group (n = 20)	Attention control education group (n = 18)	Twice weekly for 8 weeks	Significant reduction in depression scores in yoga group as compared to control group
Streeter et al., 2018[24]	MDD (BDI-II ≥ 14) n = 30 RCT: Two groups	High dose yoga group (HDG; n = 15): Three 90-minute yoga class	Low dose yoga group (LDG; n = 15): Two 90-minute yoga class	12 weeks of Iyengar yoga and coherent breathing	Both groups showed significant decline in depressive symptoms with more subjects in HDG scoring BDI ≤ 10 by week 12

Contd...

Contd...

Author/Year	Sample	Yoga technique	Control	Duration of yoga	Results
Nugent et al., 2019[25]	MDD [the 16-item Quick Inventory of Depressive Symptomatology (QIDS)— 8–17] n = 87 RCT: Two groups	Hatha Yoga (n = 48)	Healthy living workshop (n = 39)	60- to 80-minute session/weekly once or twice for 10 weeks	IL-6 concentration reduced significantly in the Yoga group relative to health education control group
Streeter et al., 2020[26]	MDD (BDI-II ≥ 14) n = 30 RCT: Two groups	High dose yoga group (HDG; n = 15): Three 90-minute yoga class	Low dose yoga group (LDG; n = 15): Two 90-minute yoga class	12 weeks of Iyengar yoga and coherent breathing	BDI-II scores improved significantly in both groups. Gamma-aminobutyric acid (GABA) levels increased significantly in the LDG and also indicated once a week yoga is necessary to maintain the elevated GABA levels
Muralidharan et al., 2020[19]	MDD (HAM-D ≥ 18) n = 70 RCT: Two groups	Yoga + antidepressant medication (n = 35)	Standard anti-depressant medication (n = 35)	12 sessions in 1st month and two sessions in 2nd and 3rd month	Both groups showed significant reduction in depression scores with more improvement and higher remission in yoga group. CSP which involves $GABA_B$ mediated cortical inhibition improved significantly in yoga group only suggestive of increased GABA activity following yoga

monotherapy for 8 weeks to patients with mild-to-moderate depression helped in reducing the severity of depression significantly in comparison to attention control education group.[23] Another clinical trial on dysthymia, the group given SKY showed remission by the end of the first month of practice, and maintained the same for next 3 months.[28] Similar trial using SKY in inpatients of major depression with melancholia, SKY was found to be as effective as antidepressant medication (imipramine), although less effective than ECT.[22] Another study comparing full SKY to partial SKY found both interventions to be effective in reducing depression scores, although the full SKY group showed a better response in comparison.[21] A relaxing posture called *Shavasana* given as monotherapy for 30 days to female university students was found to be significantly effective in lowering symptoms of depression as compared to no intervention.[20]

Most of the studies assessing efficacy of yoga in depression have used yoga practices from various schools such as *SKY, Iyengar yoga, Hatha yoga,* and *Sahaja yoga.* A content-based generic yoga module was validated at NIMHANS and the same was used in a study which included 62 patients with the Diagnostic and Statistical Manual of

Mental Disorders, 4th Edition, Text Revision (DSM-IV-TR) diagnosis of major depression. Patients received one of the three treatments as per their choice—yoga only, drugs only or both. They found significant reduction in HDRS scores and increase in brain-derived neurotrophic factor (BDNF) levels in all the three groups with greater improvement in yoga groups suggestive of the antidepressant effect of yoga through neuroplastic mechanisms.[29] A significant reduction in serum cortisol levels was reported in both the yoga groups in comparison to the medication only group, highlighting the antistress effects of yoga.[30] From the above studies, it may be concluded that yoga can be prescribed for most patients with depression as an adjunct along with standard treatments. For patients with mild-to-moderate depression without suicidal risk, yoga may be considered as a sole therapy with the consent of the patient and family.

■ CLINICAL APPLIED ASPECTS OF YOGA IN DEPRESSION

A meta-analysis of studies on yoga for depression found yoga to bring about improvement in short-term depression more than relaxation and aerobic exercise, and concluded that yoga could be considered as an ancillary treatment option for patients with depressive disorders or symptoms.[31] Recent systematic reviews have found some evidence of the positive effects of yoga in depression which is comparable to other evidence-based interventions.[32] The Canadian Network for Mood and Anxiety Treatments (CANMAT) for the management of MDD in adults (2016) stated level 2 evidence for yoga as a second-line adjunctive therapy for mild-to-moderate depression.[33] A comprehensive yoga therapy module from NIMHANS included specific practices which were included after considering the clinical symptoms of depression and validating the module with yoga experts and clinicians. As per the final module, *Surya Namaskar, Ardhachakrasana, Ustrasana, Bhujangasana, Suryanuloma-viloma, Ujjayi, Bhastrika, Kapalbhati, Pranava japa* and Yogic counseling target depressed mood while *Surya Namaskar, Paschimottanasana, Bhujangasana, Pavanmuktasana, Viparitakarani, Kapalbhati, Ujjayi, Bhastika*, and *Suryanuloma-viloma* help in dealing with somatic symptoms associated with depression such as anorexia, weight gain or loss and constipation. *Pranava japa* helps with diminished memory and concentration problems. *Shavasana* helps in regaining energy levels. Yogic counseling may help improve social and occupational functioning.[34] **Appendix 1.1** provides the validated yoga module for depression. Depression may also be a part of another severe mental illness called bipolar affective disorder (BPAD) that involves severe mood swings in the form of depression or mania (**Appendix 1.5** provides yoga module for BPAD).

■ PRECAUTIONS WHILE TEACHING YOGA THERAPY TO PATIENTS WITH DEPRESSION

Patients with depression are often found to assume a slumping posture with sinking shoulders and bowed down head. A depressed individual also feels hopeless, lethargic and dull. Practices that involve chest opening and backbends can help in correcting this as it is thought that these postures generate a sense of freshness and openness in the individual. Patients with depression often have difficulty concentrating as they are lost in their own thoughts. To engage them in yoga practices mindfully, avoid boredom and mechanical practice, the following principle given in the *Mandukya Karika* should be employed while administering yoga practices:

*"Laye sambodhayet cittam; Vikshiptam shamayet punah
Sakashayam vijaniyat samapraptam na calayet."*

i.e., *"when the mind is in a state of sleep, awaken and stimulate it, while when it is agitated, calm down the distractions and when it comes in the state of steadiness, do not disturb it again."* Based on this principle, the sequence of practices should include a fast and repetitive practice followed by slow movement and then maintaining the final posture with breath awareness. Meditation can be a beneficial practice in depression but in the initial phase of practice, to avoid brooding and too much of rumination, it should be guided and can include more of the chanting component for better outcomes.

SUMMARY AND CONCLUSION

There is tremendous interest in using and studying yoga-based interventions as a therapeutic tool in depression. The available evidence is indeed promising and is supportive of its use as monotherapy for depression of mild-to-moderate severity and as an adjuvant to conventional pharmacotherapy in other cases. However, more work is needed to understand the neurobiological basis of yoga therapy in depression. Future studies should use more objective measures to study the effects of yoga. Future studies can also employ the use of yoga for severe depression with suicidal ideations as an adjuvant. Access to standardized yoga, double-blinding and finding appropriate controls are some challenges related to yoga therapy research in depression. Current and future research in this area needs to address these issues in order to make yoga a viable addition to the therapeutic armamentarium and reduce the burden of depression.

CASE VIGNETTE

A lady aged 62 years with history of hypertension presented with complaints of low mood, anhedonia, reduced concentration, low energy levels and inability to do household activities along with disturbed sleep, irregular bowel movements, and death wishes. She also had complaints of excessive weight gain since past 3 years. On mental status examination, she was observed to have retarded psychomotor activity with reduced speech and depressed mood with active suicidal ideations with past-history of two suicidal attempts. Her score on HDRS at the time of admission was 27 and was diagnosed with severe depression without psychotic symptoms. She was started on standard antidepressant treatment and was referred to yoga therapy as well. First two yoga sessions were conducted on one-to-one basis. For the first two yoga sessions, as she lacked energy and motivation, she was not willing to do the practice but with gentle encouragement and emphasizing on the importance of the same from the family members and support from the therapist, she started attending the session regularly. As the patient had active suicidal ideations, family members were asked to accompany the patient at all times, even during the yoga sessions. Patients' husband was also asked to join the same batch of yoga along with the patient and was asked to practice with her along with other patients with similar problem. During this time period, the patient was asked by the consultant psychiatrist to undertake ECT for three cycles. Thus, yoga therapy was given to her on the alternate days (when she was not receiving ECT). With ECT sessions, though she used to feel tired initially but that did not affect her level of motivation, therapist kept encouraging her by giving positive feedback to participate in the yoga sessions. During the period of treatment with ECT, she was taught easy and gentle practices such as loosening and asanas which she could perform comfortably, along with pranayama and relaxation. She showed remarkable improvement within 10 days of this integrative treatment reporting with better moods, regaining back interest, better energy levels, good quality of sleep, and absence of death wishes. Though most of these dramatic improvements in mood were most likely due to the ECT but patient attributed her increase in energy levels especially to yoga practice. With regular practice, she started enjoying yoga sessions and the initial reluctance changed to acceptance as she started seeking yoga on her own for the subsequent sessions. Her HAM-D score reduced to 14 by the end of first month.

On follow-up after 3 months, she reported to maintain the improved state and continued to practice yoga on a regular basis with her family members using a recorded video. Patient said "Though medicine and ECT made her active again, but with these treatments she used to

	Clinical Insights: Yoga Therapy in Depression
Prior to the session	• It is important to understand that being slow, less energetic and less attentive may be a part of the patient's illness and not laziness. • Activity scheduling is important—encourage the patient to keep himself/herself busy in activities they used to enjoy earlier. • Any patient with depression should be assessed for suicidality. • Any patient with suicidal thoughts should undergo therapy in the presence of the caregiver; do not leave such patients alone. • Let the caregiver be present if the patient is of the opposite gender. • Patients with moderate to severe depression have severe fatigue, and so it is better to start the session with 30 minutes and gradually increase the duration. • In patients with severe fatigue, group sessions should be encouraged. • Patients who are on electroconvulsive therapy (ECT) may have more bodyache, headache, and drowsiness. Yoga during ECT therapy can be provided on alternate (non-ECT) days. • Medications such as tricyclic antidepressants and benzodiazepines can cause postural hypotension (dizziness while suddenly getting up from sitting or supine position), especially in elderly subjects. So practices should be modified accordingly. • Avoid fast breathing practices such as *Bhastrika* in patients having dizziness.
During the session	• Observe patience while dealing with such patients. Multiple instructions may often be required. • Do not force practices on the patient, start with simpler practices with lesser duration of each practice in the beginning. The foremost thing is to make the patient believe that he/she can do yoga. • Focus on more practice and less theory. • The intensity of practice should neither be too slow nor too fast, and the therapist should build the intensity very gradually. • Involve practices which could improve quality of sleep (e.g., humming breath, *Om* chanting, and deep breathing at bedtime). • Give lots of positive reinforcement on achieving small goals during the practice. Let the patient demonstrate the yoga in the session, if he/she has learned it well.
After the session	• Maintain professional boundaries. If a patient wants to contact, keep contact through an official channel within a fixed duration.

	Clinical Insights: Yoga Therapy for Bipolar Affective Disorder—Manic Episode
Before the session	• Assessment of any possible emergency (such as risk of harm to self or others) is mandatory. Appropriate referral must be made in that case. • *Be cautious about overdoing the yoga practices* in such patients, this may lead to side effects, excessive physical activity may cause physical exhaustion. • Therapists should have the knowledge of the clinical symptoms (e.g., oversocialization, overactivity, overfamiliarity, oversexuality, elevated or irritable mood, etc.), so that he/she understands how to deal with such patients. • One-on-one session is recommended till symptomatic stabilization to avoid disruption in group practices. • It is *preferable to match the gender of the therapist and the patient*.

Contd...

Contd...

Clinical Insights: Yoga Therapy for Bipolar Affective Disorder—Manic Episode

	• The yoga setting should be such that the therapist may seek help in case of unprovoked aggression and risk of harm to the therapist (e.g., the positioning of therapist near the door in the therapy room, absence of sharp, potential harmful objects in vicinity). • Therapists should have a calm and nonthreatening attitude while dealing with such patients. • Caregivers should be involved in practice with the patient, although more attention should be given to the patient. • Discussing on philosophy and powers of yoga should be discouraged, practice should be emphasized.
During the session	• Patients having mania should not be instructed with authority. The way to address them must be humble though firm. • *Frequently changing yoga practices of moderate intensity interspersed with very brief periods of relaxation* is a good option. • Focus should be to *dissipate the excessive energy* and activity level that is usually associated with mania. Thus, yoga practices should not be too slow. On the other hand, very fast exercises may precipitate physical exhaustion. • Patients are usually highly distractible. Thus, *repetition of instructions may be required*. Shorter duration of exercise is better than prolonged duration as the patient may not be able to sustain attention for such a long term. • *Longer meditative practices should be avoided. Mantra chants can be advised.* • Awareness regarding possible symptoms will help the therapist employ limit setting, positive reinforcement, etc., as and when necessary during the sessions (e.g., any untoward overfamiliarity can be dealt with by effective limit setting). • The caregiver should be present during the practice. • The therapy room should be designed in such a way that no object which can cause harm to the patient or anyone else is present within reach. • Patients often have hyper-religiosity. Mantra chanting may be avoided in that case to prevent exacerbating symptoms. • Yoga practices focusing on normalization of biological functions such as sleep, eating should be taught (especially sleep-inducing yoga techniques should be taught at the end, as sleep regulation is an important component of treatment of mania).
After the session	• The patient and the caregiver should be educated adequately about do's and don'ts of Yoga while practicing at home. The plan of further management including follow-ups should be discussed. • Follow-ups to be scheduled according to the clinical status and feasibility. • Every follow-up should contain repeat assessments. Supervised sessions may be conducted if required. • Appropriate referrals must be made as and when necessary and continued collaboration with the treating psychiatrist and/or clinical psychologist is mandatory.

feel that her "natural self" is getting locked up and she felt suffocated, it is the practice of yoga which helped her gain her "natural self" back."

REFERENCES

1. Ritchie H, Roser M (2018). Mental health. Our World in Data. [online] Available from https://ourworldindata.org/mental-health#data-availability-on-mental-health [Last accessed September, 2020].
2. National Mental Health Survey of India, 2015-16: Summary. National Institute of Mental Health and Neurosciences, Bengaluru. Supported by Ministry of Health and Family Welfare, Government of India.
3. Ferrari AJ, Norman RE, Freedman G, Baxter AJ, Pirkis JE, Harris MG, et al. The burden attributable to mental and substance use disorders as risk factors for suicide: findings from the Global Burden of Disease Study 2010. PLoS One. 2014;9(4):e91936.
4. Prabhupada SB. Bhagavad Gita as It Is. Intermex Publishing; 2006.
5. Dasa DG. The Vedic Personality Inventory: An Analysis of Gunas. Bhakti Vedanta College; 1999.

6. Sharma RK, Dash B. Charaka Samhita. Varanasi, India: Chowkhamba Publications; 2014.
7. Iyengar, BK. Light on the Yoga Sutras of Patanjali. London: Harper Collins; 1993.
8. Nagarathna R, Nagarathna HR, Gangadhar BN, Bhargav H. Yoga for Depression, 1st edition, Bengaluru: Vivekananda Yoga Therapy and Research Foundation, Swami Vivekananda Yoga Prakashana; 2013.
9. Kinser PA, Lyon DE. A conceptual framework of stress vulnerability, depression, and health outcomes in women: potential uses in research on complementary therapies for depression. Brain Behav. 2014;4(5):665-74.
10. Kemp AH, Quintana DS, Gray MA, Felmingham KL, Brown K, Gatt JM. Impact of depression and antidepressant treatment on heart rate variability: a review and meta-analysis. Biol Psychiatry. 2010;67:1067-74.
11. Slavich GM, Irwin MR. From stress to inflammation and major depressive disorder: a social signal transduction theory of depression. Psychol Bull. 2014;140(3):774-815.
12. Uebelacker LA, Epstein-Lubow G, Gaudiano BA, Tremont G, Battle CL, Miller IW. Hatha yoga for depression: critical review of the evidence for efficacy, plausible mechanisms of action, and directions for future research. J Psychiatr Pract. 2010;16:22-33.
13. Kalyani BG, Venkatasubramanian G, Arasappa R, Rao NP, Kalmady SV, Behere RV, et al. Neurohemodynamic correlates of 'OM' chanting: a pilot functional magnetic resonance imaging study. Int J Yoga. 2011;4(1):3-6.
14. Svatmarama. Hatha Yoga Pradipika, 4th edition. Madras, India: Adyar Library and Research Centre; 1994.
15. Chinmayanada S. Mandukya Upanishad. Mumbai, India: Sachin Publishers; 1984.
16. Brown RP, Gerbarg PL. Sudarshan Kriya yogic breathing in the treatment of stress, anxiety, and depression: part I—neurophysiologic model. J Altern Complement Med. 2005;11:189-201.
17. Sharma VK, Das S, Mondal S, Goswami U, Gandhi A. Effect of Sahaj Yoga on neuro-cognitive functions in patients suffering from major depression. Indian J Physiol Pharmacol. 2006;50:375-83.
18. Shapiro D, Cook IA, Davydov DM, Ottaviani C, Leuchter AF, Abrams M. Yoga as a complementary treatment of depression: effects of traits and moods on treatment outcome. Evid Based Complement Alternat Med. 2007;4:493-502.
19. Bhargav PH, Reddy PV, Govindaraj R, Gulati K, Ravindran A, Devaraj G, Muralidharan K, et al. Impact of a course of add-on supervised yoga on cortical inhibition in major depressive disorder: a randomized controlled trial. Can J Psychiatry. 2020;706743720953247.
20. Khumar SS, Kaur P, Kaur S. Effectiveness of Shavasana on depression among university students. Indian J Clin Psychol. 1993;20:82-7.
21. Rohini V, Pandey RS, Janakiramaiah N, Gangadhar BN, Vedamurthachar A. A comparative study of full and partial Sudarshan Kriya Yoga (SKY) in major depressive disorder. NIMHANS J. 2000;18:53-7.
22. Janakiramaiah N, Gangadhar BN, Murthy PJ, Harish MG, Subbakrishna DK, Vedamurthachar A. Antidepressant efficacy of Sudarshan Kriya Yoga (SKY) in melancholia: a randomized comparison with electroconvulsive therapy (ECT) and imipramine. J Affect Disord. 2000;57:255-9.
23. Prathikanti S, Rivera R, Cochran A, Tungol JG, Fayazmanesh N, Weinmann E. Treating major depression with yoga: a prospective, randomized, controlled pilot trial. PLoS One. 2017;12:e0173869.
24. Streeter CC, Gerbarg PL, Nielsen GH, Brown RP, Jensen JE, Silveri M. Effects of yoga on thalamic gamma-aminobutyric acid, mood and depression: analysis of two randomized controlled trials. Neuropsychiatry (London). 2018;8(6):1923-39.
25. Nugent NR, Brick L, Armey MF, Tyrka AR, Ridout KK, Uebelacker LA. Benefits of yoga on IL-6: findings from a randomized controlled trial of yoga for depression. Behav Med. 2019;1-10.
26. Streeter CC, Gerbarg PL, Brown RP, Scott TM, Nielsen GH, Owen L, et al. Thalamic gamma-aminobutyric acid level changes in major depressive disorder after a 12-week Iyengar yoga and coherent breathing intervention. J Altern Complement Med. 2020;26(3):190-7.
27. Saeed SA, Cunningham K, Bloch RM. Depression and anxiety disorders: benefits of exercise, yoga, and meditation. Am Fam Physician. 2019;99(10):620-7.
28. Janakiramaiah N, Gangadhar BN, Murthy PJ, Harish MG, Shetty KT, Subbakrishna DK, et al. Therapeutic efficacy of Sudarshan Kriya Yoga (SKY) in dysthymic disorder. NIMHANS J. 1998;16:21-8.
29. Naveen GH, Thirthalli J, Rao MG, Varambally S, Christopher R, Gangadhar BN. Positive therapeutic and neurotropic effects of yoga in depression: a comparative study. Indian J Psychiatry. 2013;55(3):S400-4.
30. Thirthalli J, Naveen GH, Rao MG, Varambally S, Christopher R, Gangadhar BN. Cortisol and antidepressant effects of yoga. Indian J Psychiatry. 2013;55(3):S405-8.

31. Ravindran AV, da Silva TL. Complementary and alternative therapies as add-on to pharmacotherapy for mood and anxiety disorders: a systematic review. J Affect Disord. 2013;150:707-19.
32. Cramer H, Anheyer D, Lauche R, Dobos G. A systematic review of yoga for major depressive disorder. J Affect Disord. 2017;213:70-7.
33. Ravindran AV, Balneaves LG, Faulkner G, Ortiz A, McIntosh D, Morehouse RL, et al. Canadian Network for Mood and Anxiety Treatments (CANMAT) 2016 Clinical guidelines for the management of adults with major depressive disorder: Section 5. complementary and alternative medicine treatments. Can J Psychiatry. 2016;61(9):576-87.
34. Naveen GH, Rao MG, Vishal V, Thirthalli J, Varambally S, Gangadhar BN. Development and feasibility of yoga therapy module for out-patients with depression in India. Indian J Psychiatry. 2013;55(7):350-6.

CHAPTER 11

Yoga for Anxiety Disorders

Pooja More, Rakesh Chander, Narayana Manjunatha, Daniel Mintie

■ INTRODUCTION TO ANXIETY DISORDERS

Fear is a natural, healthy response and a necessary warning system in humans. Anxiety, by way of contrast, is a response to irrational thinking about oneself, other people, and the world. While fear and anxiety arise from different sources, they share physiologic pathways and expressions. Anxiety disorders (ADs) are among the most common mental disorders encountered in the everyday clinical setting.[1] They are more prevalent than any other disorder and are comorbid with many medical conditions as well. The identification and diagnosis of the ADs are challenging, especially in the low- and middle-income countries (LAMICs), making it one of the "invisible" mental disorders among the general population. Many landmark epidemiological surveys have emphasized this fact, identifying high levels of medical comorbidity in persons diagnosed with ADs. Due to their "camouflaging effect", many general physicians and nonmental health experts find it difficult to detect ADs in patients. This causes a significant delay in effective management of these disorders, contributing to their high personal and social costs. ADs represent a significant disease burden through absenteeism and reduced productivity at work. This state of affairs challenges the healthcare sector to respond with appropriate, feasible, and effective treatment protocols for ADs.

■ PREVALENCE OF ANXIETY DISORDERS

The National Comorbidity Replication Survey in the United States (2001–2003) found the lifetime prevalence of any psychiatric disorder to be 46.4%, among which ADs were the most common (28.8%).[2] The last 12-month prevalence of any psychiatric disorder in adults was 26.2%; among these ADs were the most common at 18.1%.[3] At the level of primary care, prevalence of ICD-10 ADs was 16.4%[4] and the burden of ADs was high.[5]

Among all mental disorders, ADs including panic disorder with or without agoraphobia, generalized anxiety disorder (GAD), social anxiety disorder (SAD), phobias, and separation AD are the most frequent and associated with high burden of illness.[6] While psychopharmacology, particularly the administration of benzodiazepines, can alleviate anxiety symptoms, it does not address the root causes of these disorders. In addition, anxiolytic medication always brings with it issues of tolerance, dependency, and side effects, creating additional challenges for patients.[7] For this reason, cognitive behavioral therapy (CBT) has emerged as a first-line treatment for all ADs. CBT addresses the negative thinking and avoidant behavior that drive these disorders, offering an evidence-based, drug-free, and highly effective treatment protocol.[8]

Complementary and alternative approaches to treating ADs have gained traction worldwide over the last 30 years. These approaches include herbal medications, nutritional supplements, yoga therapy, mindfulness practice, and meditation.[9,10]

TREATING ANXIETY DISORDERS

Anxiety disorders comprise a spectrum that includes GAD, panic disorder, SAD, agoraphobia, and other specific phobias. All these disorders share common social, psychological, behavioral, and biological mechanisms. Apprehension about the future is a common element, as are restlessness, hyperarousal, fatigue, sleep disturbances, and avoidant behavior. While new augmenting strategies have equipped clinicians to address some of these disorders, affordability and acceptability of these newer regimens make it difficult for them to be offered at all levels of care. These barriers make such medical augmentation not feasible in a country like India. Prescribing lifestyle modifications might better address these disorders. With most ADs being mild to moderate in severity, primary care, and community healthcare centers represent first-line treatment venues and might reduce progression to severe and complex clinical presentations. It is likely that lifestyle changes for any patient will confer more benefits than risks. These lifestyle strategies include aerobic exercises, meditation, and yoga, which are all feasible and acceptable in Indian culture. Relatively little datum is available on the efficacy of these complementary and alternative approaches, but preliminary findings appear promising.

There are many research studies in the area of effectiveness of yoga on anxiety as a symptom rather than ADs. It is difficult to interpret from these studies whether they were carried out on individuals with anxiety (it is likely that it may have been on individuals with day-to-day stress of life) or on patients with ADs. ADs are established medical illnesses that need clinical attention for its management.

Against this background, this chapter will provide a narrative review of the effectiveness of yoga on both anxiety as a symptom, as well as, on ADs.

Anxiety has been referred to as *"chitta udvega"* (restless state of the mind) in Ancient *Ayurveda* texts. *Acharya Charaka*, Father of Medicine in *Ayurveda* has mentioned it as a *manasa vikara*.[11] Traditional Indian texts define *Yoga* as *"Manah prashamanopayah yoga ityabhidhiyate"* (Yoga is a technique to calm down the mind—*Yoga Vasistha*)[12] and *"Samatvam yoga uchyate"* (balanced state of body and mind—*Bhagavad Gita*).[13] The *Upanishads* also say that fear is the root cause of anxiety, and that one who knows the bliss of *brahman* does not fear anything.[14] Thus, yoga-based interventions which aim to calm and balance the mind and reduce fear, seem logically best suited to help patients with ADs. Among the complementary and alternative medicine (CAM) therapies, yoga is used very widely, especially for depression and ADs.

NEUROBIOLOGY OF ANXIETY DISORDERS AND EFFECT OF YOGA INTERVENTION

Anxiety disorders manifest with a wide range of physical and affective symptoms as well as changes in behavior and cognition, characterized by a variety of neuroendocrine, neurotransmitter, and neuroanatomical disruptions especially in emotional centers (limbic system) of the brain. The brain circuits in the amygdala are thought to comprise inhibitory networks of gamma-aminobutyric acidergic (GABAergic) interneurons and this neurotransmitter thus plays a key role in the modulation of anxiety responses both in the normal and pathological state.[15] Limbic system over activity can increase arousal and awareness of the environment leading to symptoms of anxiety.[16] Patients with AD have downregulated GABA system in occipital cortex.[17] A single session of 60-minute yoga practice increased 27% of brain GABA levels in regular yoga practitioners compared to reading.[18] Another study with 12-week *Iyengar* yoga intervention (3 sessions/week for 36 sessions, each session for 60 min) showed increased thalamic GABA levels associated with greater improvement in mood and anxiety compared to metabolically matched walking exercise.[19] Decreased parasympathetic nervous system and GABAergic activity that underlies stress-related disorders [epilepsy, depression, and post-traumatic stress disorder (PTSD)] can be corrected by yoga practices resulting in amelioration of disease symptoms.[20]

Trait anxiety (TA) which is an important risk factor for ADs and predictor of cardiovascular morbidity and mortality is associated with autonomic dysfunction.[21] Heart rate variability (HRV) may be used to assess autonomic imbalances, diseases, and mortality. Parasympathetic activity and HRV have been associated with a wide range of conditions including cardiovascular disease.[22] Increased parasympathetic activity and decreased sympathetic activity were observed in slow breathing compared to fast breathing were observed in healthy.[23] Yoga (guided relaxation) has shown to reduce perceived stress, increase high-frequency band of the HRV spectrum (parasympathetic) dominance.[24] Effortless meditation (*dhyana*) phase causes vagal modulation and brings about maximum changes in autonomic variables and breath rate suggestive of reduced sympathetic activity among school children.[25]

Regular practice of meditation has neuroprotective effects and reduces the cognitive decline associated with normal aging.[26] Attention training programs have helped to lower anxiety levels, as the subjects are able to shift their attention away from the threatening stimulus. Practice of meditation triggers neurotransmitters that modulate psychological disorders such as anxiety.[27] Physical exercise and breathing training are effective in improving cardiac autonomic control (CAC) in patients with affective spectrum disorders.[28] Based on Yoga techniques, it has been consistently shown that breathing exercises have beneficial effects on CAC and breathing function.[29]

LITERATURE REVIEW OF YOGA AND ANXIETY
Effects of Yoga on Anxiety

Yoga has come to be recognized, by researchers and clinicians, as a complementary treatment for ADs. Yoga-based interventions offer a promising lifestyle intervention for anxiety which are increasingly popular worldwide, with the primary components of *asana*, *pranayama*, and meditation.[30]

Ten months of yoga practice in healthy individuals has been shown to increase parasympathetic activity, increase musculoskeletal flexibility, reduce anxiety and depression, improve learning and psychomotor ability, and produce better mental function.[31] Yoga helps reduce anxiety, increase feelings of well-being and relaxation, and improve concentration, self-confidence, and efficiency.[32] Research has begun to identify ways in which meditation and yoga provide endocrine system benefits, increasing neurotransmitter activity that modulates anxiety.[33] Sixty minutes of yoga practice has been shown to raise brain GABA levels by 27%, an increase in line with that produced by benzodiazepine medication.[18]

Yoga and Performance Anxiety

A controlled study demonstrated the benefits of one session each of yoga and meditation (*Kripalu yoga*) (once weekly) on performance anxiety in young adult professional musicians. This study demonstrated that yoga and meditation techniques could reduce performance anxiety and mood disturbances among young professional musicians.[34]

Yoga and Examination Anxiety

A study of class X students appearing for board examinations reported the beneficial effects of 2 hours of daily *yoga, asana* and *pranayama* practice for 6 weeks. Yoga training helped to reduce examination anxiety, depression, and academic stress.[35] Another study demonstrated the significant improvement in anxiety and group performance in a mathematics examination among class IX students following 6 weeks of breath regulation practices, laughter technique, development of alternate emotion responses to the threatening stimulus and super brain yoga practice.[36]

Yoga and State Anxiety

A two group prepost interventional study found that a combination of yoga postures and supine rest improved memory scores and decreased state anxiety immediately after the practice.[37] Another two group prepost interventional study reported the effect of yoga practice and theory sessions on state anxiety in healthy individuals. Following a 2-hour yoga session, both the practice and theory groups showed significant decreases in state anxiety levels, with a greater reduction in state anxiety in the yoga practice group compared to the yoga theory group.[38] A systematic review also supports the effectiveness of yoga as a viable therapeutic option for reducing state anxiety in a variety of settings.[39]

YOGA FOR SPECIFIC ANXIETY DISORDERS

Yoga and Generalized Anxiety Disorder

Meditation has been found to be as effective as pharmacotherapy in controlling symptoms of GAD. A preliminary study examined the effect of 6 weeks of *Kundalini* yoga-enhanced cognitive behavioral therapy (Y-CBT) on GAD. Y-CBT produced improvements in state and trait anxiety, and in depression, panic, sleep, and quality of life.[40] Another study compared the effect of *yogic* practices (*asana* and *pranayama*) and naturopathic procedures (full body massage, steam, diaphragmatic breathing, and acupressure) in patients with GAD.[41] Twenty-one days of intervention showed decreases in anxiety in the yoga group compared to the naturopathy group, though there was no significant difference between the groups. A pilot study showed the efficacy and tolerability of *Sudarshan Kriya Yoga* (SKY) in outpatients with GAD. There was a significant reduction in anxiety; the response rate was 73% and the remission rate 41%.[42] Another clinical trial found significant reduction in anxiety and depression after 2 weeks, and after 3 and 6 months of SKY practice in patients with GAD.[43]

A pilot study with self as control design noted a reduction in state anxiety and enhanced psychomotor performance measured by Digit letter substitution task immediately after the practice of *mind sound resonance technique (MSRT)* in patients with GAD compared to supine rest.[44] Many mindfulness-based programs have been studied, including mindfulness-based stress reduction (MBSR), and found to significantly reduce stress, anxiety symptoms, and worry. Mindfulness-based cognitive therapy (MBCT), a protocol shown to be effective in reducing relapse in patients with major depression, has also been useful in reducing anxiety in patients with GAD and panic disorder. A randomized controlled trial (RCT) found MBSR to correlate with symptom improvement[45] and changes in frontal limbic areas associated with emotional regulation, as well as increased functional connectivity between the amygdala and prefrontal cortex as seen in functional magnetic resonance imaging (fMRI).[46]

Yoga and Panic Disorder

A comparison study demonstrated the effectiveness of MBSR program in reducing symptoms of anxiety and panic, and these gains were maintained at 3-month follow-up in patients with GAD and panic disorder[47] compared to nonstudy participants who met the initial screening criteria for entry into the study.

A controlled observational study in patients with panic disorder showed significant improvements in panic symptomatology following the practice of *Hatha yoga* techniques including *asana*, *pranayama*, relaxation or *yoga nidra*, and meditation or mindfulness practice (50 min twice weekly for 2 months), either alone or in combination with CBT.[48]

Yoga and Post-traumatic Stress Disorder

Post-traumatic stress disorder often brings with it hypervigilance, panic, and other anxiety symptoms. Yoga therapies for PTSD are now being offered globally, either as monotherapy or in conjunction with approaches such as CBT.

The RCT studied the effect of *Kripalu* yoga in military veterans diagnosed with PTSD. They found significant decreases in symptoms of PTSD after a 10-week yoga intervention.[49] A review on the effects of yoga including meditation in trauma survivors noted improvement in PTSD symptoms as a result of yoga practice.[50] Another clinical trial showed that 1 week of yoga practice (stretching exercises, physical postures, regulated breathing, and yoga-based guided relaxation) resulted in significant reductions in fear, anxiety, sadness, disturbed sleep, and breath rate in tsunami survivors in the Andaman islands.[51] The RCT studied the effects of 1 week of yoga practice among survivors of floods in the Indian state of Bihar and found that 1 hour of daily yoga practice for 1 week (including *Shithilikarana vyayama*, *asana*, *pranayama*, and guided relaxation in *shavasana*) correlated with significant decreases in sadness. They concluded that yoga has potential to reduce sadness and prevent anxiety in survivors of natural disasters.[52]

The RCT has found that women with chronic, treatment-resistant PTSD experienced reductions in PTSD symptoms and maintenance of these improvements after 10 weeks of practice of *Hatha yoga* postures, breathing practices, and meditation.[53] Similarly, another RCT noted the effectiveness of SKY in treatment-resistant PTSD.[54] A systematic review and meta-analysis on RCTs found yoga to be an effective adjunctive intervention for PTSD.[55] Another study reported yoga therapy as an adjunctive PTSD therapy in military combat veterans.[56] The program, which included a 6-week yoga intervention held twice a week, noted significant improvements in hyperarousal symptoms of PTSD and also improved overall sleep quality. A single group trial studied the effects of an 8-week *Kundalini* yoga and CBT program for 3 hours per week. Total PTSD symptom scores were significantly improved following the program, as were PTSD cluster symptoms (intrusion, arousal, avoidance, and negative alterations in mood). Improvements in all PTSD scores were maintained at follow-up. Participants' total sleep quality improved, as did sleep disturbance and daytime dysfunction due to sleepiness. All these improvements were maintained at 8-week follow-up.[57]

Yoga and Phobia

One comparison study compared the effectiveness of two relaxation procedures (modified progressive relaxation training and *Agni yoga*) in treating snake phobia. After four training sessions, approach distance, subjective fear, and pulse rates were measured during a snake approach test; a snake fear scale was administered before and after approaching the snake. The results supported the effectiveness of yoga in reducing both cognitive and somatic symptoms of phobia.[58]

Yoga and Anxiety Neurosis

A study demonstrated the efficacy of yoga meditation for patients with short history of the illness and the efficacy of flooding therapy in those with a longer history.[59]

YOGA: AN EMERGING THERAPY FOR ANXIETY

Patients with ADs especially those suffering from milder forms of these disorders, often prefer yoga therapy to pharmacotherapy. This preference may be driven by increasing awareness of the efficacy of yoga therapy and by the absence of undesirable side effects associated with it. The three most common types of yoga utilized in anxiety are SKY, *Vinyasa yoga* and *Iyengar's yoga*. SKY has been widely studied as an intervention for anxiety and typically involves a seated posture and 45 minutes of various breathing patterns. These patterns include 2–3 cycles/min of slow breathing (*Ujjayi*), 20–30 cycles of rapid breathing through a partially closed glottis (*Bhastrika*), and cyclical breathing with frequency increasing from 20 to 80 cycles/min (*Kriya*). SKY studies have been carried out on subjects with nonsyndromal and syndromal anxiety symptoms. Parameters studied include remission rates, quality of life, and adverse effects. Findings note improved quality of life and few side-effects, yet overall the response rate of yoga therapy for anxiety has been mixed.[60]

LIMITATIONS OF RESEARCH

Studies of *yoga's* effectiveness as a therapy for ADs have been limited by small sample size, lack of specificity regarding the yoga performed, lack of randomization, heterogeneous populations, varying severity of illnesses, and varied treatment durations. Studies have run for an average of 3–4 months and few have been replicated by other researchers. There are no definitive safety data on yoga as a therapy, save a few anecdotal reports of exacerbation of underlying medical conditions such as glaucoma and hyponatremia. These side effects seem to be associated with specific *asanas* or *pranayama* which involve headstand, shoulder stand, inversion postures, and advanced breathing techniques.

PRACTICE TIPS, CHALLENGES AND RECOMMENDATIONS

A suggested yoga module for anxiety disorders is provided in **Appendix 1.2**.

Individuals with physical disability may have difficulty in practicing certain styles of yoga, although modifications can often be made to address such disabilities. A considerable challenge to this emerging field is access to trained yoga therapists. Self-help books and online classes (*Tele-Yoga*) are proving effective approaches to improving access to care. It is recommended that patients always practice yoga therapy under the supervision of a trained yoga therapist. While practicing, mindfulness is very important. Patients should synchronize their breath with the body movements and give themselves time to relax into poses. Breath should not be held in any posture or while doing any *pranayama* techniques (unless this is specifically called for). Patients must listen to their bodies and not overstrain. If pain is experienced, it is best to stop and notify the therapist or teacher. Practice is best done in loose clothing and in a quiet, undisturbed setting with mobile phones turned off. The ideal times for yoga practice are mornings between 5 and 7 AM and evenings between 5 and 7 PM. Practice should be avoided after heavy meals. Strong perfumes or drinking too much tea or coffee are best avoided. A *sattvic* diet is recommended, as are inspirational books and encouraging lectures. Yoga and CBT agree on one final point: positive thinking is an essential ingredient for any practice, setting the stage for true physical, psychological, and spiritual development.

CONCLUSION

Yoga's role in the treatment of anxiety is both new and promising. Available data are preliminary and can serve as a foundation upon which to build new research in this field. New studies ought to focus on specific styles of yoga, test hypotheses regarding mechanisms of action and include larger sample sizes. Much remains unknown regarding the neurobiology of specific styles of yoga and their effects on specific diagnoses. So too, many questions remain unanswered regarding the efficacy of yoga therapy for anxiety in acute versus chronic cases. Nevertheless, yoga continues to be a culturally acceptable form of treatment for psychiatric disorders in countries throughout the world. Datum is rapidly accumulating in support of yoga's efficacy in improving anxiety symptoms and supporting physical and emotional wellness. It is safe to say that this ancient, drug-free, low-cost approach to human well-being deserves consideration by providers and patients across the mental health spectrum.

■ CASE VIGNETTE

A 35-year-old lady (Miss C) presented to the Department of Integrative Medicine (IMD), National Institute of Mental Health and Neuro Sciences (NIMHANS) with complaints of continuous stress and worry about the health of her son, who was suffering from leukemia (blood cancer). She described herself as a "worrier" from the beginning but her anxiety had become much worse in the past 2–3 years since her son became unwell and her husband was working abroad, and she no longer feels that she can control these thoughts. She also complained that the feeling of stress was persisting all the time and she worried about "almost everything".

Some other complaints associated with anxiety were excessive burping and acidity, poor concentration, breathing difficulty, increased heart rate, and muscle stiffness. Her sleep was poor and she was having trouble falling asleep and frequent disturbances at night. She often felt "restless" or "on edge", which she associated with her poor quality of sleep.

She stated that she felt tired and irritable throughout the day. She had been diagnosed with GAD by a psychiatrist at NIMHANS and had been on medications since 1 year.

With medications, she was able to control her anxiety and was able to carry out her day-to-day activities with relatively lesser difficulty, although history revealed poor drug compliance, resulting in flaring up of the symptoms.

She was referred to IMD by her psychiatrist for further management through yoga. After assessment by a resident at the department, she was advised to undergo regular yoga therapy for ADs. Yoga therapy proposed for her included breathing practices, pranayama, asana, chanting, relaxation techniques, and yogic counseling. After 1 week of practice, it was observed that pranayama, chanting, and relaxation techniques were specifically beneficial to her. Instructions for physical practices such as asana were revised to ensure more emphasis on connecting body and breath. Further chants were also mixed with bodily movements in the form of breathing practices. By this time, her apprehensiveness toward yoga had decreased and she was able to overcome the initial difficulties in understanding the practices.

Among pranayama practices, she was initiated with nadi shuddhi, bhramari, and vibhagiya pranayama. Further, chandra anuloma viloma and sheetali pranayama were added considering symptoms of hyperacidity. She was also advised to have a brief 5 minutes practice of pranayama at home as per need. For relaxation, nadanusandhana and deep relaxation techniques were offered, which according to her, gave deep rest to her agitated mind and body. Discussion regarding her understanding of yoga therapy was promoted at the end of yoga sessions. These discussions focused on conceptual understanding of the panchakosha model and yogic diet.

Her assessments were repeated on Day 7, 14, and 21. During these assessments, apart from the improvement in her symptoms, she also reported changes made by her in lifestyle and diet as per yogic understanding. She reported that yoga therapy sessions made her

	Clinical Insights: Yoga Therapy in Anxiety Disorders
Prior to the session	• Have a clear idea of the patient's history, clinical status, medical comorbidities (such as hyperthyroidism, anemia, cardiac problems, bronchial asthma, hypoglycemia in diabetes), medications he/she is on and any other nonpharmacological methods (such as psychotherapy) they have used previously before coming to the yoga sessions. • Elicit patient's understanding of the referral and what their expectations are during and after the yoga sessions. • If patients are on medicines, emphasize the need to continue medicines and the role of yoga as an add-on to their current treatment. Instruct not to stop medicines without the psychiatrist's advice. • Establish a good rapport but clarify the professional boundaries such as what are the Do's and Don'ts during, after, and also once the session ends.
During the session	• Orient the patient to the different practices of yoga and how each practice would be beneficial for the improvement of their symptoms (e.g., relationship between breath and mind should be explained). • Preferably start as one-on-one session (especially in cases with social anxiety) and later, as the patient becomes more comfortable, he/she can be introduced into the group session. • *Do not focus on perfection in postures or techniques initially* as they may become anxious of the practices itself and that may hinder the process. • *Focus more on practices which bring about relaxation* (e.g., left nostril breathing, gentle humming breath, chanting *Om*, and sectional breathing with prolonged exhalations) as these patients have a high sympathetic arousal. • Later on, *focus should be on increasing the awareness of bodily sensations during practices*. The patient should be encouraged to feel the changes in the body and mind after each practice with a brief pause between the practices. It may help them feel more in control of their body. • As the sessions progress, and once the patient becomes familiar with the different *asanas*, the therapist can gradually stop doing the practices along with the patient. Instead, instruct them verbally, as necessary, to *make them more self-reliant*. • It is wise to instruct *not to overdo breathing practices (hyperventilation-inducing practices such Kapalabhati and Bhastrika)* since it is possible that dizziness secondary to excessive carbon dioxide washout may result in patients misinterpreting it as a side effect due to sessions. • In patients with GAD, it may help to *give the schedule to the patients prior to the sessions*. This will help to address the anticipatory anxiety and make them prepared for the next session. • In cases of dissociative disorders, the therapist must be aware that the patient can have a dissociative spell while in the session. The therapist should remain calm during this episode. • Make sure that the patient is safe, but be cautious about giving excessive attention to the symptoms as this may reinforce such behavior (e.g., if a patient has dissociative seizures during the session, then such patient may be asked to take rest briefly, but the session should be continued and the patient should be asked to join the session back as soon as he/she feels better).
After the session	• At least a week prior to the termination of sessions, groom the patient for the same. • Clarify any doubts related to any practice. • Explain about the frequency of follow-up sessions and the subsequent assessments. • Explain to the patient that the therapeutic benefits of yoga can be perceived only on regular practice. • Encourage them to see yoga as a lifestyle rather than a prescribed medicine to their illness.

feel relaxed, her anxiety levels had reduced, and her sleep had improved. Other symptoms like palpitations, breathing difficulty, stiffness, and tiredness also had reduced. For this improvement, she gave maximum credit to relaxation and chanting practices. Over a period of time, her interest in yoga increased, and she used to look forward to her therapy session every day.

REFERENCES

1. Locke AB, Kirst N, Shultz CG. Diagnosis and management of generalized anxiety disorder and panic disorder in adults. Am Fam Physician. 2015;91(9):617-24.

2. Kessler RC, Berglund P, Demler O, Jin R, Merikangas KR, Walters EE. Lifetime prevalence and age-of-onset distributions of DSM-IV disorders in the National Comorbidity Survey Replication. Arch Gen Psychiatry. 2005;62(6):593-602. Erratum in: Arch Gen Psychiatry. 2005;62(7):768. Merikangas, Kathleen R [added].
3. Kessler RC, Chiu WT, Demler O, Merikangas KR, Walters EE. Prevalence, severity, and comorbidity of 12-month DSM-IV disorders in the National Comorbidity Survey Replication. Arch Gen Psychiatry. 2005;62(6):617-27. Erratum in: Arch Gen Psychiatry. 2005;62(7):709. Merikangas, Kathleen R [added].
4. Toft T, Fink P, Oernboel E, Christensen K, Frostholm L, Olesen F. Mental disorders in primary care: prevalence and comorbidity among disorders. Results from the functional illness in primary care (FIP) study. Psychol Med. 2005;35(8):1175-84.
5. Spitzer RL, Williams JB, Kroenke K, Linzer M, deGruy FV 3rd, Hahn SR, et al. Utility of a new procedure for diagnosing mental disorders in primary care. The PRIME-MD 1000 study. JAMA. 1994;272(22):1749-56.
6. Bandelow B, Michaelis S. Epidemiology of anxiety disorders in the 21st century. Dialogues Clin Neurosci. 2015;17(3):327-35.
7. Lader M. Long-term anxiolytic therapy: the issue of drug withdrawal. J Clin Psychiatry. 1987;48 Suppl:12-6.
8. Kaczkurkin AN, Foa EB. Cognitive-behavioral therapy for anxiety disorders: an update on the empirical evidence. Dialogues Clin Neurosci. 2015;17(3):337-46.
9. Sarris J, Moylan S, Camfield DA, Pase MP, Mischoulon D, Berk M, et al. Complementary medicine, exercise, meditation, diet, and lifestyle modification for anxiety disorders: a review of current evidence. Evid Based Complement Alternat Med. 2012;2012:809653.
10. Bystritsky A, Hovav S, Sherbourne C, Stein MB, Rose RD, Campbell-Sills L, et al. Use of complementary and alternative medicine in a large sample of anxiety patients. Psychosomatics. 2012;53(3):266-72.
11. Acharya YT (Ed). Agnivesha, Charaka Samhita, Ayurveda Dipika commentary by Chakrapāṇi. Vimana sthana, 6/5, 254. Varanasi, India: Chaukhamba Surbharati Prakashan; 2000.
12. Venkateshananda S. Vashishtha's Yoga. 3.9.32. New York, Albany: State University of New York Press; 1993.
13. Shivanada S. Bhagavad Gita. Chapter 2/48th Shloka. Uttar Pradesh: A Divine Life Society Publications; 2000. [online] Available from: http://www.SivanandaDlshq.org/ [Last accessed September, 2020].
14. Sethumadhavan TN. Taittiriya Upanishad. Kartika Shukla Pratipada (Bali Pratipada). Chapter 12, Section 9. 2011. p. 48. Nagpur. [online] Available from Esamskriti.com [Last accessed September, 2020].
15. Martin EI, Ressler KJ, Binder E, Nemeroff CB. The neurobiology of anxiety disorders: brain imaging, genetics, and psychoneuroendocrinology. Psychiatr Clin North Am. 2009;32(3):549-75.
16. Gray JA. A theory of anxiety: the role of the limbic system. Encephale. 1983;9(4 Suppl 2):161B-6B.
17. Goddard AW, Mason GF, Almai A, Rothman DL, Behar KL, Petroff OA, et al. Reductions in occipital cortex GABA levels in panic disorder detected with 1 hour-magnetic resonance spectroscopy. Arch Gen Psychiatry. 2001;58(6):556-61.
18. Streeter CC, Jensen JE, Perlmutter RM, Cabral HJ, Tian H, Terhune DB, et al. Yoga asana sessions increase brain GABA levels: a pilot study. J Altern Complement Med. 2007;13(4):419-26.
19. Streeter CC, Whitfield TH, Owen L, Rein T, Karri SK, Yakhkind A, et al. Effects of yoga versus walking on mood, anxiety, and brain GABA levels: a randomized controlled MRS study. J Altern Complement Med. 2010;16(11):1145-52.
20. Streeter CC, Gerbarg PL, Saper RB, Ciraulo DA, Brown RP. Effects of yoga on the autonomic nervous system, gamma-aminobutyric acid, and allostasis in epilepsy, depression, and post-traumatic stress disorder. Med Hypotheses. 2012;78(5):571-9.
21. Miu AC, Heilman RM, Miclea M. Reduced heart rate variability and vagal tone in anxiety: trait versus state, and the effects of autogenic training. Auton Neurosci. 2009;145(1-2):99-103.
22. Thayer JF, Yamamoto SS, Brosschot JF. The relationship of autonomic imbalance, heart rate variability and cardiovascular disease risk factors. Int J Cardiology. 2010;141(2):122-31.
23. Pal GK, Velkumary S, Madanmohan. Effect of short-term practice of breathing exercises on autonomic functions in normal human volunteers. Indian J Med Res. 2004;120(2):115-21.
24. Satyapriya M, Nagendra HR, Nagarathna R, Padmalatha V. Effect of integrated yoga on stress and heart rate variability in pregnant women. Int J Gynaecol Obstet. 2009;104(3):218-22.
25. Telles S, Singh N, Bhardwaj AK, Kumar A, Balkrishna A. Effect of yoga or physical exercise on physical, cognitive and emotional measures in children: a randomized controlled trial. Child Adolesc Psychiatry Ment Health. 2013;7(1):37.
26. Pagnoni G, Cekic M. Age effects on gray matter volume and attentional performance in Zen meditation. Neurobiol Aging. 2007;28(10):1623-7.

27. Krishnakumar D, Hamblin MR, Lakshmanan S. Meditation and yoga can modulate brain mechanisms that affect behavior and anxiety: a modern scientific perspective. Anc Sci. 2015;2(1):13-9.
28. Brown RP, Gerbarg PL. Sudarshan Kriya yogic breathing in the treatment of stress, anxiety, and depression: part I-neurophysiologic model. J Altern Complement Med. 2005;11(1):189-201. Erratum in: J Altern Complement Med. 2005;11(2):383-4.
29. Santaella DF, Devesa CR, Rojo MR, Amato MB, Drager LF, Casali KR, et al. Yoga respiratory training improves respiratory function and cardiac sympathovagal balance in elderly subjects: a randomised controlled trial. BMJ Open. 2011;1(1):e000085.
30. Hofmann SG, Curtiss J, Khalsa SB, Hoge E, Rosenfield D, Bui E, et al. Yoga for generalized anxiety disorder: design of a randomized controlled clinical trial. Contemp Clin Trials. 2015;44:70-6.
31. Ray US, Mukhopadhyaya S, Purkayastha SS, Asnani V, Tomer OS, Prashad R, et al. Effect of yogic exercises on physical and mental health of young fellowship course trainees. Indian J Physiol Pharmacol. 2001;45(1):37-53.
32. Malathi A, Damodaran A. Stress due to exams in medical students—role of yoga. Indian J Physiol Pharmacol. 1999;43(2):218-24.
33. Krishnakumar D, Hamblin MR, Lakshmanan S. Meditation and yoga can modulate brain mechanisms that affect behavior and anxiety: a modern scientific perspective. Anc Sci. 2015;2(1):13-9.
34. Khalsa SB, Shorter SM, Cope S, Wyshak G, Sklar E. Yoga ameliorates performance anxiety and mood disturbance in young professional musicians. Appl Psychophysiol Biofeedback. 2009;34(4):279-89.
35. Pant G, Shete BT, Uddhav SS. Yoga for controlling examination anxiety, depression and academic stress among students appearing for Indian board examination. Int J Recent Sci Res. 2013;4(20):1216-9.
36. Singh P. Management of mathematics phobia among ninth standard students. Int J Indian Psychol. 2016;3(2):69-76.
37. Pailoor S, Telles S. Effect of two yoga-based relaxation techniques on memory scores and state anxiety. Bio Psycho Social Med. 2009;3:8.
38. Telles S, Gaur V, Balkrishna A. Effect of a yoga practice session and a yoga theory session on state anxiety. Percept Mot Skills. 2009;109(3):924-30.
39. Chugh-Gupta N, Baldassarre FG, Vrkljan BH. A systematic review of yoga for state anxiety: considerations for occupational therapy. Can J Occup Ther. 2013;80(3):150-70.
40. Khalsa MK, Greiner-Ferris JM, Hofmann SG, Khalsa SB. Yoga-enhanced cognitive behavioural therapy (Y-CBT) for anxiety management: a pilot study. Clin Psychol Psychother. 2015;22(4):364-71.
41. Gupta K, Mamidi P. A pilot study on certain yogic and naturopathic procedures in generalized anxiety disorder. Int J Res Ayurveda Pharm. 2013;4(6):858-61.
42. Katzman MA, Vermani M, Gerbarg PL, Brown RP, Iorio C, Davis M, et al. A multicomponent yoga-based, breath intervention program as an adjunctive treatment in patients suffering from generalized anxiety disorder with or without comorbidities. Int J Yoga. 2012;5(1):57-65.
43. Doria S, de Vuono A, Sanlorenzo R, Irtelli F, Mencacci C. Anti-anxiety efficacy of Sudarshan Kriya yoga in general anxiety disorder: a multicomponent, yoga-based, breath intervention program for patients suffering from generalized anxiety disorder with or without comorbidities. J Affect Disord. 2015;184:310-7.
44. Dhansoia V, Bhargav H, Metri K. Immediate effect of mind sound resonance technique on state anxiety and cognitive functions in patients suffering from generalized anxiety disorder: a self-controlled pilot study. Int J Yoga. 2015;8(1):70-3.
45. Hoge EA, Bui E, Marques L, Metcalf CA, Morris LK, Robinaugh DJ, et al. Randomized controlled trial of mindfulness meditation for generalized anxiety disorder: effects on anxiety and stress reactivity. J Clin Psychiatry. 2013;74(8):786-92.
46. Hölzel BK, Hoge EA, Greve DN, Gard T, Creswell JD, Brown KW, et al. Neural mechanisms of symptom improvements in generalized anxiety disorder following mindfulness training. Neuroimage Clin. 2013;2:448-58.
47. Kabat-Zinn J, Massion AO, Kristeller J, Peterson LG, Fletcher KE, Pbert L, et al. Effectiveness of a meditation-based stress reduction program in the treatment of anxiety disorders. Am J Psychiatry. 1992;149(7):936-43.
48. Vorkapic CF, Rangé B. Reducing the symptomatology of panic disorder: the effects of a yoga program alone and in combination with cognitive-behavioral therapy. Front Psychiatry. 2014;5:177.
49. Reinhardt KM, Noggle TJ, Johnston J, Zameer A, Cheema S, Khalsa SB. Kripalu yoga for military veterans with PTSD: a randomized trial. J Clin Psychol. 2018;74(1):93-108.
50. Telles S, Singh N, Balkrishna A. Managing mental health disorders resulting from trauma

through yoga: a review. Depress Res Treat. 2012;2012:401513.
51. Telles S, Naveen KV, Dash M. Yoga reduces symptoms of distress in tsunami survivors in the Andaman islands. Evid Based Complement Alternat Med. 2007;4(4):503-9.
52. Telles S, Singh N, Joshi M, Balkrishna A. Post-traumatic stress symptoms and heart rate variability in Bihar flood survivors following yoga: a randomized controlled study. BMC Psychiatry. 2010;2(10):18.
53. van der Kolk BA, Stone L, West J, Rhodes A, Emerson D, Suvak M, et al. Yoga as an adjunctive treatment for post-traumatic stress disorder: a randomized controlled trial. J Clin Psychiatry. 2014;75(6):e559-65.
54. Carter J, Gerbarg PL, Brown RP, Ware RS, D'Ambrosio C, Anand L, et al. Multi-component yoga breath program for Vietnam veteran post traumatic stress disorder: randomized controlled trial. J Trauma Stress Disor Treat. 2013;2(3).
55. Cramer H, Anheyer D, Saha FJ, Dobos G. Yoga for post-traumatic stress disorder: a systematic review and meta-analysis. BMC Psychiatry. 2018;18(1):72.
56. Staples JK, Hamilton MF, Uddo M. A yoga program for the symptoms of post-traumatic stress disorder in veterans. Mil Med. 2013;178(8):854-60.
57. Staples JK, Mintie D, Khalsa SB. Evaluation of a combined yoga and cognitive behavioral therapy program for post-traumatic stress disorder. J Altern Complement Med. 2016;22(6):A94.
58. Norton GR, Johnson WE. A comparison of two relaxation procedures for reducing cognitive and somatic anxiety. J Behav Ther Exp Psychiatry. 1983;14(3):209-14.
59. Girodo M. Yoga meditation and flooding in the treatment of anxiety neurosis. J Behav Ther Exp Psychiatry. 1974;5(2):157-60.
60. Cramer H, Lauche R, Haller H, Dobos G. A systematic review and meta-analysis of yoga for low back pain. Clin J Pain. 2013;29(5):450-60.

CHAPTER 12

Yoga in Obsessive Compulsive Disorder

Sanchari Mukhopadhyay, Nishitha Jasti, Shubha Bhat, Shubham Sharma

INTRODUCTION

Obsessive compulsive disorder (OCD) is characterized by recurrent intrusive thoughts, impulses, images or urges, and is often accompanied by some other thoughts or actions to neutralize, ignore or suppress them. They tend to persist despite attempts to resist and often cause significant distress in the person.[1] The National Mental Health Survey conducted by the National Institute of Mental Health and Neuro Sciences (NIMHANS), Bengaluru in 2015–2016 found a point prevalence for OCD of 0.8% in the Indian population.[2] Conventional treatments for OCD include pharmacotherapy and psychotherapy. Among pharmacological interventions, selective serotonin reuptake inhibitors (SSRIs) and clomipramine (a tricyclic antidepressant) are most commonly used. Of the psychotherapeutic interventions, cognitive behavioral therapy and exposure response prevention are best supported by evidence.[3]

However, studies have found that around one-third of patients with OCD do not respond to drug treatment, and conventional treatment modalities only produce a maximum improvement of 40–60%.[4] Yoga can help in filling this gap, as yoga-based interventions have shown significant promise in improving symptoms, functioning, and quality of life in patients with psychiatric disorders such as depression and schizophrenia.[5] Yoga has been noted, albeit not extensively, to have some beneficial effects in patients with OCD.[4]

UNDERSTANDING PSYCHOPATHOLOGY OF OCD: YOGA PHILOSOPHY PERSPECTIVE

The classical text, Patanjali's Yoga Sutras describe the following mental afflictions *(Kleshas): Avidya* (confusion), *Asmita* (self-centeredness), *Raga* (strong desire/attachment), *Dwesha* (hatred), and *Abhinivesha* (fear).[6] Of which, *Asmita* is observed to be heightened in patients with OCD, which results in self-centric projections in the mind. *Asmita* leads to excess speed of thoughts in mind that manifests as high *Rajas* (one of the three attributes of the mind: *Sattva, Rajas,* and *Tamas*). *Rajas* (overactivity of the mind) creates a split in the *Asmita*, from which *Raga* (strong desire to act toward obsession in this context) and *Dwesha* (resistance to compulsion in this context) arise, conflict with each other, and finally result in *Abhinivesha* (fear). *Abhinivesha* deranges one's ability to perceive things the way they are, resulting in *Avidya* (chronic confusion). *Avidya* leads to development and strengthening of *Viparyaya vritti* (one of the five *vrittis* mentioned by Sage Patanjali). *Viparyaya* is the state of mind in which a false projection is veiled on a true object, which can be observed in terms of obsessions, intrusive thoughts, and images in patients with OCD. Further, *Viparyaya vritti* fuels *Asmita* of the individual, thus continuing this vicious cycle **(Fig. 1)**. On the other hand, increased *Rajas* at the mind causes hyperactivity in the Sun channel (*Surya nadi*) that manifests as increased sympathetic activity, stress, and

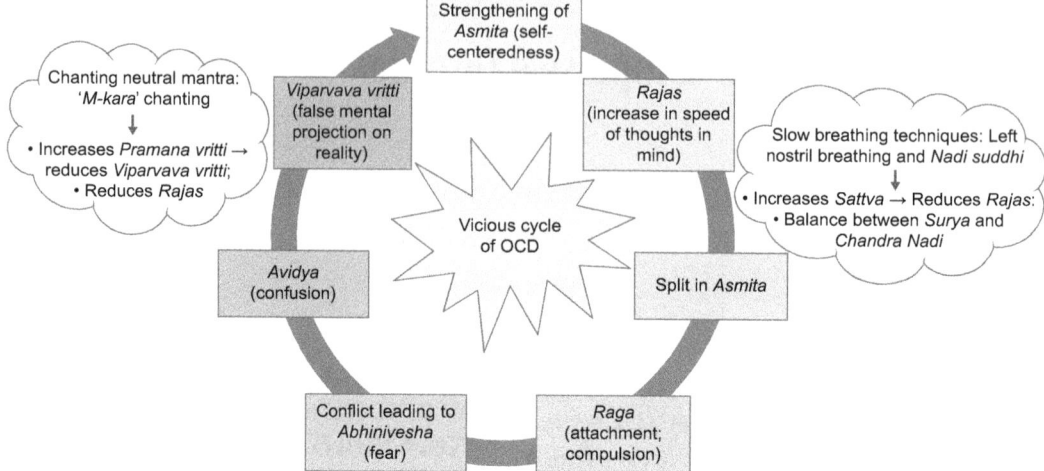

Fig. 1: Vicious cycle of obsessive compulsive disorder from yoga philosophy perspective.

anxiety. As per the recommendations of Sage Vasistha, yoga is a skillful way of calming down the mind (*manah prashamanopayah yoga ityabhidhiyate*).[7] Therefore, yoga therapeutics shall aim at transcending the mind from *Viparyaya vritti*-dominance to *Pramana vritti*-dominance (*Pramana vritti* refers to the mental state characterized by right perception), reducing the *Rajo guna*, and balancing the Moon (*Chandra nadi*) and the Sun energy channels. To achieve these objectives, a neutral chant (not suggestive of any specific subject) such as humming sound or "*M-kara*" component (in *Bhramari*) can be advised to bring the mind to *Pramana vritti*-dominance, reduce *Rajo guna* and allow the internalization of consciousness.[8] This will ultimately result in reduced speed of mind, reduction in obsessive intrusive thoughts, and anxiety. Further, left nostril breathing (*Chandra anuloma viloma pranayama*) can be advised to increase the energy in the *Chandra nadi* to bring a balance between *Surya* and *Chandra nadi* in addition to reduction in *Rajas*. From the above, it can be said that techniques such as *Bhramari pranayama* (humming bee breath), *Nadi shuddhi pranayama* (alternate nostril breath), and *Chandra anuloma viloma pranayama* play as core components in yoga therapy for treating OCD.

EVIDENCE FOR YOGA IN OCD

The type of yoga most studied in OCD is *Kundalini Yoga* (KY). One small open-label pilot study and two randomized controlled trials (RCTs) on its effects in OCD have been published.[9-11] KY was evidenced to have beneficial effects on patients with OCD in all of the studies. In the former, five patients completed the 12-month trial, showing significant positive outcome in their clinical symptoms and severity. Though all of them had improved on fluoxetine, an SSRI, for at least 3 months prior to this study, it was seen that dose reduction and cessation of the medicine were possible in them after incorporation of the Yoga practice.[9]

One RCT by Shannahoff-Khalsa et al. showed that KY was more effective as a monotherapy or adjunct to pharmacotherapy as compared to relaxation response and mindfulness meditation techniques.[10] Each group had seven participants who were given the particular mode of treatment for 3 months. Those receiving KY had significant improvement in all the outcome measures including clinical symptoms, stress and mood, and the other group showed no improvement. When all the patients were merged to receive KY, there was improvement in the measures mentioned above after 1 year. In this study also, dose reduction or elimination of the medication was possible in many patients by the end of the study.[10] Another RCT also compared the effect of KY to relaxation response meditation in patients with OCD, in addition to their ongoing medications. Patients receiving KY reported significant improvement after approximately 1.5 years of treatment.[11]

In a single-blind RCT, which used *Hatha Yoga*, women with OCD showed significant reduction in their anxiety with supervised Yoga practice twice a week for 12 sessions, as compared to the control group who watched television for the same duration. Both the groups continued the same dose of medications that they were already on. However, the groups did not differ in terms of obsessive and compulsive symptoms.[12]

The qualities of the RCTs, as assessed by Jadad scoring,[13] are given in **Table 1**. It denotes superior quality of one (total score ≥ 3) and inferior quality of two trials.[14] Overall, the evidence is promising but not unequivocal.

In the absence of a validated and standardized yoga module for OCD, a recent pilot study was done to develop and validate a module, and to examine its effects on patients with OCD. The module was developed and validated after extensive review of Yoga texts and opinions of ten independent yoga experts. Content validity was checked for the practices. Those practices with the best agreement among raters were retained in the final module. The final module was then tested for feasibility and preliminary efficacy in patients with OCD, and it was found that patients obtained significant improvement in terms of anxiety and distress with thrice a week 1-hour supervised yoga sessions for 2 weeks.[15]

■ NEUROBIOLOGY OF YOGA AND POSSIBLE MECHANISMS OF ACTION

Yoga has been shown to reduce cortisol by downregulation of the hypothalamic-pituitary-adrenal axis (HPA-axis), decrease proinflammatory markers and hormones related to sympathetic overdrive and these may be the probable mechanisms leading to alleviation of anxiety. Yoga practice was also shown to improve response to SSRIs in those with susceptible 5-HTTLPR and MTHFR polymorphisms.[16] This is of interest as SSRIs are the most commonly used and safest medications for patients with OCD. Yoga practices have been demonstrated to reduce sympathetic activity levels and induce a state of parasympathetic dominance. Greater connectivity among caudate, frontal and temporal regions of the brain is seen with yoga.[17,18] The upregulation of frontoparietal attention networks and frontolimbic emotional networks has also been hypothesized as possible mechanisms for the psychological and cognitive effects.[19] It has been seen that gamma-aminobutyric acid (GABA) levels in plasma, anterior cingulate cortex (ACC) and orbitofrontal cortex (OFC) are lower in patients with OCD. The GABA level in the OFC region is also found to have a negative correlation with the psychopathology in OCD.[20] Thus, OCD can be considered as a condition with impaired inhibitory regulation of brain, especially the OFC and ACC areas. Since yoga is known to increase GABA levels, it may be hypothesized to have a beneficial effect on symptoms of

TABLE 1: Jadad score for quality assessment of randomized controlled trials.

Study	Randomization score	Blinding score	Patient accounts score	Total Jadad score
Shannahoff-Khalsa DS et al., 1999	1	0	1	2
Shannahoff-Khalsa DS et al., 2019	2	0	1	3
Ranjbar F et al., 2013	1	1	–	2

OCD as well. These findings add some insight into possible ways in which yoga can improve OCD. However, more systematic research is required to delineate the effects of yoga on neurobiology of OCD.

LACUNAE IN THE AVAILABLE RESEARCH

The studies on KY were methodologically limited and sample sizes were very small.[21] In addition, KY can have adverse effects when practiced inappropriately. For example, it is usually not recommended in case of cardiac illnesses as it may precipitate dysrhythmia and bradycardia.[22] We also found no studies conclusively evaluating the safety and efficacy of other types of yoga in OCD. The biological underpinnings of yoga therapy in OCD are also unclear. Thus, there are many areas that need to researched further to establish the efficacy of yoga in OCD as well as to delineate the mechanisms of its action.

IMPLICATIONS AND FUTURE DIRECTIONS

Yoga has proved to be effective in several psychiatric disorders. However, how exactly yoga acts on the symptoms and biology of OCD is not yet clear. Although a few studies have mentioned the effectiveness of yoga in OCD, they all have considerable methodological limitations. Future research is necessary to substantiate the role of yoga as an adjunct or stand-alone treatment in the treatment of OCD. Some of the areas that need clarification include the profile of OCD symptoms, which respond best to yoga, patient profile suitable for yoga therapy, specific practices targeting symptoms, and the neurobiological effects of particular yoga practices in patients with OCD.

RECOMMENDATIONS

Based on our clinical experience at the NIMHANS Integrated Centre for Yoga (NICY), we have attempted to give a general outline of recommendations for yoga therapy in patients with OCD. The validated yoga module for OCD is provided in **Appendix 1.3**.[14]

- It is crucial to build a very good rapport with the patients suffering from OCD. Usually, patients will have a chain of thoughts leading to a compulsion to reduce their anxiety and it then turns into a vicious cycle. The target of yoga therapy is to break this chain at the level of thoughts.
- If the patient has obsession of dirt, certain logistic difficulties may present. Therapist must be assertive in the delivery of instructions to the patient to make sure not to reinforce the obsessions and maintain the protocol. However, the approach toward the patient should not be rude and confrontational.
- Therapist should advise the corrections in the yoga practices according to the mood state and receptivity level of the patient.
- Therapist should not emphasize on strict principles such as punctuality for at least initial 2 or 3 sessions. Such principles should be gradually introduced into the yoga session on the basis of patient's state of illness and therapist's rapport with the patient.
- The duration of a session should not exceed the recommended time of an hour, particularly due to repeated practicing or multiple reassurance seeking by the patient, which can be presentations of the illness.
- Extreme perfection should not be attempted in yoga practice as it can exacerbate symptoms.
- If the patient prefers, he/she should be allowed to be accompanied by their caregiver.

CONCLUSION

There is preliminary evidence for the positive effects of yoga in patients with OCD. Research into the deficient areas can help us understand the nuances in detail and develop tailor-made approaches for OCD. If proven to be efficacious and safe, yoga can be an immensely useful modality to improve obsessions and compulsions, particularly in patients partially responding or resistant to conventional treatments and to enhance their quality of life.

CASE VIGNETTE

A 28-year-old lady presented with an illness of 1-year duration, insidious onset, and continuous course, characterized by repeated intrusive thoughts about mathematical formulae and morality, interpersonal issues with husband, sadness, and anxiety. She could not resist mathematical vectors or figures and thoughts of moral wrongdoings from coming to her mind despite her best efforts. She started compulsively washing her hands whenever she

Clinical Insights: Yoga Therapy for Obsessive Compulsive Disorder

Prior to the session	• Realistic expectations must be set by discussion with the patient and family members, regarding what yoga can and cannot help with. • Assessment of any possible emergency like suicidality is mandatory. Appropriate referral must be made in that case. • Knowledge of the clinical symptoms is important to design yoga practices accordingly. Severe cases may require one-on-one session in the beginning. • Severe cases may not cooperate much, whatever possible and feasible should be taught (probably focusing more on breathing and standing practices in the beginning) and rapport should be built. • Preferably, it should be a collaborative work of the yoga therapist, psychiatrist, and psychotherapist if the patient is also on other modes of treatment.

During the session	• *Punctuality and perfection may not be stressed upon in the very first session.*
	• While providing relaxations, *it is better to provide relaxation of the whole body in general rather than naming part by part.*
	• *In case attention and concentr*ation are not sustained, shorter duration of practice is a good way to start and ensure compliance. Gradually, the duration can be increased to reach the desired level.
	• The therapist should take care not to reinforce any symptom and the hindrances must be dealt with tactfully. Examples of hindrances may be:
	   – *Obsessive doubt of contamination*: The patient may not consent to practice the yoga in the provided mat or in the therapy room.
	   – *Checking compulsion*: The patient may have difficulty in moving ahead with the practice and may continue checking one particular pose for a long time.
	• The optimum duration of 1 hour of session should not be exceeded to accommodate the excessive reassurance seeking or checking compulsions of the patient. If required, the patient may be reassured once or twice and then encouraged to move on with the practice.
	• The yoga practice should be customized to suit the patient's symptoms. The symptoms should be assessed at baseline as well as before every session. *Any worsening should be thoroughly evaluated.* If a practice is likely causing the worsening, that must be modified appropriately. For example, mantra chanting may worsen symptoms in those with musical/humming obsessions. It is imperative to deal with caution.
	• Group sessions may be useful, at least in the later part of the sessions.
	• Caregivers are to be allowed to accompany the patient depending on clinical severity and patient's wish.
	• *Self-efficacy should be encouraged and therapist-dependence to be minimized.*
	• Any positive or negative countertransference in part of the therapist should be managed accordingly so that it does not come in the way of the professional therapist–patient relationship.
	• The therapist may be emotionally exhausted and so it may be a good idea to change the therapist with every new batch of patients.

After the session	• Termination of sessions should be discussed for at least two to three sessions prior to the last one, to prepare the patient • The patient should be educated adequately about do's and don'ts of yoga at home. The plan of further management including follow-ups should be discussed. • Follow-ups to be scheduled according to the clinical status and feasibility. • Every follow-up should contain repeat assessments. Supervised sessions may be conducted if required.

had these repetitive thoughts. The time spent in the obsessions and compulsions gradually increased to a total of 5–6 hours in a day. She tried to distract herself with various activities but to no avail, and her distress continued to increase. There was also significant socio-occupational decline. When she presented to NICY, NIMHANS for yoga therapy, she had been on 20 mg of escitalopram daily for the past 6 weeks.

Yoga therapy was started according to a validated module.[15] After 2 weeks (10 sessions) of individual supervised yoga therapy sessions, she was asked to continue the same for another 20 days at home. After this, she reported significant improvement in multiple domains. Her anxiety reduced considerably and her concentration and confidence improved. In the physical domains, she reported of significantly better flexibility. According to her, yoga practice helped her be calm and gain sufficient motivation to work. She specifically mentioned about ustrasana, ardhachakrasana and all backward bending asanas which helped her get rid of the obsessive thoughts. Nadi shuddhi pranayama was found to reduce her obsessional thoughts, initially only during the session and then up to 2 hours after end of the sessions. Further, she reported improvement in mood and pleasure while practicing the postures and went on to say that yoga contributed to 35% of her improvement. Her preference for yoga was based on her experience of reductions in her obsessions and anxiety, and positive energy inside her body.

Objectively, her scores on the Clinical Global Impression (CGI) scale reduced from 5 to 2, Yale–Brown Obsessive Compulsive Scale (Y-BOCS)-obsession scores from 10 to 4, Y-BOCS-compulsion scores from 10 to 5, Y-BOCS-overall rating from 20 to 9, Hamilton anxiety rating scores from 26 to 11, and Hamilton depression rating scores from 20 to 10. There were also improvements in her yoga self-efficacy scale score (48–92), yoga performance assessment score (19–32) and visual analog score. To summarize, her obsessive symptoms, illness severity, anxiety, sadness, and subjective well-being improved with 1 month of yoga therapy.

REFERENCES

1. Substance Abuse and Mental Health Services Administration (2016). Impact of the DSM-IV to DSM-5 changes on the National Survey on Drug Use and Health: Table 3.13, DSM-IV to DSM-5 obsessive-compulsive disorder comparison. [online] Available from: https://www.ncbi.nlm.nih.gov/books/NBK519704/table/ch3.t13/ [Last accessed September, 2020].
2. Gautham MS, Gururaj G, Varghese M, Benegal V, Rao GN, Kokane A, et al. The National Mental Health Survey of India (2016): prevalence, socio-demographic correlates and treatment gap of mental morbidity. Int J Soc Psychiatry. 2020;66(4):361-72.
3. Pittenger C, Kelmendi B, Bloch M, Krystal JH, Coric V. Clinical treatment of obsessive compulsive disorder. Psychiatry (Edgmont). 2005;2(11):34-43.
4. Shannahoff-Khalsa DS. An introduction to Kundalini yoga meditation techniques that are specific for the treatment of psychiatric disorders. J Altern Complement Med. 2004;10(1):91-101.
5. Varambally S, George S, Gangadhar BN. Yoga for psychiatric disorders: from fad to evidence-based intervention? Br J Psychiatry J Ment Sci. 2020;216(6):291-3.
6. Iyengar B. Light on the Yoga Sutras of Patanjali. London: Aquarian/Thorsons; 1993.
7. Sureshananda S. Yoga Vasishta Sara. Tiruvannamalai: Sri Ramanasramam; 1976.
8. Chinmayananda S. Mandukya Upanishad. Mylapore, Madras: Sri Ramakrishna Math; 1984.
9. Shannahoff-Khalsa DS, Beckett LR. Clinical case report: efficacy of yogic techniques in the treatment of obsessive compulsive disorders. Int J Neurosci. 1996;85(1-2):1-17.
10. Shannahoff-Khalsa DS, Ray LE, Levine S, Gallen CC, Schwartz BJ, Sidorowich JJ. Randomized controlled trial of yogic meditation techniques for patients with obsessive-compulsive disorder. CNS Spectr. 1999;4(12):34-47.
11. Shannahoff-Khalsa D, Fernandes RY, Pereira CA, March JS, Leckman JF, Golshan S, et al. Kundalini yoga meditation versus the relaxation response meditation for treating adults with obsessive-compulsive disorder: a randomized clinical trial. Front Psychiatry. 2019;10:793.

12. Ranjbar F, Broomand M, Akbarzadeh A. The effect of yoga on anxiety symptoms in women with obsessive compulsive disorder. Life Sci J. 2013;10:565-8.
13. Jadad AR, Moore RA, Carroll D, Jenkinson C, Reynolds DJ, Gavaghan DJ, et al. Assessing the quality of reports of randomized clinical trials: is blinding necessary? Control Clin Trials. 1996;17(1):1-12.
14. Balasubramanian SP, Wiener M, Alshameeri Z, Tiruvoipati R, Elbourne D, Reed MW. Standards of reporting of randomized controlled trials in general surgery. Ann Surg. 2006;244(5):663-7.
15. Bhat S, Varambally S, Karmani S, Govindaraj R, Gangadhar BN. Designing and validation of a yoga-based intervention for obsessive compulsive disorder. Int Rev Psychiatry (Abingdon England). 2016;28(3):327-33.
16. Tolahunase MR, Sagar R, Faiq M, Dada R. Yoga- and meditation-based lifestyle intervention increases neuroplasticity and reduces severity of major depressive disorder: a randomized controlled trial. Restor Neurol Neurosci. 2018;36(3):423–42.
17. Bhargav H, George S, Varambally S, Gangadhar BN. Yoga and psychiatric disorders: a review of biomarker evidence. Int Rev Psychiatry. 2020. pp. 1-8.
18. Gard T, Taquet M, Dixit R, Hölzel BK, Dickerson BC, Lazar SW. Greater widespread functional connectivity of the caudate in older adults who practice kripalu yoga and vipassana meditation than in controls. Front Hum Neurosci; 2015. [online] Available from: https://www.frontiersin.org/articles/10.3389/fnhum.2015.00137/full [Last accessed September, 2020].
19. Rubia K. The neurobiology of meditation and its clinical effectiveness in psychiatric disorders. Biol Psychol. 2009;82(1):1-11.
20. Zhang Z, Fan Q, Bai Y, Wang Z, Zhang H, Xiao Z. Brain gamma-aminobutyric acid (GABA) concentration of the prefrontal lobe in unmedicated patients with obsessive-compulsive disorder: a research of magnetic resonance spectroscopy. Shanghai Arch Psychiatry. 2016;28(5):263-70.
21. Sarris J, Camfield D, Berk M. Complementary medicine, self-help, and lifestyle interventions for obsessive compulsive disorder (OCD) and the OCD spectrum: a systematic review. J Affect Disord. 2012;138(3):213-21.
22. Joshi A, De Sousa A. Yoga in the management of anxiety disorders. Sri Lanka J Psychiatry. 2012;3(1):3-9.

CHAPTER 13

Yoga Therapy for Schizophrenia

Elizabeth Visceglia, Rashmi Arasappa, Ramajayam Govindaraj

■ INTRODUCTION

In 1908, Eugen Bleuler coined the term "schizophrenia", which literally means split mind, for an illness previously known as *dementia praecox*. Bleuler closely observed many individuals suffering from this illness and witnessed a loss of unity within their psychic functions and within the personality itself. This disconnect is a fundamental feature of schizophrenia, with patients experiencing a lack of congruence between thought and mood, and between internal experiences and external "reality", resulting in hallucinations and delusions which are pathognomonic of this disorder.

Bleuler could not have imagined how deep these "fissures" go. Currently, schizophrenia is understood as a neurodevelopmental disorder of aberrant connectivity between different networks and areas of the brain, which can result in disordered thought, movement, and perceptual patterns. Recent research has shown that this disconnection exists on multiple levels in schizophrenia—from the neuronal networks, to mental processes, to interpersonal relationships—leading to its description as a "connectopathy".[1] A person with schizophrenia suffers a cascade of disconnectedness: on the cellular/neuronal level, the personal/emotional level, and the social/interpersonal level. Internal and external splitting mirror each other.

Thus, on both a literal and symbolic level, the experience of Yoga (the term is derived from the Sanskrit word *"yuj"* which means to "yoke together" or "unite")—for such patients seems perfectly therapeutic. One of the earliest descriptions of Yoga as per the Ahirbudhnya Upanishad is *"Samyoga yoga ityukto jivatma paramatmanah"* (roughly translated as "Yoga is the union between individual soul and the universal soul"). The *Brihadaranyaka Upanishad* states that in Yoga ".... having become calm and concentrated, one perceives the Self (Atman) within oneself". The ultimate aim of yoga practice as designed by the ancients is to unite the body, mind and the universal consciousness. As a part of this process, achieving unity of body and mind through yoking the breath to the body and mind is a much-needed addition to our current, pharmaceutically-focused approach to schizophrenia. Thus, yoga can begin to heal many divisions and disconnections found in people suffering from schizophrenia.

■ YOGIC PERSPECTIVE OF DISORDER AND MANAGEMENT

In the *Atharva Veda*, health is described as balance between the five elements, *panchabhutas*, which in combinations of two, create the three tendencies or *doshas*. The three *doshas*, *Vata*, *Pitta*, and *Kapha*, control physical and mental function, and an imbalance can manifest in physical or mental illness. Moreover, the three *gunas*, or qualities of personality, *Sattva* (harmony, goodness), *Rajas* (passion, action), and *Tamas* (darkness, chaos), are also present in all things and beings in the world. From a Yogic perspective, schizophrenia can be conceptualized as two aspects of imbalance in the *gunas*: (1) excessive *rajasic* energy, leading to confusing and chaotic mental perceptions, restlessness, and agitation; and (2) excessive *tamasic* energy, resulting in the disconnection, apathy, and depression found in this disorder. The *sattvic guna* of balance is overwhelmed by these imbalances, and the result is an array of "positive symptoms" (hallucinations, delusions, and disorganized speech or behavior) and "negative symptoms" (anhedonia, social withdrawal, flattened affect, and avolition) used as diagnostic criteria in the Diagnostic and Statistical Manual of Mental Disorders, 5th Edition (DSM-5).[2]

From a chakra or yogic energetic perspective, lack of sufficient energy in the grounding lower chakras and excessive energy in the imaginative, creative, perceiving upper chakras can literally pull the energetic body in competing directions, rather than allowing it to function as a unified whole.[3] Patanjali's Yoga Sutras describe vrittis called "viparyaya" and "vikalpa" which can be understood as delusions and loss of touch with reality.

As an antidote to this splitting on multiple levels, Yoga invites mind and body to engage in the same task, with constant attention to the breath, and may begin to heal these internal divisions. Furthermore, many people with schizophrenia suffer from a variety of other mental and physical difficulties, including depression, anxiety, post-traumatic stress disorder (PTSD), hypertension, and diabetes, and there is ample evidence showing the effectiveness of yoga in these disorders.[4-6]

■ YOGA FOR SCHIZOPHRENIA: THE RATIONALE

Schizophrenia is a disorder with dysfunction at cognitive, emotional, and behavioral levels. Disconnect between thoughts, emotions, and action is the hallmark of patients with severe symptoms of schizophrenia.

According to yogic understanding, disease (including schizophrenia) begins as conflict at the level of the mind[7] leading to functional and structural changes in the body including the brain. The final expression of the disease is as symptoms that we come across, such as impaired attention, memory, and executive functions; impaired emotion regulation and social interactions; and poor self-care, hallucinatory behavior, etc.

As per the yogic understanding, the first three layers of consciousness—(1) *Annamaya kosha*, (2) *Pranamaya kosha*, and (3) *Manomaya kosha*, connected with behavior (actions), emotions, and thoughts, respectively, are poorly integrated in schizophrenia. Seen through this paradigm, yoga practice could help in improving the integration of these layers; asana, pranayama, and yoga-based relaxation techniques may help in integrating thoughts, emotions, and behavior through their effect on the three layers of consciousness-mentioned above.

Asana

Asana which involves physical postures, has a definite role in keeping patients engaged with a meaningful physical activity, who otherwise may be lost in their own world of thoughts. Mindful practice of asana involves the individual at all the three levels—(1) thoughts, (2) emotions, and (3) behavior, which are disconnected in patients with schizophrenia. For example, some of the inverted poses (such as *sarvangasana* or shoulder stand, *shashankasana* or rabbit pose) when done comfortably with or without support, help the patient to shunt the excess accumulated prana at the face level (*mukhaprana* which is thought to be excess in patients with schizophrenia) to the floor, leading to balanced prana and hence emotion regulation, giving a sense of good feeling which in turn reflexively regulates thoughts and behavior.

Another key component in asana is mindfulness of changes in body and breath while performing the asana. As per psychological understanding, one of the common problems leading to psychotic symptoms, especially delusion, is the cognitive bias[8] caused by jumping to conclusions. The mindfulness component of asana serves to check this cognitive bias in a generic form, which might get generalized to other areas of functioning. For example, when one holds an asana/posture, usually the reflex mechanism starts immediately to counter the asana/posture secondary to pain or discomfort. But when the mindfulness component is added to asana, the subject develops cognitive control gradually, to hold the pose in spite of the involuntary reflex mechanisms that pushes the body to come out of the asana. Instead of jumping to conclusion and coming out of the posture due to discomfort signaled by the body, one develops the will to resist and hold the pose. This capacity to resist the discomfort and the resulting cognitive flexibility slowly spills over to other spheres of social life also, leading to better social functioning. This is substantiated by some of the recent studies[9,10] with improvement in variables (psychological and biological) related to social cognition.

Pranayama

In healthy volunteers, even simple deep breathing done slowly and mindfully has the capacity to modulate emotions.[11,12] Although many patients find it difficult initially to learn pranayama, once learnt it has profound effects on emotions and thoughts. For patients with schizophrenia, apart from balancing pranayama like *nadi shuddhi*, high-frequency yoga breathing such as *kapalabhati* or *bhastrika*, which improves frontal blood flow, is also helpful to counter the hypofrontality and related cognitive deficits which are common in schizophrenia. Regular practice of pranayama also improves vagal tone, leading to calmness of mind which helps further to regulate thoughts, emotions, and actions.

Yoga-based Relaxation with a Positive Resolve

Thoughts and emotions that are not expressed get accumulated in the form of prana and it gets manifested in the form of dysfunctional behavior (e.g., anger, aggression, etc.). One of the easiest ways to relax physically, emotionally, and mentally is to vocalize some resonating sounds as prescribed in yogic literature. One such common practice is *nadanusandhana* or chanting, A, U, M, and AUM in a tone that the patient feels comfortable. This practice also stimulates the vagal nerve through the auricular branch and has a calming effect on the mind and emotions. Also, adding a positive resolve postrelaxation has deep effect on one's thought process. Positive resolve could be chosen appropriately as per the patients' symptom profile (e.g., "I am competent to ignore the hallucinatory voices and focus on my work" could be a positive resolve).

REVIEW OF LITERATURE

The last decade has seen a substantial increase in research studying the effects of yoga-based interventions in schizophrenia, many of them being randomized controlled trials (RCTs). In one RCT, patients with schizophrenia stabilized on antipsychotics showed improvement in their negative symptoms and social functioning with yoga as compared to exercise or waitlist. Also, improvement in the yoga group was about five times greater than that in the exercise or waitlist groups in terms of negative symptoms.[13] In another RCT, inpatients with schizophrenia in the yoga group showed improvement in severity of illness, and associated symptoms such as anxiety/insight (general psychopathology) and depression. There was an advantage of yoga over exercise in reducing the severity of illness and depression.[14] In another pilot study, improvements in positive symptoms were seen along with the other symptoms improvements as mentioned in above studies.[15] Yoga as an add-on intervention to pharmacotherapy in patients with chronic schizophrenia resulted in greater improvement in items of the Positive and Negative Syndrome Scale (PANSS) compared to pharmacotherapy alone.[16] A review (2012) concluded that yoga helped in reducing psychopathology and also had a positive impact on reducing stress and anxiety symptoms in patients with schizophrenia.[17] Yet another RCT found that the yoga therapy group showed significant improvements in socio-occupational functioning, facial emotion recognition deficits, and increase in oxytocin levels as compared with the waitlist group.[10]

From the above studies, we can conclude that yoga not only helps in improvement of psychotic symptoms but also helps in improving social cognition and socio-occupational functioning. A recent review of eight studies which examined the effects of yoga as compared to standard care in patients with schizophrenia concluded that yoga may be beneficial in improving symptoms, social functioning, and quality of life. However, they added that available evidence was insufficient to draw strong conclusions and called for more systematic research.[18]

Yoga has also been shown to have a positive effect on cognitive functions in patients with schizophrenia. In an RCT conducted among patients with early psychosis, both yoga and aerobic exercise groups demonstrated significant improvements in verbal encoding, short-term memory, long-term memory, and working memory, with moderate to large effect sizes compared to control groups (waitlist). In addition, the yoga group showed significantly enhanced attention and concentration. Significant increases in the thickness of the left superior frontal gyrus and the right inferior frontal gyrus (pars triangularis) were seen in the aerobic exercise group; whereas increased thickness of the postcentral gyrus and the posterior corpus callosum were seen in the yoga group. There was a statistically significant correlation between improvements in working memory and changes in the postcentral gyrus. Both interventions improved memory in patients with early psychosis, with yoga having a superior effect on attention. They also concluded that the observed increments in cortical thickness and volume may indicate increased neurogenesis.[19,20]

In another RCT, speed index (speed of mental processing) of attention domain in the yoga group showed greater improvement than in the physical exercise group after 6 months of training. However, the physical exercise group showed improvement in the accuracy index of attention domain compared to treatment as usual, again after 6 months of intervention. The domains that improved at the 21-day assessment showed continued improvement at the 3- and 6-month assessment points, supporting the notion of a sustained effect from relatively brief interventions. Some domains like abstraction and mental flexibility in the yoga therapy group and spatial memory in the physical exercise group, showed statistically significant improvement only at the 6-month assessment, suggesting incremental improvement. The improvement in cognitive functions at the 6-month assessment with yoga therapy and physical exercise was remarkable, as it was sustained during the unsupervised, post-training period, when compliance was likely to be irregular.[21]

However, there are several practical barriers to yoga as a therapy for patients with schizophrenia. In an RCT conducted by Varambally et al.,[13] more than half of the patients eligible for yoga did not consent to the study. Logistic factors such as the need for daily training under supervision in a specialized center for long periods were the most important barrier that prevented patients with schizophrenia from receiving yoga therapy. Alternative models/schedules that are patient-friendly need be explored further to benefit more patients with schizophrenia.[22]

POSSIBLE MECHANISMS OF ACTION

As discussed above, yoga-based interventions have shown improvements in patients with schizophrenia, and we can postulate why. It seems likely that the regulatory effects of Yoga on the autonomic nervous system are central. People with schizophrenia have a higher baseline level of physiological arousal, where, even under normal conditions, the body is chronically agitated.[23,24] Simultaneously, and related to the splitting characteristic of this disorder, the parasympathetic nervous system is underactive.[25] This hyper-responsiveness to stress can chronically overactivate the sympathetic-adrenal-medullary axis and the hypothalamic-pituitary-adrenal axis. This leads to high rates of production and release of cortisol and epinephrine, the so-called stress hormones, which increase the body's state of alert, heart rate, and respiratory rate. When these hormones are persistently released, they strain the entire mind and body, and can cause ongoing mental and physical distress. Elevated cortisol levels have been found to exacerbate psychotic symptoms in schizophrenia[26] and can interfere with cellular function, leading to dopamine dysregulation,[27] long considered a hallmark of the pathophysiology of schizophrenia.

Yoga, with its lengthened breath cycle and especially its emphasis on longer exhalation, strengthens the parasympathetic nervous system. Breathing with increased airway resistance, as in ujjayi breathing, and with lengthened exhalations are hypothesized to stimulate the vagus nerve[28] and thus activate the parasympathetic nervous system. Breathing exercises alone have been found to be helpful in women with schizophrenia,[29] and yoga may regulate the dysfunctional autonomic system mainly through slower, conscious, and diaphragmatic breathing. Furthermore, Yoga has been shown to improve depressive symptomatology[4] so these practices may also contribute to improvements in the depressive and negative symptoms common in schizophrenia, which are typically worsened by some antipsychotics.[30,31]

Both yoga asana and pranayama are mindful practices, where attention is focused nonjudgmentally on the actions and sensations of the body. Coordination of breath and movement requires ongoing awareness by the practitioner and cultivates the development of interoceptive skills, or the felt sense of the internal body state. Poor interoceptive skills have been linked to low stress resilience,[32] and it can be inferred that improving these skills through cultivating ongoing attention to inner sensations will improve stress resilience, much needed in this often-traumatized population of patients with schizophrenia.[33] The embodied cognition view of Yoga similarly suggests that the felt experience of the body deeply affects the mind, its emotions, and its thoughts.[34]

Other possible mechanisms of action may involve the act of copying the movements and breathing patterns of the instructor during asana practice. Mehta et al. surmise that the activation of the mirror neuron system—as the student follows the teacher and to some extent the other students in the class, creates a connected and resonant state with others.[1] This shared experience may well activate release of oxytocin, the "bonding hormone", important in mother-infant bonding, social relationships, trust and attachment.

A review article looking at putative neurobiological mechanisms of effects of yoga proposed that (1) various styles of meditation may help in strengthening the lateral and medial prefrontal brain networks, thus improving neurocognition and mentalizing abilities, and (2) learning and performing coordinated physical postures with a teacher facilitates imitation and the process of being imitated, which can improve social cognition and empathy through reinforcement of the premotor and parietal mirror neuron system. It was suggested that oxytocin may play a role in mediating these processes leading to better social connectedness and social outcomes.[1,10]

While none of these mechanisms has yet been proven, it is clear from our patients' experiences that Yoga can be an important addition to the treatment of schizophrenia. A student in one of the yoga sessions once said, "Yoga helps me feel my feet touch the ground more", a clear expression of yogic embodiment as an important tool for greater health and well-being in schizophrenia.

PRACTICAL GUIDELINES REGARDING YOGA THERAPY FOR PATIENTS WITH SCHIZOPHRENIA

Although patients with schizophrenia have impairments at thought, emotions, and action levels, it is better to focus more on physical activity-based practices such as asana and pranayama as it would be difficult to manage these patients with only subtle practices such as meditation as one cannot monitor what goes on in the patient's mind. Moreover, patients with schizophrenia have increased levels of dopamine in certain brain areas, and meditation also has been shown to increase brain dopamine levels. Hence it is better to avoid practices which involve intense focusing such as long periods of meditation that might further increase dopamine and worsen psychotic symptoms. If there is a need to learn meditation, it is advisable to practice only under the supervision of the treating psychiatrist and a trained yoga instructor.

Although the term Yoga implies a comprehensive lifestyle rather than a set of prescribed practices, in a therapeutic setting it is good to have a defined set of practices as per the patient's need. Of course, it has to be flexible to be modified as and when required. Practices must be chosen carefully after considering other medical and psychiatric comorbidities which tend to be common in these patients. **Appendix 1.4** provides a validated yoga module for schizophrenia.

CASE VIGNETTE

Mr A, 27-year-old, was brought to the psychiatric hospital, because on several occasions he had become violent toward his father. For a few weeks he had reported hearing of voices when nobody was around. The voices eventually ceased, but he then adopted a strange way of living. He would sit up all night, sleep all day, and become very angry when his father tried to get him out of his bed. He did not shave or wash for weeks, smoked continuously and ate very irregularly.

In the hospital, he showed a complete lack of concern for anything that happened around him. He kept himself alone as much as possible and conversed very little with patients or the staffs. He was described as careless, disinterested in everything including eating, dressing, sleep, personal hygiene. He refused to participate in any kind of regular activity.

Working strategy:
For patients like Mr A in the case vignette, it is important to assess how cooperative the patient would be to practice yoga. If the patient poses a threat to self and others due to their symptoms, it is advised to teach yoga after stabilization with antipsychotic medications for 3–4 weeks. Even if the patient is cooperative, it is common for patients with schizophrenia to slip into their inner world easily. So, keeping them grounded physically with Surya namaskar and asana is important, before one starts teaching pranayama and yoga-based relaxation techniques. As the patient makes progress in practice, the component of mindfulness during yoga practice can be emphasized gradually. For reasons explained earlier, intense and long meditation practices are best avoided for patients with schizophrenia.

A suggested yoga module for patients with schizophrenia:
Loosening practices, Surya Namaskar, Vakrasana, Ustrasana, Bhujangasana, Shalabhasana, Dhanurasana, Viparitakarani/sarvangasana, Matsyasana, Bhastrika, Nadi shuddhi, Quick relaxation technique, Nadanusandhana.

Clinical Insights: Yoga Therapy for Schizophrenia

Prior to the session	• Patients with schizophrenia may get angry or disruptive without external provocation or show unprovoked aggression. The therapist should understand that this is a part of their illness and needs to be very patient while dealing with this population. • Suicidal ideas should be assessed. The caregiver should be encouraged to accompany the patient and preferably to practice with the patient. • Avoid talking to caregivers separately in front of the patient. Let the patient feel that he/she is important. This may improve adherence. • Critical comments from caregivers should not be encouraged and the patient should be given positive reinforcement on his efforts to practice yoga. • Some medications may cause postural hypotension which may lead to dizziness on suddenly getting up from sitting or lying down postures. Patients should be asked whether they have such symptoms. If yes, the practices should be modified accordingly.
During the session	• *The therapist should never touch the patient without prior consent.* • The therapist should always give clear instructions to a patient by addressing him/her by name. • Due to medications, the patient may be drowsy and thus *loud, slow, and clear instructions should be given using the name of the patient* to keep them aware of the practice. • Practices involving long-term closure of the eyes, sitting without doing anything for a longer time, focused meditations should be avoided. • Some medications may cause stiffness and trembling of hands. In such cases, the initial yoga practice should aim toward joint-loosening, and postures that require extra flexibility must be avoided. • Some patients may show inappropriate behavior or gestures during the sessions. The therapist should understand that this is a part of the illness and should not take offence.
After the session	• The patient should be encouraged to learn the practices by slowly focusing on self-practice with prompting only when necessary. • Caregivers should ideally be taught the same module and should be asked to motivate the patient by practicing with him/her.

*These practices have been validated for content by experts from Yoga philosophy, Yoga therapy, Psychology, and Psychiatry, and found feasible as well as efficacious in patients with schizophrenia. Full details on the validated yoga module may be found in the article by Govindaraj et al.[35] The validated yoga module for schizophrenia is provided in **Appendix 1.4**.*

REFERENCES

1. Mehta UM, Keshavan MS, Gangadhar BN. Bridging the schism of schizophrenia through yoga: review of putative mechanisms. Int Rev Psychiatry. 2016;28(3):254-64.
2. American Psychiatric Association. Diagnostic and Statistical Manual of Mental Disorders: DSM-5. Arlington, VA: American Psychiatric Association; 2013.
3. Judith A. Eastern Body, Western Mind: Psychology and the Chakra System As a Path to the Self. Berkeley, CA: Celestial Arts; 2004.
4. Cramer H, Lauche R, Langhorst J, Dobos G. Yoga for depression: a systematic review and meta-analysis. Depress Anxiety. 2013;30(11):1068-83.
5. Justice L, Brems C. Bridging body and mind: case series of a 10-week trauma-informed yoga protocol for veterans. Int J Yoga Ther. 2019;29(1):65-79.
6. Tyagi A, Cohen M. Yoga and hypertension: a systematic review. Altern Ther Health Med. 2014;20(2):32-59.
7. Nagendra HR. Yoga for Promotion of Positive Health. Bengaluru, India: Swami Vivekananda Yoga Prakashana; 2004.
8. Dudley R, Taylor P, Wickham S, Hutton P. Psychosis, delusions and the "jumping to conclusions" reasoning bias: a systematic review and meta-analysis. Schizophr Bull. 2016;42(3):652-65.
9. Govindaraj R, Naik S, Manjunath NK, Mehta UM, Gangadhar BN, Varambally S. Add-on yoga therapy for social cognition in schizophrenia: a pilot study. Int J Yoga. 2018;11(3):242-4.
10. Jayaram N, Varambally S, Behere RV, Venkatasubramanian G, Arasappa R, Christopher R, et al. Effect of yoga therapy on plasma oxytocin and facial emotion recognition deficits in patients of schizophrenia. Indian J Psychiatry. 2013;55(Suppl 3):S409-13.
11. Homma I, Masaoka Y. Breathing rhythms and emotions. Exp Physiol. 2008;93(9):1011-21.

12. Boiten FA. The effects of emotional behaviour on components of the respiratory cycle. Biol Psychol. 1998;49(1-2):29-51.
13. Varambally S, Gangadhar BN, Thirthalli J, Jagannathan A, Kumar S, Venkatasubramanian G, et al. Therapeutic efficacy of add-on yogasana intervention in stabilized outpatient schizophrenia: randomized controlled comparison with exercise and waitlist. Indian J Psychiatry. 2012;54(3):227-32.
14. Manjunath RB, Varambally S, Thirthalli J, Basavaraddi IV, Gangadhar BN. Efficacy of yoga as an add-on treatment for in-patients with functional psychotic disorder. Indian J Psychiatry. 2013;55(Suppl 3):S374-8.
15. Visceglia E, Lewis S. Yoga therapy as an adjunctive treatment for schizophrenia: a randomized, controlled pilot study. J Altern Complement Med. 2011;17(7):601-7.
16. Paikkatt B, Singh AR, Singh PK, Jahan M, Ranjan JK. Efficacy of yoga therapy for the management of psychopathology of patients having chronic schizophrenia. Indian J Psychiatry. 2015;57(4):355-60.
17. Tsui MC. Review of the effects of yoga on people with schizophrenia. J Yoga Phys Ther. 2012; S1-001.
18. Broderick J, Knowles A, Chadwick J, Vancampfort D. Yoga versus standard care for schizophrenia. Cochrane Database Syst Rev. 2015;(10):CD010554.
19. Lin J. The impacts of aerobic exercise and mind-body exercise (yoga) on neuro-cognition and clinical symptoms in early psychosis: a single-blind randomized controlled clinical trial (Thesis). Pokfulam, Hong Kong SAR: University of Hong Kong; 2013.
20. Lin J, Chan S, Lee E, Chang WC, Tse M, Su W, et al. Aerobic exercise and yoga improve neurocognitive function in women with early psychosis. NPJ Schizophr. 2015;1:15047.
21. Bhatia T, Mazumdar S, Wood J, He F, Gur RE, Gur RC, et al. A randomised controlled trial of adjunctive yoga and adjunctive physical exercise training for cognitive dysfunction in schizophrenia. Acta Neuropsychiatr. 2017;29(2):102-14.
22. Baspure S, Jagannathan A, Kumar S, Varambally S, Thirthalli J, Venkatasubramanain G, et al. Barriers to yoga therapy as an add-on treatment for schizophrenia in India. Int J Yoga. 2012;5(1):70-3.
23. Zahn TP, Carpenter Jr WT, McGlashan TH. Autonomic nervous system activity in acute schizophrenia: I. method and comparison with normal controls. Arch Gen Psychiatry. 1981;38(3):251-8.
24. Zahn TP, Carpenter WT Jr, McGlashan TH. Autonomic nervous system activity in acute schizophrenia: II. relationships to short-term prognosis and clinical state. Arch Gen Psychiatry. 1981;38(3):260-6.
25. Toichi M, Kubota Y, Murai T, Kamio Y, Sakihama M, Toriuchi T, et al. The influence of psychotic states on the autonomic nervous system in schizophrenia. Int J Psychophysiol. 1999;31(2):147-54.
26. Walker E, Mittal V, Tessner K. Stress and the hypothalamic pituitary adrenal axis in the developmental course of schizophrenia. Annu Rev Clin Psychol. 2008;4:189-216.
27. Mizoguchi K, Shoji H, Ikeda R, Tanaka Y, Tabira T. Persistent depressive state after chronic stress in rats is accompanied by HPA axis dysregulation and reduced prefrontal dopaminergic neurotransmission. Pharmacol Biochem Behav. 2008;91(1):170-5.
28. Brown RP, Gerbarg PL, Muskin PR. Yogic breathing, Sudarshan Kriya for treatment of depression, anxiety, stress, PTSD, aggression, and violence. In: Tasman A, Kay J, Lieberman J (Ed). Psychiatry, 2nd edition. New York: John Wiley and Sons; 2003.
29. Sageman S. Breaking through the despair: spiritually oriented group therapy as a means of healing women with severe mental illness. J Am Acad Psychoanal Dyn Psychiatry. 2004;32(1): 125-41.
30. Bressan RA, Costa DC, Jones HM, Ell PJ, Pilowsky LS. Typical antipsychotic drugs—D2 receptor occupancy and depressive symptoms in schizophrenia. Schizophr Res. 2002;56(1):31-6.
31. Artaloytia JF, Arango C, Lahti A, Sanz J, Pascual A, Cubero P, et al. Negative signs and symptoms secondary to antipsychotics: a double-blind, randomized trial of a single dose of placebo, haloperidol, and risperidone in healthy volunteers. Am J Psychiatry. 2006;163(3):488-93.
32. Haase L, Stewart JL, Youssef B, May AC, Isakovic S, Simmons AN, et al. When the brain does not adequately feel the body: links between low resilience and interoception. Biol Psychol. 2016;113:37-45.
33. Read J, van Os J, Morrison AP, Ross CA. Childhood trauma, psychosis and schizophrenia: a literature review with theoretical and clinical implications. Acta Psychiatr Scand. 2005;112(5):330-50.
34. Varela FJ, Thompson E, Rosch E. The Embodied Mind: Cognitive Science and Human Experience. Cambridge, MA: MIT Press; 1991. p. 308.
35. Govindaraj R, Varambally S, Sharma M, Gangadhar BN. Designing and validation of a yoga-based intervention for schizophrenia. Int Rev Psychiatry. 2016;28(3):323-6.

CHAPTER 14

Evidence for Efficacy of Yoga in Geriatric Psychiatry

Palanimuthu T Sivakumar, Shiva Shanker Reddy Mukku, Hariprasad VR, BV Kathyayani

■ INTRODUCTION

Geriatric psychiatry is the branch of psychiatry which deals with the mental health care of older adults (aged 60 years and above). The number of older adults is increasing globally. The population of older adults in India grew from 25 million in 1950 to 104 million in 2011. Furthermore, it is projected to reach 150 million by 2025 and 300 million by 2050.[1] Psychiatric disorders are common in older adults. Nearly one-fourth of older adults suffer from either common or severe mental health problems.[2] The prevalence of psychiatric morbidity in rural older adults was found to be 23.7%, with mood disorders being the most common (7.6%), followed by mild cognitive impairment (MCI) (4.6%), mental and substance use disorders (4.0%), and dementia (2.8%).[2] In urban areas, the prevalence ranges from 19.3 to 49.2%.[2,3] A much higher proportion of older adults have subsyndromal illness or only a few symptoms. Mental health issues in older adults could either be of late-onset (after 60 years of age) or early-onset beginning in younger age and persisting into late-life. They are likely to result in significant disability, poor quality of life, increased dependency, high caregiver burden, and increase the risk for institutionalization. Mental health issues in older adults are under-recognized and undertreated due to decreased awareness and misattribution of symptoms as part of normal aging. They require comprehensive and holistic management to improve the health and well-being of older adults. Yoga is emerging as a potentially useful therapeutic tool in the management of mental health issues in older adults.

■ YOGA FOR THE TREATMENT OF GERIATRIC PSYCHIATRIC DISORDERS

Tracing its origins to early Vedic texts, Yoga as a metaphysical practice is revered in most of Indian classical literature. From rudimentary ideas or practices found in Indus Valley civilization artifacts, over the years, Yoga has evolved into a systematic practice of psychophysical healing, leading one to liberation, guiding the practitioners in ethics, diet, health, and progress toward enlightened embodiment.[4] With the human body and mind as a means to reach higher states of consciousness, ensuring its health meant success in the spiritual journey. Yoga was hence transformed into a therapeutic tool to ensure a healthy body and mind. The Yogic therapeutic paradigm encompasses teachings from various classical and medieval Hathayogic texts, viz., *Patanjali's Yoga Sutra, Bhagavad Gita, Upanishads, Hatha Ratnavali, Hatha Yoga Pradipika, Gheranda Samhita,* and *Yoga Rahasya*. While the *Yoga Sutras of Patanjali* provide a framework for this comprehensive system of psychosomatic healing, *Upanishads and Bhagavad Gita* advise a yogic way of life with virtues emphasizing detachment, devotion, nonviolence, austerity, compassion, sensory withdrawal, cleanliness, contentment, hard work, and other ethical actions to overcome the agitated mind. Similarly, *Shatkarma* practices (six purificatory techniques) detoxify the body, *asana* (bodily postures) provides strength to the body; *mudra* (yogic gestures), *pranayama* (breathing practices), *pratyahara* (sensory withdrawal), *dhyana* (meditation), and *samadhi* give steadiness, lightness, calmness, perception of self and freedom, respectively.

Classical Indian literature emphasizes aging as a natural and inevitable part of one's life, affecting physical, psychological and social dimensions of health, equating it with the natural disease (*Swabhavaja vyadhi*). Terms *Jara* or *Vardhakya* etymologically denote all-round degeneration under the influence of aging. The *Vriddhavastha* is characterized by decay in *dhatus* (bodily tissues), declining ability of sensory and motor organs, decreasing digestion and metabolism, loss of luster of the skin, appearance of wrinkles on the skin, graying of hairs, deteriorating mental and cognitive abilities, osteoporosis, diminishing immunity, potency and strength. Aging changes may also appear untimely under the influence of imbalanced bioenergies (*dosha*) as a result of illness affecting growth and immunity (e.g., *Rajayakshma*), excessive indulgence in improper diet, unhealthy sleep practices, and not adhering to health promoting daily and seasonal regimens. Ayurveda, an ancient medicinal system dedicates a therapeutic specialization known as "*Rasayana*" to prevent untimely aging, restore youth, provide positive health and help prolong life.[5,6]

Although there is no explicit yoga practice recipe for healthy aging in yogic texts, the achievements underlined for the dedicated practice of Hatha yoga highlights its importance in healthy and successful aging. In addition, some of the practices, viz., *Viparita karani, Paschimottanasana, Matsyendrasana, Surya Bhedana pranayama*, etc., were revered classically for their ability to restore youth and delay aging.

■ RATIONALE FOR USE OF YOGA IN THE MANAGEMENT OF GERIATRIC PSYCHIATRIC DISORDERS

Lifestyle measures such as regular physical activity, cognitive activities, and social engagement are considered useful and effective therapeutic interventions for mental health conditions in older adults such as depression, anxiety, and neurocognitive disorders. Recent studies have indicated the efficacy of multidomain interventions including physical and cognitive activity for improving the cognitive function in those at high risk for dementia.[7] Yoga as a mind-body intervention has demonstrated its clinical effectiveness in mental health conditions such as depression, anxiety, schizophrenia, and MCI.[8-11] Yoga is also found useful in the management of diabetes, hypertension, and cardiovascular diseases in addition to standard treatments.[12,13]

Older adults have high rates of chronic medical conditions such as diabetes, hypertension, cardiovascular diseases, osteoarthritis, etc., and they are likely to be on multiple medications, contributing to significant risk for drug interactions. They also have high sensitivity for adverse effects to psychotropic medications. In view of this, yoga can be considered as a potentially useful nonpharmacological intervention in the management of mental health conditions in older adults. In patients with moderate and severe mental illness, yoga can be used as an adjuvant intervention along with other standard mental health interventions. In patients with mild mental health disorders and symptoms below the clinical threshold, yoga could be considered as a monotherapy if the patient prefers this treatment method. Yoga also has a potential role in promoting positive mental health and preventing mental health issues in older adults.

EVIDENCE BASE FOR YOGA IN OLDER ADULTS WITH PSYCHIATRIC ILLNESS

The evidence for yoga in older adults with psychiatric illness comes mostly from observational studies and a few controlled studies. A study by Manjunath et al. looked at the effectiveness of yoga in sleep among older adults compared to waitlist group. Yoga intervention was given for 6 months and assessments were done at the end of 3 and 6 months. Patients who received the Yoga intervention showed improvements in sleep latency, total sleep duration, and self-rated sleep quality.[14] In an intervention study by Krishnamurthy et al., yoga was used as a treatment for geriatric depression in 69 older adults. Yoga was compared to ayurveda and waitlist control group. The geriatric depression scores improved in the Yoga group compared to Ayurveda group and waitlist group.[10] In another observational study, Siddarth et al. reported that older adults who received Yoga intervention showed improvement in mood state, mental health, and sleep compared to those who received aerobic exercises.[15] Hariprasad et al. developed a yoga module for older adults based on traditional and contemporary literature. This Yoga module was reviewed by experts in yoga and appropriate modifications were done.[16] Details of this module of yoga-based intervention is provided in **Appendix 1.6**. In a randomized controlled study, yoga-based intervention was found to be effective in improving cognitive functions in residents of elderly homes. In this randomized controlled trial (RCT), older adults were randomized to yoga ($n = 62$) and waitlist groups ($n = 43$). Subjects were assessed pre- and postintervention using neuropsychological tests. Yoga-based intervention was given for 6 months. The study reported improvements in verbal memory, visual memory, fluency, working memory, and executive functions compared to waitlist group.[9] In another study from the same sample, it was also reported that older adults in the yoga group showed improvements in quality of life and sleep quality compared to the waitlist group.[17]

One of the first RCTs related to yoga in older adults was by Oken et al. comparing yoga, exercise, and waitlist groups in 135 patients. There were improvements in quality of life, energy levels, and fatigue levels. However, there was no improvement in cognition, with either yoga or exercise.[18] In another study, yoga was compared with exercise in older adults and they found improvements in depressive symptoms, pain and fatigue in both groups with greater improvement in the yoga group.[19] A systematic review analyzed the impact of yoga in physical mobility of older adults. This review included six trials and a total of 307 older adults and noted that yoga improved physical mobility and balance with moderate effect size.[20] In an RCT, yoga was investigated as a treatment for depression in older adults compared to waitlist group. They demonstrated improvement in depression, anxiety, and self-esteem scores in the yoga group as compared to the waitlist group.[21] In another systematic review combining 27 studies on the effects of yoga on physical health and related quality of life found improvements in physical health as well as health-related quality of life.[22] A recent study looked at the experiences of older adults with depression participating in mindful Yoga. The prominent themes which emerged were "improved in physical status", "actively involved in the community", "positive psychological effects", and "perceived therapeutic ingredients".[23] Another ongoing RCT, is comparing yoga with cognitive behavioral therapy (CBT) for late-life worry, anxiety symptoms, and sleep disturbances.[24] **(Table 1).**

POSSIBLE MECHANISMS OF YOGA

Yoga is a holistic and multidimensional practice involving specific body postures (asana), breathing techniques (pranayama),

TABLE 1: Studies on yoga and elderly.

Author	Design and setting	Objective	Sample size	Intervention	Results
Manjunath NK et al., 2005	Observational study	Effect of yoga vs. ayurveda vs. waitlist group on sleep in older adults	Total no. = 120 Assessed at 3 and 6 months	Yoga group shown significant decrease in sleep latency, hours slept	Improvement in self-rated sleep
Oken BS et al., 2006	Randomized controlled trial (RCT)	To determine the effect of yoga on cognition, mood, quality of life, and fatigue	N = 135 Yoga vs. exercise vs. waitlist group	There was no effect on cognition with yoga or exercise	Improvement in quality of life and energy level
Krishnamurthy MN and Telles S, 2007	RCT in elderly homes	Effects of yoga and ayurveda on geriatric depression	N = 69 (three groups—yoga, ayurveda, and waitlist control)	Physical postures, relaxation techniques, regulated breathing, devotional songs, and lectures	Depression scores significantly reduced in Yoga group at 3 and 6 months compared to other groups
Hariprasad VR et al., 2013	RCT, elderly homes	Compared the effect of yoga vs. waitlist group on sleep and quality of life	Yoga (n = 62) Waitlist (n = 58) Duration of 6 months	Yoga module developed for older adults delivered as group intervention for 6 months	Yoga group shown improvement in quality of life and sleep quality
Hariprasad VR et al., 2013	RCT, elderly homes	Compared the effect of yoga vs. waitlist group on cognitive function	Yoga (n = 62) Waitlist group (n = 58) Duration of 6 months	Yoga module developed for older adults delivered as group intervention for 6 months	Improvement in verbal, visual memory, working memory, executive function, processing speed in yoga group
Siddarth D et al., 2014	Observational study in community dwelling middle aged and older adults	Effect of Yoga or Tai chi vs. aerobic exercise on mental health and sleep	Yoga (n = 8) Tai chi (n = 12) Aerobic exercise (n = 22)	Twice a week group intervention for 60 minutes	Participants in Yoga and Tai chi have better mood, mental health and sleep compared to aerobic exercise group
Yagli NV et al., 2015	Interventional	Compare yoga vs. exercise	N = 10 in each group	Yoga—8 sessions Exercise—8 sessions	Quality of life, Nottingham health profile, depression, pain, fatigue improved postintervention in both the group. But more reduction of scores in yoga group

Contd...

Contd...

Author	Design and setting	Objective	Sample size	Intervention	Results
Youkhana S et al., 2016	Systematic review	To study the impact of yoga on physical mobility in older adults	Six trials N = 307	Yoga-based exercise had a medium effect on balance performance (g = 0.40, 95% CI: 0.15–0.65)	Medium effect on physical mobility (Hedges' g = 0.50, 95% CI: 0.06–0.95)
Ramanathan M et al., 2017	RCT	Yoga vs. waitlist group	Total no. = 40	Yoga—60-minute session twice weekly for 12 weeks	There was reduction in HAS, HRDS score and improvement in self-esteem scores
Sivaramakrishnan D et al., 2019	Systematic review	Effect of yoga on physical and health related quality of life	27 studies	Yoga improved physical function	Health-related quality of life outcomes
Lee KC et al., 2019	Qualitative study, outpatients	To explore the experiences of older adults with depression participating in a mindful yoga intervention group	N = 9	Themes emerged are—"improved physical status", "actively involved in the community", "positive psychological effects", "perceived therapeutic ingredients", "facilitators of practicing mindful yoga", and "barriers to practicing mindful yoga	

(HAS: Hamilton Anxiety Scale; HDRS: Hamilton Depression Rating Scale)

yogic gestures and energy locks (bandha and mudra), meditative techniques (dharana and dhyana), chanting (mantra), devotion (bhakti), and selfless service (seva). It is aimed at treating the person as a whole and empowering the individual toward positive health. As per traditional texts, the mechanism by which these yogic practices work may be summarized as: (1) restoring homeostasis in state of bioenergies, digestion and metabolism, bodily tissues, and excretory functions which get deranged due to disease, unhealthy lifestyle, and aging; (2) reducing agitations of the mind and improving a sense of well-being; (3) removing obstructions in subtle pranic channels (aka nadis) and promote healthy circulation of bioenergies; and (4) nourishing and strengthening the body tissues and promoting *Ojas* (immunity).

Kuntsevich and colleagues (2010) provide a similar rationale behind the mechanisms of action of yoga, which include: (1) assisting restoration of physiological imbalance to normality postinjury or disease; (2) promoting homeostasis in molecular and cellular interactions; (3) quenching abnormal "noise" in cellular and molecular signaling networks due to biological and environmental stress. This is said to be achieved through influencing various cell signaling molecules, nervous system functions, modulating psychoneuroimmunological responses, and bioelectromagnetism.

The ability of yoga/yogic practices to improve strength, balance, and flexibility is very important especially in the elderly for improving gait and reducing the risk of falls. This in turn instils confidence and imparts a sense of well-being in the elderly, eliciting positive psychoneuroimmunological responses. Studies have shown that physical activity, relaxation, and CBTs augment cell immune competence in elderly.[25,26] While Yogic practices such as breathing exercises improve natural killer cells, mindfulness-based stress reduction programs restore natural killer activity, and cytokine levels to healthy levels among patients affected by immune dysregulation. This is important as immune functions are badly affected due to aging, stress, and depression, resulting in greater susceptibility to diseases especially infections, autoimmune disorders, and neoplasm in elderly.[27,28] Effects of yoga and its effect on nervous system activity have been widely studied. Heart rate variability studies have shown that yogic practices, especially pranayama and meditation increase vagal tone. This effect could play a crucial role in modulating the body's inflammatory response to infections, physical and psychosocial stress. Also, evidence suggests that yogic practices reduce sympathetic outflow, promote parasympathetic activation, and improve baroreflex sensitivity thus helping to restore cardiovascular functions in the elderly.[27,28]

Aging leads to a decline in cognitive functioning. Memory functions (working memory, long-term memory, associative, spatial, prospective memory), processing speed, and executive functions (attention, inhibition, and interference) undergo age-related decline. Reduction in brain volume, cortical thickness, ventricular dilatation, loss of neural bodies in the neocortex, hippocampus, cerebellum, reduction in synaptic density, and neurofibrillary tangles are often associated with aging. Yoga and similar mind-body practices are known to improve various cognitive functions such as memory, executive functions and processing speed and neuroimaging studies such as functional magnetic resonance imaging (fMRI) confirm the increased activity of corresponding brain regions. Structural imaging studies have shown the ability of yoga to improve age-related volumetric changes in the brain, especially the hippocampus, a key part of the brain involved in memory encoding which is often affected in elderly with MCI and Alzheimer's disease.[29-31] Both in health and in illness, signaling molecules such as hormones, neurotransmitters, growth factors, neuropeptides, eicosanoids, cytokines, chemokines, and adipokines play a key role in transmitting information between cells and tissues. Studies in recent years have tried eliciting the effects of yogic practices on such signaling molecules. Brain-derived neurotrophic factor (BDNF) is one such growth factor which has been extensively studied with reference to cognition in elderly. Serum BDNF levels are found to increase with yoga, meditation, and other body-mind exercises.[32,33] Due to its ability to facilitate neural repair, promote synaptic plasticity, neurogenesis and enhance memory and learning, improving BDNF levels in the elderly could contribute to preserving cognition. Another signaling molecule of importance is melatonin, which is a hormone released by the pineal gland. In addition to maintaining circadian rhythm, melatonin acts as an antioxidant and prevents cell damage in metabolic, neurodegenerative, and aging conditions. Yogic practices and meditation have been found to activate the pineal gland and increase levels of circulating melatonin.[27,28] It is evident from both traditional and conventional understandings that yoga through its different psychosomatic and social components works simultaneously at multiple levels to evoke comprehensive psychophysiological and biochemical responses toward overall well-being.

YOGA MODULE FOR OLDER ADULTS

*A simple, easy-to-do and yet comprehensive yoga program designed exclusively for the older adults is shown in **Appendix 1.6** of the book.* The program is designed based on the teachings of traditional Yogic texts, validated by experts and customized to the needs and abilities of older adults. The program takes cues from yogic practices which are revered in classical treatises for their ability to slow down the effects of aging including cognitive decline; promote emotional and mental calmness; improve metabolism, overall health, and quality of life. The module incorporates all key elements of yoga, viz., *Sukshma vyayama* (loosening/warm up exercises), *Asana* (physical postures), *Pranayama* (breathing exercises), and *Dhyana* (meditation) for promoting well-being across different spheres of existence (*Pancha kosha*), from gross to transcendental. Emphasis is laid on following the given sequence, ease into postures with comfort, synchronized breathing and self-awareness in order to avoid injuries, elevate the experience and maximize the benefit. The Yoga program avoids complex, advanced, and balancing postures, as well as yogic practices generally avoided in cardiovascular, cerebrovascular, and uncontrolled hypertension conditions. The suitability of the yogic practices is further ensured by modifying some of the postures and by encouraging the use of appropriate props to overcome physical limitations experienced by the older adults.[16]

This Yoga module has undergone rigorous scrutiny and validation by experts belonging to different schools of yoga, for its appropriateness and usefulness in older adults. Further, study using this yoga program has confirmed its usefulness in improving several domains of cognitive function, sleep, and quality of life among elderly living in residential care.

CHAIR YOGA

Some of the older adults are likely to have physical limitations to practice usual practices of yoga. Recent studies have systematically evaluated *"Chair Yoga"* as a practice of yoga with suitable adaptations that are usually required in older adults with physical limitations. It is practiced using a chair as a support, either seated or standing, it aims to simplify the yoga practice without the need for any specialized equipment or large space. Though different Yoga schools have designed own unique way of practice, but generally most of the chair yoga routines encompass basic tenets of yogic practices involving physical postures, breathing exercises, deep relaxation, meditation, and self-awareness.[34]

Chair yoga has demonstrated clinical benefits on several physical measures that are relevant for mental health and well-being of older adults. Improvement in gait speed, pain interference and fatigue in older adults with osteoarthritis has been shown with chair yoga.[35] Studies have also shown positive benefits of chair yoga on measures such as reduced fear of falling, physical fitness, stress hormones levels, improvement in handgrip strength, muscle strength in upper and lower limb, static balance, agility, dynamic balance, sense of well-being, and prevention of functional decline.[36-38] Few studies have indicated the benefits of chair yoga on behavioral measures such as stress frequency and severity, anxiety, depression, and quality of life in older adults.[39,40] The benefits of chair yoga to improve physical measures in older adults with Alzheimer's dementia have also been demonstrated.[41]

SPECIAL INSTRUCTIONS FOR ELDERLY

- Consult your doctor before taking up yoga sessions.
- Discuss with the yoga therapist about your existing health conditions.
- Customization may be needed for individuals, especially those suffering from herniated disk, glaucoma, arthritis, and heart problems.

- Know your limits and do not exert undue pressure or push yourself too hard while attempting yoga postures.
- Do not hurry; take enough time to complete yogic postures.
- Follow the sequence of yogic practices as advised.
- Place of practice should be preferably quiet and well-ventilated.
- Wear loose fitting and comfortable clothing. Remove spectacles (if possible), wristwatches, and jewelry.
- Empty your bladder and bowel before the practice.
- Yoga may be practiced at anytime of the day. Morning practice on empty stomach, helps invigorate and prepares for the entire day. However, yoga practice at evenings comes easier and helps to relax and energize from day's stress and strain. Choose a suitable time for your practice as per your convenience.
- Do not practice Yoga, especially asana and pranayama immediately after food. Give at least 3–4 hours of gap after major meal.
- If there is excessive pain in any part of the body, practice should be terminated immediately and medical advice should be sought.

CHALLENGES IN YOGA FOR OLDER ADULTS

There are a few challenges in effectively utilizing Yoga among older adults. Older adults with severe or decompensated physical illness cannot practice Yoga similar to any other physical activity. Yoga requires maintaining postures and asanas. Many older adults usually have stiffening of spine and joints due to osteoarthritis and other age-related changes, which might increase the difficulty initially. Apart from this, many older adults have giddiness and balance-related problems which again increase the difficulty of practicing yoga initially. Older adults may also have sensory impairments such as hearing loss and visual impairment which can interfere with learning yoga by observation and listening to instructions. Among other relevant things, cognitive impairment which if moderate to severe will interfere with learning Yoga. Finally, the learning curve for yoga may last from few weeks to months and might be even longer in older adults. The benefits of yoga may not be apparent in the initial few sessions. This might lead to early drop out in older adults with yoga. These are some of the challenges with yoga in older adults. However, the Yoga module can be successfully adapted to suit older adults with use of additional support and props. Selected components of the Yoga module that are feasible can be used in older adults having limitations for some of the components. The limitations and challenges for Yoga therapy are equally applicable to other forms of physical exercise and other mind-body interventions.

CONCLUSION

Increase in older adult population is worldwide phenomenon, which is also becoming evident in India. Older adults due to their various vulnerable factors are at higher risk of mental illnesses. Mental illnesses in older adults are related to cerebral neurodegeneration, medical comorbidities, and psychosocial factors. Mental illnesses in older adults lead to decreased quality of life, higher utilization of health services, increased dependency and institutionalization, and premature mortality. Apart from standard methods of treatment for mental illness in older adults, there is felt need for methods for holistic management in older adults. In this pursuit, many cultural-based traditional systems of therapy were tried and one among them is yoga. Yoga is a mind-body based therapy with its origins traceable to ancient Vedic literature. Positive impact of yoga in practicing older adults reported with chronic medical illness. Research on older adults with mental health issues reported effectiveness in preventing mental health issues in older adults. It is also reported to have therapeutic effects on depression and sleep in older adults. Few studies reported improvement in cognitive functioning in older adults at risk of dementia. Evidence shows that yoga regularizes the neuroendocrine systems, circadian rhythm, increases the parasympathetic activity and protects certain regions from neurodegeneration. Yoga due to wider availability and acceptability has the potential to be used for treatment of subsyndromal disorders and as an add treatment to standard therapy in severe mental illness in older adults.

■ CASE VIGNETTE

Mr S, a 62-year-old retired banker, presented with symptoms of feeling low and fatigued on

	Clinical Insights: Yoga Therapy for the Elderly with Mild Cognitive Impairment (MCI) or Early Stages of Dementia
Prior to the session	• Make a note of comorbid medical conditions such as hypertension, heart diseases, diabetes, arthritis, etc., avoid contraindicated practices. • Make a note of medications which a patient may be taking. Remain aware of the fact that the geriatric population is more prone to develop side effects due to the medications. Modify practices accordingly (e.g., antihypertensives, antidepressants or benzodiazepines may cause adverse effects such as electrolyte imbalance or postural hypotension, etc.). Dizziness may be a presenting complaint. In that case, sudden standing up from sitting or lying down practice should be avoided, forward-backward bending should be avoided, fast breathing practices should be avoided. • *Avoid raising the hands above the head level* and acute forward bends for patients with *known cardiac disorders*. • *Avoid forward bends* in patients with *low back pain*. • *Avoid raising the hands up and down during Bhastrika in patients with neck pain*. • *Kapalabhati practice should be done cautiously* not exceeding 40 strokes per minute. • Keep a gentle but firm attitude, become a student of your elderly patient in order to teach him/her and try to avoid authoritative instructions. • Patients with dementia may sometimes become aggressive, may start blaming and doubting the people around them. Understand this as part of their illness, and be patient. • You may have to give the same instructions repeatedly as the patient may not be able to grasp easily. • If possible, let the caregiver be with the patient during the practice. This will help overcome the language barrier (if any) and improve understanding.
During the session	• Instructions should be slow, simple, and clear. • Be a bit louder as many of the elderly patients may have a hearing impairment. • Try to follow the same sequence of practices each time, add practices very gradually. • Consider *Chair Yoga, Bedside Yoga*, etc., for the patients to make it more feasible and acceptable. • *Trataka practice and mantra chants may be emphasized for enhancement of cognitive functions*. • Practices should be milder in intensity. • Let the patient perform standing practices beside the wall for support. • Do not ask the patient to close his/her eyes during standing poses and other standing practices, this may cause imbalance and fall. • It is a good practice for the therapist to introduce himself/herself every time he meets a patient with dementia and orient them to day, time, and place. This 2-minute reorientation should become a part of yoga class. • *Multisensory approach and imitation should be encouraged* for patients with dementia. The therapist may actually touch the patient (in the presence of a caregiver) and let the patient assume a posture passively and then encourage them to do it actively on their own. Similarly, adding music and sounds into the practice would be a good idea. • The therapist may also add a practice of giving cues toward positive memories. • Never show frustration or impatience in front of the patient while teaching the practices. • Especially in the case of patients with dementia, never let the patient go back alone after the session. Always make sure that the patient is accompanied by a caregiver.
After the session	• It is always better to give the patient a book and a video which has exact details of the yoga practices with necessary illustrations. It will help them memorize and continue the practices post-cessation of the supervised sessions. • Caregivers should be taught the same module and encouraged to practice at home with the patient.

and off for the last 1 year. He had intermittent sleep disturbances. He also had worries about his health as his diabetes and hypertension were not controlled despite being on medications. He also had occasional forgetfulness but was able to do all activities independently. He did not engage in any regular physical activity nor did he have any social engagement. His family members had persuaded him to come for a mental health evaluation. He was reluctant to take additional medications as he was already taking four different medications every day. He agreed to explore Yoga as a treatment for his mental health problems. He joined the Yoga program in his residential community and started attending group sessions every day. He noticed improvements in his mood symptoms over the next 3-4 weeks. He also felt better as he could improve his social interaction as part of the group activity. He also noticed better control of his diabetes and hypertension over this period.

Yoga therapy is acceptable to many older adults in Indian settings as it is a familiar and culturally appropriate mind-body intervention.

REFERENCES

1. Ministry of Statistics and Programme Implementaton, Government of India (2016). Elderly in India - profile and programmes 2016. [online] Available from: http://mospi.nic.in/sites/default/files/publication_reports/ElderlyinIndia_2016.pdf [Last accessed September, 2020].
2. Tiwari SC, Srivastava G, Tripathi RK, Pandey NM, Agarwal GG, Pandey S, et al. Prevalence of psychiatric morbidity amongst the community dwelling rural older adults in northern India. Indian J Med Res. 2013;138(4):504-14.
3. Chowdary R, Kumar P, Wander GS, Mishra BP, Sharma A. Psychiatric manifestations among cardiac patients: a hospital based study. Delhi Psychiatry J. 2014;17:253-7.
4. Fields GP. Religious Therapeutics: Body and Health in Yoga, Ayurveda, and Tantra. New York: State University of New York Press; 2001. p. 222.
5. Newton KG. The biology of aging (JARA): an ayurvedic approach. Bull Indian Inst Hist Med Hyderabad. 2001;31(2):161-79.
6. Devi V, Jain N, Valli K. Importance of novel drug delivery systems in herbal medicines. Pharmacogn Rev. 2010;4:27-31.
7. Kivipelto M, Solomon A, Ahtiluoto S, Ngandu T, Lehtisalo J, Antikainen R, et al. The Finnish Geriatric Intervention Study to Prevent Cognitive Impairment and Disability (FINGER): study design and progress. Alzheimers Dement. 2013;9(6):657-65.
8. Gangadhar BN, Varambally S. Yoga therapy for schizophrenia. Int J Yoga. 2012;5(2):85-91.
9. Hariprasad VR, Koparde V, Sivakumar PT, Varambally S, Thirthalli J, Varghese M, et al. Randomized clinical trial of yoga-based intervention in residents from elderly homes: effects on cognitive function. Indian J Psychiatry. 2013;55(Suppl 3):S357-63.
10. Krishnamurthy MN, Telles S. Assessing depression following two ancient Indian interventions: effects of yoga and ayurveda on older adults in a residential home. J Gerontol Nurs. 2007;33(2):17-23.
11. Rao NP, Varambally S, Gangadhar BN. Yoga school of thought and psychiatry: therapeutic potential. Indian J Psychiatry. 2013;55:S145-9.
12. Desveaux L, Lee A, Goldstein R, Brooks D. Yoga in the management of chronic disease: a systematic review and meta-analysis. Med Care. 2015;53(7):653-61.
13. Yang K. A review of yoga programs for four leading risk factors of chronic diseases. Evid Based Complement Alternat Med. 2007;4(4):487-91.
14. Manjunath NK, Telles S. Influence of yoga and ayurveda on self-rated sleep in a geriatric population. Indian J Med Res. 2005;121(5):683-90.
15. Siddarth D, Siddarth P, Lavretsky H. An observational study of the health benefits of yoga or tai chi compared with aerobic exercise in community-dwelling middle-aged and older adults. Am J Geriatr Psychiatry. 2014;22(3):272-3.
16. Hariprasad VR, Varambally S, Varambally PT, Thirthalli J, Basavaraddi I, Gangadhar BN. Designing, validation and feasibility of a yoga-based intervention for elderly. Indian J Psychiatry. 2013;55(Suppl 3):S344-9.
17. Hariprasad VR, Sivakumar PT, Koparde V, Varambally S, Thirthalli J, Varghese M, et al. Effects of yoga intervention on sleep and quality-of-life in elderly: a randomized controlled trial. Indian J Psychiatry. 2013;55(Suppl 3):S364-8.
18. Oken BS, Zajdel D, Kishiyama S, Flegal K, Dehen C, Haas M, et al. Randomized, controlled, six-month trial of yoga in healthy seniors: effects on cognition and quality of life. Altern Ther Health Med. 2006;12(1):40-7.

19. Yagli NV, Ulger O. The effects of yoga on the quality of life and depression in elderly breast cancer patients. Complement Ther Clin Pract. 2015;21(1):7-10.
20. Youkhana S, Dean CM, Wolff M, Sherrington C, Tiedemann A. Yoga-based exercise improves balance and mobility in people aged 60 and over: a systematic review and meta-analysis. Age Ageing. 2016;45(1):21-9.
21. Ramanathan M, Bhavanani AB, Trakroo M. Effect of a 12-week yoga therapy program on mental health status in elderly women inmates of a hospice. Int J Yoga. 2017;10(1):24-8.
22. Sivaramakrishnan D, Fitzsimons C, Kelly P, Ludwig K, Mutrie N, Saunders DH, et al. The effects of yoga compared to active and inactive controls on physical function and health related quality of life in older adults: systematic review and meta-analysis of randomised controlled trials. Int J Behav Nutr Phys Act. 2019;16(1):33.
23. Lee KC, Tang WK, Bressington D. The experience of mindful yoga for older adults with depression. J Psychiatr Ment Health Nurs. 2019;26(3-4):87-100.
24. Brenes GA, Divers J, Miller ME, Danhauer SC. A randomized preference trial of cognitive-behavioral therapy and yoga for the treatment of worry in anxious older adults. Contemp Clin Trials Commun. 2018;10:169-76.
25. Senchina DS, Kohut ML. Immunological outcomes of exercise in older adults. Clin Interv Aging. 2007;2(1):3-16.
26. Reig-Ferrer A, Ferrer-Cascales R, Santos-Ruiz A, Campos-Ferrer A, Prieto-Seva A, Velasco-Ruiz I, et al. A relaxation technique enhances psychological well-being and immune parameters in elderly people from a nursing home: a randomized controlled study. BMC Complement Altern Med. 2014;14:311.
27. Kuntsevich V, Bushell WC, Theise ND. Mechanisms of yogic practices in health, aging, and disease. Mt Sinai J Med. 2010;77:559-69.
28. McCall MC. How might yoga work? An overview of potential underlying mechanisms. J Yoga Phys Ther. 2013;3:130.
29. Cahn BR, Polich J. Meditation states and traits: EEG, ERP, and neuroimaging studies. Psychol Bull. 2006;132(2):180-211.
30. Hariprasad VR, Varambally S, Shivakumar V, Kalmady SV, Venkatasubramanian G, Gangadhar BN. Yoga increases the volume of the hippocampus in elderly subjects. Indian J Psychiatry. 2013;55(7):S394.
31. Zhang Y, Li C, Zou L, Liu X, Song W. The effects of mind-body exercise on cognitive performance in elderly: a systematic review and meta-analysis. Int J Environ Res Public Health. 2018;15(12):2791.
32. Halappa N, Thirthalli J, Varambally S, Rao M, Christopher R, Nanjundaiah G. Improvement in neurocognitive functions and serum brain-derived neurotrophic factor levels in patients with depression treated with antidepressants and yoga. Indian J Psychiatry. 2018;60(1):32-7.
33. Čekanauskaitė A, Skurvydas A, Žlibinaitė L, Mickevičienė D, Kilikevičienė S, Solianik R. A 10-week yoga practice has no effect on cognition, but improves balance and motor learning by attenuating brain-derived neurotrophic factor levels in older adults. Exp Gerontol. 2020;138:110998.
34. Coffin N. Chair Yoga For Seniors: A Gentle Sequence to Get You Started; 2013. [online] Available from: https://www.goodreads.com/book/show/20442123-chair-yoga-for-seniors [Last accessed September, 2020].
35. Park J, McCaffrey R, Newman D, Liehr P, Ouslander JG. A pilot randomized controlled trial of the effects of chair yoga on pain and physical function among community-dwelling older adults with lower extremity osteoarthritis. J Am Geriatr Soc. 2017;65(3):592-7.
36. Furtado GE, Uba-Chupel M, Carvalho HM, Souza NR, Ferreira JP, Teixeira AM. Effects of a chair-yoga exercises on stress hormone levels, daily life activities, falls and physical fitness in institutionalized older adults. Complement Ther Clin Pract. 2016;24:123-9.
37. Yao CT, Tseng CH. Effectiveness of chair yoga for improving the functional fitness and well-being of female community-dwelling older adults with low physical activities. Top Geriatr Rehabil. 2019;35(4):248-54.
38. Kertapati Y, Sahar J, Nursasi AY. The effects of chair yoga with spiritual intervention on the functional status of older adults. Enferm Clin. 2018;28(Suppl 1):70-3.
39. Bonura KB, Pargman D. The effects of yoga versus exercise on stress, anxiety, and depression in older adults. Int J Yoga Therap. 2009;19(1):79-89.
40. Litchke LG, Hodges JS, Reardon RF. Benefits of chair yoga for persons with mild to severe Alzheimer's disease. Act Adapt Aging. 2012;36(4):317-28.
41. McCaffrey R, Park J, Newman D, Hagen D. The effect of chair yoga in older adults with moderate and severe Alzheimer's disease. Res Gerontol Nurs. 2014;7(4):171-7.

CHAPTER 15

Yoga for Childhood and Adolescent Psychiatric Disorders

Shalu Abraham, Rashmi Arasappa, Kankan Gulati, Umesh Chikkanna

■ INTRODUCTION

Globalization has exposed children and adolescents to various new technologies, opportunities, and options. With novel resources available, better performance is expected of them resulting in significant stress in their lives. Many of these life stressors are known risk factors for the development of mental health disorders.[1,2]

The National Mental Health Survey 2016 estimated that about 9.8 million Indians aged 13–17 years suffer from serious mental illnesses, which would be greater in number if the entire age spectrum of childhood and adolescence is considered. The most common prevalent problems were depressive episode and recurrent depressive disorder (2.6%), agoraphobia (2.3%), intellectual disability (1.7%), autism spectrum disorder (ASD; 1.6%), phobic anxiety disorder (1.3%), and psychotic disorder (1.3%).[3]

Despite such a great burden of Child and Adolescent Mental Health (CAMH) disorders, significant treatment gap exists in provision of mental health care due to several reasons.[4] One major reason is that childhood psychiatric illnesses often require multimodal interventions including pharmacological, behavioral, family and school involvement, for effective outcomes. There are several shortcomings in the existing treatments as many are long-term illnesses. Also, there is a significant shortage of workforce to deliver the necessary services. In this scenario, complementary and alternative medicine (CAM) interventions are also now being increasingly explored for its effectiveness in the prevention and treatment of psychiatric problems in children and adolescents. Yoga is known for improving overall health and fitness. There is a progressive trend towards the use of yoga as a mind-body CAM intervention to improve specific physical and mental health conditions in the child and adolescent population.[5] The Diagnostic and Statistical Manual of Mental Disorders (DSM)-5 classification of childhood mental health disorders is shown in **Table 1**.

■ A TRADITIONAL INDIAN MEDICINE PERSPECTIVE OF DEVELOPMENTAL DISORDERS

Ayurveda

According to *Vedic* principles, growth and development is a synchronized and coordinated program through biological factors. Growing period is marked by the dominance of *Kapha dosha* which is controlled and coordinated by other *doshas* (bioforces or humors mainly *Vata*). Any error or imbalance in this coordinated program results in developmental disorders in children. ASD and attention deficit hyperactivity disorder (ADHD) come under the developmental disorders.

Autism has *Kapha* and *Vata*-dominant clinical presentation. The restricted and repetitive behavior in autism very well suggests the hypoactivity and hyperactivity of *Manovaha srotas* (channels of mind). Delay in development of mental faculties is mainly

TABLE 1: Child and Adolescent Mental Health (CAMH) disorders.

Neurodevelopment disorders	Intellectual disability, communication disorder, autism spectrum disorder (ASD), attention deficit hyperactivity disorder (ADHD), specific learning disorder (SLD), and motor disorders
Schizophrenia spectrum	Very early-onset and early-onset schizophrenia
Mood disorders	Depressive disorder, early-onset bipolar disorder, and disruptive mood dysregulation disorder
Anxiety disorders of infancy, childhood, and adolescents	Separation anxiety disorder, generalized anxiety disorder (GAD), social anxiety disorder, and selective mutism
Obsessive compulsive and related disorders	Obsessive-compulsive disorder (OCD), trichotillomania, skin excoriation disorder, and body dysmorphic disorder
Trauma and stress-related disorders	Reactive attachment disorder, disinhibited social engagement disorder, acute stress disorder, adjustment disorder, and post-traumatic stress disorder (PTSD)
Feeding and eating disorders	Pica, rumination disorder, and avoidant/restrictive food intake disorder
Elimination disorders	Encopresis and enuresis
Gender dysphoria	In children and adolescents
Disruptive, impulse control and conduct disorders	Oppositional defiant disorder, conduct disorder, pyromania, kleptomania, and others
Substance use disorders	Mainly in adolescents—caffeine, alcohol, tobacco, cannabis, opium, stimulants, and hallucinogens

This is just an overview of CAMH disorders, current chapter focuses on some common disorders where yoga has been applied. Interested readers can further look up in DSM-5 for more details.

due to the lack of a *Prasada kapha* (normal state of *kapha*) with good *Sara* (essence/nourishment). *Tamo guna* is more prominent in autism.

In ADHD, *Vata* dominates the condition resulting in hyperactivity of *Manovaha srotas* (channels of mind). Here *Rajas dosha* operates with *Vata* to bring the psychosomatic disturbances. Both *Vata* and *Rajas* are the derivatives of *Vayu mahabhuta*. The *Chala guna* (unstable quality) of *Vata* is more predominant in the pathogenesis of ADHD. Thus, *Vata* combining with *Rajas guna* results in clinical presentation characterized by hyperactivity.

Yoga

Yoga is believed to have an influence on the evolution of human mind. It can transform the quality of consciousness and create receptive minds. In the book "Yoga Education for Children" by Swami Satyananda Saraswati, he explains the necessity of introducing yoga in children and the advantages of doing so early on in life. The advantages of introducing yoga early on in life:

- *Probable role in delaying puberty*: Early age of puberty is associated with greater psychological distress in children especially girls.[5-7] Melatonin is a hormone secreted by pineal gland which has a role in delaying puberty apart from its main function of regulating the circadian rhythm.[8] Regular practice of yoga has been shown to increase the melatonin levels in adults,[9] but studies in children are lacking as of now. It can be hypothesized that in children, practice of yoga can result in similar effects, which in turn can prevent the early puberty.
- *Balance of the autonomic system through pranayama*: According to yogic philosophy, there are 72,000 subtle energy channels in the body, of which the most important ones are: the sun channel (*pingala*) and the moon channel (*ida*). If there is blockage in these channels, brain could be working

suboptimally. This could be tackled by rejuvenating the respective *nadi* or channel through *pranayama*. Studies have shown that breathing selectively through either nostril could have an activating effect (right) or a relaxing effect (left) on the sympathetic nervous system.[10-12] Thus, through practice of *pranayama*, an optimal balance in the autonomic system can be obtained **(Fig. 1)**.

- *Correcting of hormonal imbalances*: Dullness of brain may be caused due to hormonal imbalances, which can be improved by proper practice of yoga.[13]
- *Enhancing memory*: The practice of sun salutations, *pranayama*, and *mantra* may help in developing a clear memory in children.[14]

BENEFITS OF YOGA IN HEALTHY CHILDREN

Yoga therapy can help children cope with stress and anxiety. It thus contributes positively to their physical and mental health **(Table 2)**. Yoga practice can be started as early as 5–6 years of age in healthy children.[15] Children can start practicing meditation by the age of 13 or 14, but the preparation can start from the age of 5–8 by reading out stories aloud or singing songs and then letting them close their eyes and imagine the characters they have been hearing or singing about.[16] An increasing number of studies are providing evidence for the same.

Mindfulness component in yoga is shown to be effective in enhancing self-regulatory capacities and reducing worry in youth.[17,18]

In a randomized controlled trial (RCT), which also included qualitative assessments, Conboy et al. (2013) found that the participants experienced stress reduction, along with improvement in their academic and athletic performance after 12 weeks of *Hatha Yoga* intervention (30-minute session).[19]

Khalsa and Butzer (2016) in a systematic review addressing yoga in the school setting concluded that it is a viable and potentially efficacious strategy for improving child

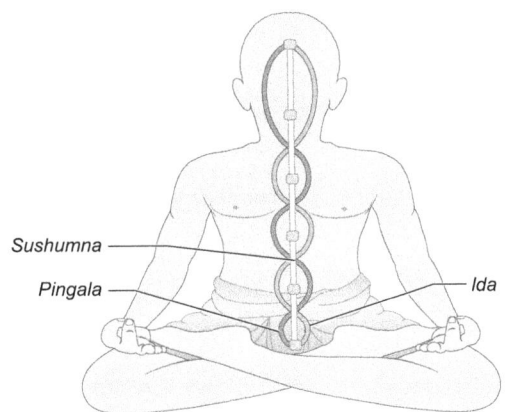

Fig. 1: The three main *nadis*, according to *Hatha Yoga Pradipika* (Chapter I, *Sloka* 15).[59]

TABLE 2: Proposed effects of yoga therapy on the different systems in children.

Systems of the human body	Effects of yoga therapy
Cardiorespiratory system[21-23]	Improves cardiorespiratory efficiency and decreases heart rate and respiratory rate
Nervous system[22,24-26]	Balances the autonomic nervous system (ANS) with a predominance of parasympathetic system, improves memory, improves central nervous system (CNS) processing as shown by improve visual and auditory reaction time and motor tapping, and improves executive functions
Musculoskeletal system[27-29]	Improves skeletal muscles strength and endurance, improves physical fitness (promotes weight loss), and improves running performance
Endocrine system[8,13]	Regulates the endocrine activities and increases melatonin
Reproductive system[30,31]	Improves dysmenorrhea in female adolescents
Mental health[17,18,20,32]	Decreases stress, depression and anxiety, improves cognition, attention, thinking, and reasoning, decreases reaction time and improves hand-eye coordination

and adolescent health.[2] A control study by Saxena et al. (2020) concluded that hatha yoga and meditation sessions carried out for 25 minutes (18 min of poses and 7 min of meditation) twice a week for 12 weeks resulted in significant reduction in self-reported scores of inattention and hyperactivity in high school children. In clinical context, hatha yoga, if practiced consistently, might serve as a tool that could delay or potentially prevent onset of a clinical diagnosis of ADHD.[20]

How does Yoga Help Improve Well-being?

Yoga is a unique practice with which the practitioner can increase self-regulation, which results in physical and psychological well-being. It can be broken down into a skill set of four tools for self-regulation: (1) ethical precepts, (2) sustained postures, (3) breath regulation, and (4) meditation techniques.

The integrative systems network model (**Fig. 2**) proposes that yoga may function through top-down and bottom-up mechanisms (of the brain) for the regulation of cognition, emotions, behaviors, and peripheral physiology, as well as for improving efficiency and integration of the processes that help in self-regulation.[33]

The higher-level brain networks include the central executive network (attention control and working memory), frontoparietal control network (meta-awareness and response inhibition), and the moral cognition network (reappraisal and goal setting).

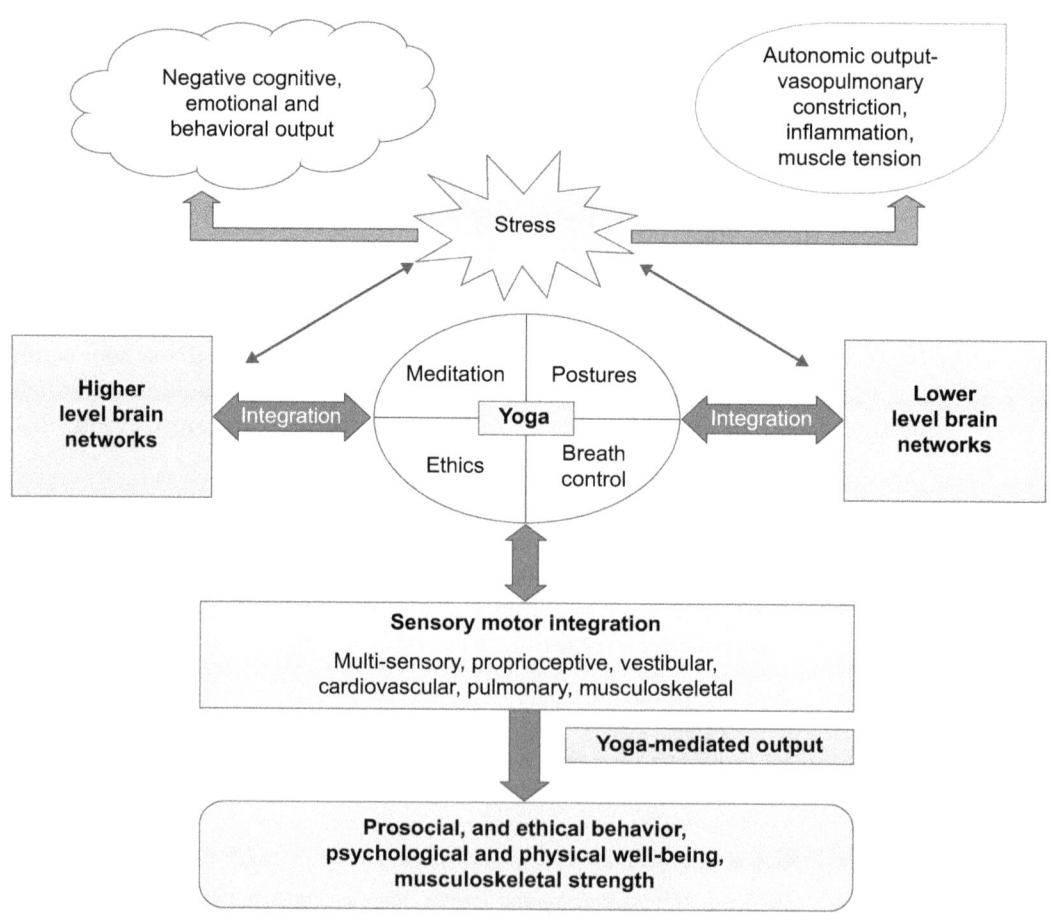

Fig. 2: Systems network model of yoga for optimizing self-regulation (simplified version).[33]

The lower-level brain networks include dorsal attention network (attention orienting), autonomic nervous system (ANS) vagal complex, and striatopallidal-thalamocortical network.

In the context of *stress*, there will be initiation of maladaptive cognitive, emotional, and behavioral output (e.g., negative appraisal, emotional reactivity, rumination) as well as physiological output initiated by lower-level brain systems, which disrupts the balance of body systems.

By the regular practice of yoga, there is increased integration between the higher and lower brain networks, which helps in improvement of accuracy in the prediction, and error correction mechanisms associated with the stress response across domains. It results in improvement in the detection and efficient response to perceived threats and also in reducing consequences of prolonged stress exposure. It is understood that placebo-related mechanisms may also operate to fuel effective top-down control and motivation; however, such mechanisms remain unclear.

ANCIENT LITERATURE ON YOGA PRACTICES FOR CHILDREN

Yoga was always known as a means to self-realization according to the ancient texts on yoga. However, now research is being conducted at different levels to find an evidence base for the health benefits of regular yoga practice. Recent studies have reported its benefits not only in normally developing children but also in children with psychiatric disorders.[2,17,18] Yogic practices may have a wide range of benefits in the development of a child in different domains such as cognitive, emotional, physical, behavioral, inter- and intrapersonal relationships[1,34] **(Fig. 3)**.

EVIDENCE FOR ROLE OF YOGA IN CHILDHOOD PSYCHIATRIC DISORDERS

Most of the scientific literature on the therapeutic application of yoga in childhood psychiatric disorders has been in areas of ADHD, followed by ASDs. However, research is now being done even in other disorders such as depression and anxiety.

Yoga for Attention Deficit Hyperactivity Disorder

Attention deficit hyperactivity disorder is one of the most common neurodevelopmental disorders in children and adolescents and affects nearly 6–7% of children and adolescents. **Table 3** depicts symptoms in a child with ADHD.

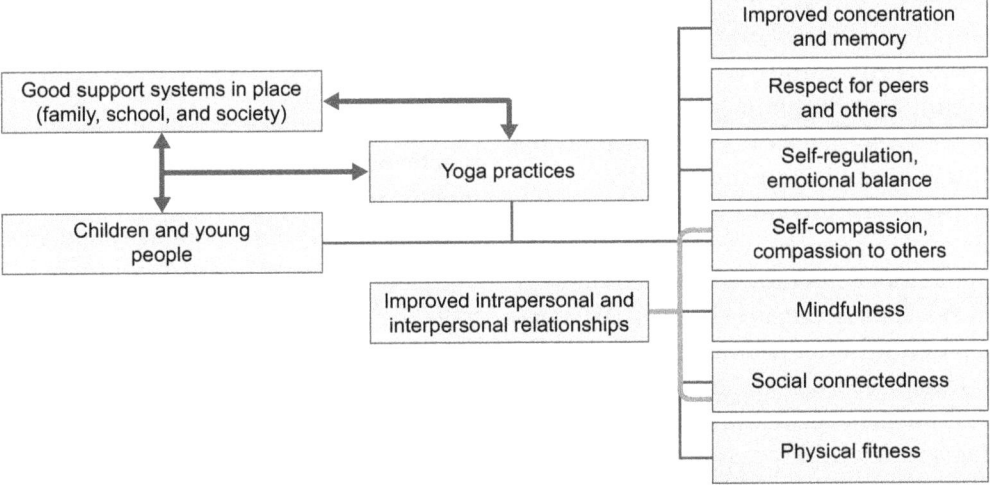

Fig. 3: Potential outcomes of yoga practice in children.[1,34]

TABLE 3: Symptoms and its corresponding behavior in a child with attention deficit hyperactivity disorder.[35]

Symptom	How a child with this symptom may behave?
Inattention	• Often has a hard time paying attention, daydreams • Often does not seem to listen • Is easily distracted from work or play • Often does not seem to care about details, makes careless mistakes • Frequently does not follow through on instructions or finish tasks • Is disorganized • Frequently loses a lot of important things • Often forgets things • Frequently avoids doing things that require ongoing mental effort
Hyperactivity	• Is in constant motion, as if "driven by a motor" • Cannot stay seated • Frequently squirms and fidgets • Talks too much • Often runs, jumps, and climbs when this is not permitted • Cannot play quietly
Impulsivity	• Frequently acts and speaks without thinking • May run into the street without looking for traffic first • Frequently has trouble taking turns • Cannot wait for things • Often calls out answers before the question is complete • Frequently interrupts others

An RCT by Jensen and Kenny (2004) showed significant benefits of yoga therapy on medication stabilized boys with ADHD ($n = 11$) compared with a control group performing cooperative activities ($n = 8$) on the Conners' Parent and Teacher Rating Scale. The 20 weekly 1-hour group sessions consisted of respiratory training, postural training, relaxation training, and concentration training (*Trataka*). They concluded that yoga might have merit as a complementary treatment for boys with ADHD already stabilized on medication. The study had limitations of having small sample size, low statistical power, and probable inconsistencies of home practices.[36]

A 6-week multimodal peer-mediated behavioral program that included yoga, meditation, and play therapy conducted on 6–11 years old children diagnosed with ADHD ($n = 76$) showed 90.5% reductions in performance-impairment score. This improvement was sustained through 12 months in 85% of students with a weekly session. About 92% of the students also had improvements on the Vanderbilt ADHD parent rating scale scores.[37]

An open-label exploratory study looked at nine patients with moderate-to-severe ADHD (eight were on medications) admitted in a child psychiatry ward. A specific yoga intervention was taught daily for six sessions during in-patient stay and they were followed up consecutively for 3 months. Significant improvement in ADHD scores was noted at the time of discharge[38] but no further reductions during follow-up were noticed.

A quasi-experimental and interventional research conducted on 80 school-age children through a pretest-posttest design showed practicing super brain yoga for 2 min/day for a month reduced the symptoms of hyperactivity disorder among the school-age children.[39]

In 2019, an RCT conducted by Cohen et al. showed that a 6-week yoga intervention using a manualized curriculum from "If I was a Bird Yoga" for preschoolers with ADHD showed modest improvements on an objective measure of attention [Kinder Test of Attentional Performance (KiTAP)] and selective improvements on parent ratings.[40]

A recent systematic review done by Barranco-Ruiz et al. (2019) concluded that mind-body therapies (MBTs), such as yoga or mindfulness, could mitigate ADHD symptoms in children and adolescents. However, further research with high-quality designs, randomization, greater sample sizes, and more intensive supervised practice programs are needed.[41]

Yoga for Autism Spectrum Disorders

Autism spectrum disorder is characterized by two major areas of difficulty: (1) social communication and (2) repetitive stereotyped behaviors **(Fig. 4)**. There has been a recent increase in the number of children diagnosed with ASD, although the cause for this is not clear.

The awareness and diagnosis of ASD, along with the limitations of current therapies, has necessitated more research for better treatments to improve lifelong outcomes. In the past decade, many researchers have investigated the effects of yoga in children with ASD.[42]

Efficacy of integrated approach to yoga therapy (IAYT) along with applied behavior analysis (ABA) was explored in six children with ASD using a 10-month program of five times/week sessions. The program began with breathing exercises (*pranayamas*), physical postures and exercises (*asanas*), deep relaxation (*yoga nidra*), and chanting (*kirtan*). Postures were in a developmental sequence and each pose was repeated twice. This study suggests that IAYT may be an effective tool to increase imitation, cognitive skills, and social-communicative behaviors in children with ASD.[44]

A study conducted by Koenig et al. (2012) tested the efficacy of the Get Ready to Learn (GRTL) yoga program among children with ASD. The GRTL program was implemented on school days for 16 weeks. The participants showed significant differences in total Aberrant Behavior Checklist (ABC) Community score compared with the control arm. There was improvement in classroom management over 16 weeks as measured by off-task behaviors and teacher redirection. Hence, it can be

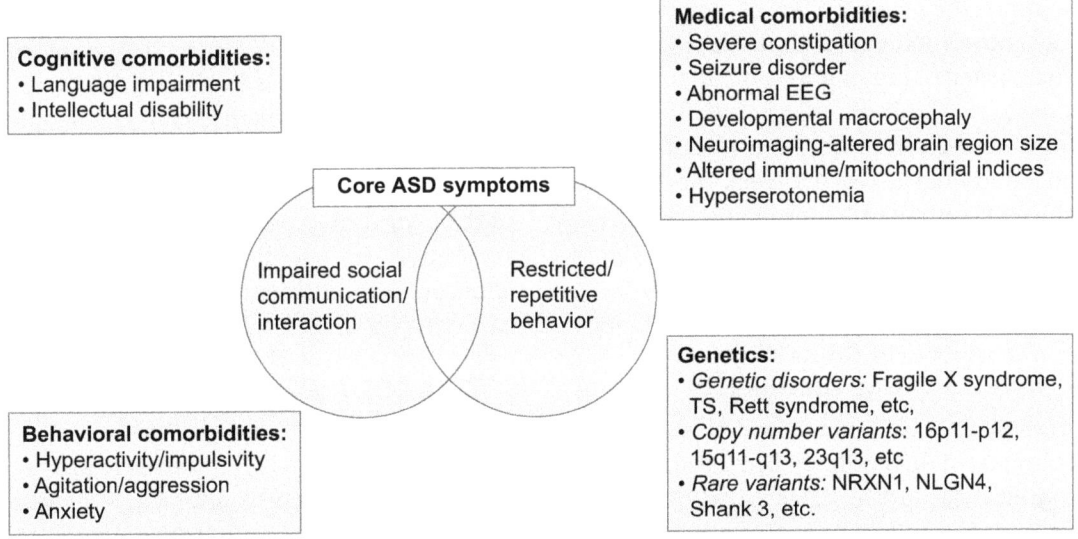

Fig. 4: Autism symptoms, comorbidities, and biomarkers. The core symptoms of autism are represented in the center and represent the common features required to receive a diagnosis. Around the periphery of Figure are symptoms or biomarkers that are not required for an autism diagnosis but are more common in autism than in the general populations.[43]

said that GRTL could be used by classroom personnel as part of their daily routine or preparatory curriculum to get their students "ready to learn".[45]

In another study, 30 children with ASD were given 1-hour yoga intervention for a period of 3 months. Pre- and post-values of the Childhood Autism Rating Scale (CARS) showed statistically significant reduction in symptoms of autism.[46]

A Cochrane-based review of evidence for improvement in core and related symptoms in patients with ASD concluded that there was minimal evidence that yoga interventions may improve core symptoms of ASD, with an Oxford Centre for Evidence-Based Medicine (CEBM) Score of Level 5.[47]

An RCT conducted by Sotoodeh et al. (2017) examined the effect of an 8-week (24-session) yoga training program (YTP) on the severity of autism in children with high-functioning autism (HFA) ($n = 29$). The results of the analysis showed that there were significant differences between the two groups with regards to all Autism Treatment Evaluation Checklist (ATEC) subscores except in domain of (speech/language/communication), which supports the positive effect of yoga training.[48]

A novel multimodal *Mandala yoga practice* comprising of group poses, color and tracing sheets, rhythmic chanting and yogic games (delivered given to children with autism on an hourly basis, twice a week for 4 weeks), showed enhanced mood and emotional expression, increased empathy toward others and improved teamwork skills **(Fig. 5)**.[49]

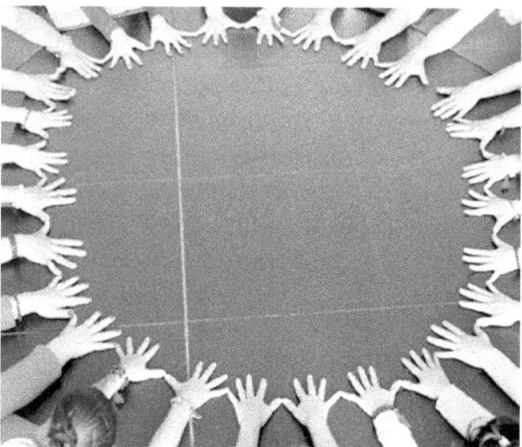

Fig. 5: Mandala yoga.

intervention, it was found that there was a significant improvement in the intelligence quotient (IQ) and social adaptation parameters in the yoga group as compared to the control. However, there is need for further studies to validate this finding.[50]

In a study done on intellectually disabled adolescents, Bhavanani et al. (2012) showed decrease in visual reaction time (VRT) and auditory reaction time (ART) after nine rounds of *Mukha bhastrika*. Decrease in reaction time (RT) signifies improved central neuronal processing ability and hence concluded that it can be used as an effective means of improving neuromuscular abilities in special children.[51]

Functional fitness often declines for people with IDD at a faster rate than the general population. Reina et al. (2020) conducted a study of yoga intervention to enhance functional fitness for people with IDD. It showed significant improvement in upper and lower body strength, and also agility and balance.[52]

■ YOGA IN CHILDREN WITH INTELLECTUAL DISABILITY

Uma et al. (1989) conducted a case control study on children with intellectual and developmental disability (IDD) aged 6–16 years ($n = 90$ vs. $n = 45$), where they were provided yoga sessions (*pranayama*, loosening exercises, *Surya Namaskar*, *yogasanas*, and meditation) for one academic year (5 hours/week). Post

■ YOGA FOR ANXIETY AND DEPRESSION IN CHILDREN

James-Palmer et al. (2020) reviewed 27 studies on yoga as an intervention for the reduction of symptoms of anxiety and depression in children and adolescents. Intervention characteristics varied greatly across studies; however, 70% of the studies overall showed improvements. For studies assessing anxiety and depression, 58% showed reductions in both symptoms, while 25% showed reductions in anxiety only. Additionally, 70% of studies assessing anxiety alone showed improvements and 40% of studies only assessing depression showed improvements.

From the above literature, the immense potential for yoga to be an effective CAM intervention for childhood mental disorders cannot be denied.[53]

YOGA THERAPY

Yoga therapy can be defined as "the application of yogic principles to a particular person with the objective of achieving a particular spiritual, psychological or physiological goal". Yoga therapy respects individual differences in age, culture, religion, philosophy, occupation, and mental and physical health.[54]

The *Bhagavad Gita* defines "Yoga" as *samatvam,* meaning that yoga is equanimity at all levels.

This may be also understood as a perfect state of health wherein physical homeostasis and mental equanimity occur in a balanced and healthy harmony.[55]

Yoga Therapy for Attention Deficit Hyperactivity Disorder

An ideal yoga module for children with ADHD should consist of yogic practices that are challenging and in turn promote relaxation, concentration and balance, and improve attention, breath and body awareness. Hariprasad et al. (2013) conducted a study to explore the feasibility and efficacy of yoga as an add-on intervention in ADHD. After the intervention, significant improvement was seen in the ADHD scores of children.[38] This module consisted of *asanas* such as *Tadasana, Vajrasana, Ustrasana, Shashankasana, Sarvangasana,* and *pranayama* such as *Kapalabhati, Suryaanuloma-viloma, Ujjayi,* and *Bhramari* followed by *Nadanusandhana.*

Yoga therapy module for ADHD is provided in **Appendix 1.7** at the end of this book.

Yoga Therapy for Autism Spectrum Disorder

The IAYT module for autism designed by Radhakrishna et al. (2010) consists of *yogasanas* and breathing exercises selected to improve cognitive, social, and communication skills. In their view, combining physical exercises with speech and language stimulation increases recall ability, imitation skills, verbal receptive skills, and expression.[44]

Few of the *asanas* include *Ardha shirshasana* (half inverted position), *Ardha chakrasana* (half wheel position) and *Trikonasana* (triangular position) which stimulate vestibular and proprioceptive senses. *Parivrtta trikonasana* (modified triangular position) and its variations seem to stimulate parasympathetic activity, calming the nervous system. They conclude that this module is feasible and even those with extreme attention deficit can slow their breath and use breath regulation to control unwanted movement of body and mind.[44]

Similarly, the National Institute of Mental Health and Neurosciences (NIMHANS) has proposed a module for ASD which is yet to be validated in further studies.

Yoga therapy module for autism spectrum disorder is provided in **Appendix 1.8** at the end of this book (based on our clinical experience).

PRACTICAL TIPS FOR YOGA THERAPY IN CHILDREN

The key to keeping children's attention and making the yoga class flow smoothly is to have challenging *asanas* in a fun and playful way. It is important to give a lot of positive reinforcement and encouragement throughout the class.[56] Even if students never get the poses absolutely right, the concepts and techniques which are taught will help them to become more balanced, peaceful, and compassionate young adults.

Precautions for Yoga Class

- The one thing that should be considered when placing a child in a yoga class is the size of the class.
- More attention has to be given to teach children and it is advisable to take one-on-one sessions for children with psychiatric disorders.
- Help students find the best alignment and show them how to get the most out of the position without getting hurt.
- The first few sessions the instructor should concentrate more on rapport building as such children take time accustomed to changes.
- Slow and steady practice will result in greater and better outcomes.

CONCLUSION

Yoga therapy for childhood psychiatric disorders is feasible and effective. It can be done in any setting and may be used as a sole or an add-on treatment along with medications as a part of a multimodal intervention.[58] The potential benefits of yoga practice in children include improved concentration/memory, respect for others, self-regulation, self-confidence, feeling of well-being, emotional regulation, and physical fitness.[1] Yoga-based interventions have been shown to help cognition and emotional control in healthy children and adolescents as well as children with ADHD[36] and ASD, although more research is needed in this important area.[58] Finally, teaching yoga to this age group is a challenging task which requires patience, adaptation, and creativity from the instructor.

Future directions for research:

- Studies with larger samples and robust study designs are required.
- There is a need to standardize the module with the most effective yoga techniques, which may be effective for individual disorders.
- Long-term follow-up studies need to be planned to see if the improvement plateaus or has a consistent improving outcome.
- Further studies need to be done with at-risk children to see if yoga can alter the course (severity) of the illness if administered early on in life.

CASE VIGNETTE

A 12-year-old boy [body mass index (BMI) = 14.74 kg/m², diagnosed with ASD underwent 3 months of yoga training as a part of a group. Diagnosis of ASD was based on Childhood Autism Rating Scale (CARS). He was cooperative enough to do yoga and had not practiced yoga in the past 6 months, before the commencement of the study. Assessment was done using Autism Treatment Evaluation Checklist (ATEC)[57] which is used to track the efficacy of a treatment. Higher scores indicate more severity of the symptoms. The ATEC assess the child on the basis of four subtest scales: Scale I. Speech/Language/Communication (14 items); Scale II. Sociability (20 items); Scale III. Sensory/Cognitive Awareness (18 items); and Scale IV. Health/Physical Behavior (25 items).

In the first month, the child attended 12 one-on-one sessions (3 sessions/week) under the supervision of the yoga therapist and then was asked to practice at home for the remaining 2 months. The first few sessions were spent on building a good rapport with the child. Following the module, yoga practices were taught in the same order, adding new practices slowly. The sessions were conducted at the same time of the day in the same yoga room, maintaining uniformity of other conditions such as lighting of the room, placement of the mats, and positioning of yoga therapist and the parent/caretaker. This was done to make the child more comfortable and avoid any kind of confusion. Initially it was very difficult for the child to adhere to the instructions given by the yoga therapist or even differentiate between the process of inhalation and exhalation (this also depends on the severity of the condition). Therefore, teaching breathing practices and pranayama was a bit of challenge. The yoga therapist had to be very patient and made the child practice asanas by providing physical assistance and pranayama and other breathing practices were practiced passively in the beginning. Slowly and gradually as the child started learning and differentiating, he was encouraged to practice on his own.

As many of the asanas are named after animals, a very practical and interesting way of teaching asanas is narrating a story to the child, i.e., by building a relationship between characters of the story to particular asanas, an example being the hare and the tortoise story. Once upon a time a hare (Shashankasana) was making fun of a tortoise (Kurmasana) for being slow and challenged him to run a race with him. The tortoise agrees, the snake (Bhujangasana) becomes the referee, gives a go, and the race begins. Soon, the hare was way ahead of the tortoise and he thought of taking a nap under a tree (Vrikshasana) which was next to a big river with many beautiful fishes (Matsyasana) swimming in it. In the meantime, the tortoise slowly and steadily passes the hare, crosses the finishing line and wins the race. Therefore, the moral of the story is that slow and steady wins the race. This will not only make the yoga session interesting but it will also provide the child with a sense of confidence that he may be a little slow as compared to his peers but he will definitely excel with consistent efforts.

After 3 months of yoga intervention, his scores decreased from 9 to 6 on Scale I, 21 to 18 on Scale II, 22 to 18 on Scale III, and 29 to 25 on Scale IV. His class teacher and the yoga therapist both reported improvement in his behavior as he was able to sit at one place for a longer

---

Clinical Insights: Yoga for Child and Adolescent Psychiatric Disorders

Prior to the session
- Therapists must be aware of the clinical diagnosis, the medications and the current status of the child. It is preferable to keep in contact with the treating consultant to have a clear idea of the do's and don'ts prior to deciding the treatment plan.
- Keep in mind that children with autism are not like other children. *Avoid touching, hugging or patting them without a good rapport*. This may generate anxiety in the child and reduce adherence to yoga.
- Talking to the caregiving parent and observing the child may give the therapist an idea about the likes, dislikes, and the general behavior of the child.
- Develop a good rapport with the child and, if possible, try to converse with the child in his/her mother tongue.
- *The instructor's, child's, and caregivers' positioning in yoga sessions should more or less remain the same* because if changed with every session, it may cause confusion to the child.
- The rationale for add-on yoga therapy and the expectations from the sessions must be discussed with parents/caregivers and a realistic treatment plan should be made.
- If the child appears very restless, try to understand the cause behind it. A child with autism may be very sensitive and slight discomforts such as tight fighting clothes, rough texture of the yoga mat or loud instructions/mantra chantings may make these children restless.

Additional points to be considered in structuring the environment:
1. Autism spectrum disorder:
   - Ensure a safe environment for practice (e.g., furniture with sharp edges, slippery floors, etc., should be avoided)
   - Ideally, a regular space and a regular time should be made for yoga with mats setup in the same place
   - Preferably *choose a sensory neutral environment* (e.g., excessively noisy fan or heaters, sound from cafeteria/traffic should be avoided, etc.)
2. Attention deficit hyperactivity disorder:
   - A space with lowlights, plain walls with minimum distractions should be considered
   - Introduce yoga to them like a fun activity.

Contd...

Contd...

	Clinical Insights: Yoga for Child and Adolescent Psychiatric Disorders
During the session	• *Try to weave a story into your yoga practice*. This will make it very interesting to the child and easy for him/her to remember. • More attention has to be given to teach children and it is advisable to take one-on-one sessions in the beginning for children with psychiatric disorders. • The first few sessions the instructor should concentrate more on rapport building as such children take time to get accustomed to change. • Practices should be adjusted for each child as each child has different needs and sensitive areas. • Teach visually and speak verbally about the modification options for each pose. In children with autism, it may be required to give instructions to children by coming down to their eye level (this will improve their eye contact as well). • Give time to adopt or release the postures. • Help students find the best alignment and show them how to get the most out of the position without getting hurt. • Use a multisensory approach, emphasize hands-on assistance, music, play, sound, and breath. • Keeping children's attention and making the yoga class flow smoothly is to have challenging *asanas* in a fun and playful way. • It is important to give a lot of positive reinforcement and encouragement throughout the class. • *Practices should be taught one by one slowly in the same order repeatedly*, adding new practices one by one, may be once or twice a week. Teaching too many practices at one go may irritate the child and he/she may lose interest. • *Yogic games (krida yoga) can be included* as a part of the yoga therapy program as it helps in the overall development of a child. It will help in improving social and communication skills, motor skills, cognition, awareness, balance, emotional growth, and channelizes energy in hyperactive children. • *Mandala yoga (forming geometries, simple pyramids, postures in circles along with other children) can be introduced later* in the practice in children diagnosed with autism. It helps in improving their emotional expression and positive mood. • Add-on preparatory tools such as massage and music may be useful, especially in children with autism. • Children may be asked to physically touch the body parts and feel the sensations of touch, sound vibrations, etc., this may help enhance body awareness in them.
After the session	• It is usually good to train the parents also, so that they can make the child practice at home, as and when feasible. It also helps in reducing the stress levels of the parents. • Parents should be educated that slow and steady practice will result in greater and better outcomes.

duration of time and started responding better to verbal instructions given in the classroom. His parents felt that his gastrointestinal problems, i.e., having frequent episodes of indigestion also showed mild improvement.

REFERENCES

1. Hagen I, Nayar US. Yoga for children and young people's mental health and well-being: research review and reflections on the mental health potentials of yoga. Front Psychiatry. 2014;5:35.
2. Khalsa SB, Butzer B. Yoga in school settings: a research review. Ann N Y Acad Sci. 2016;1373(1):45-55.
3. Murthy RS. National Mental Health Survey of India 2015-2016. Indian J Psychiatry. 2017;59(1):21-6.
4. Shastri P. Promotion and prevention in child mental health. Indian J Psychiatry. 2009;51(2):88.
5. Davison KK, Werder JL, Trost SG, Baker BL, Birch LL. Why are early maturing girls less active? Links between pubertal development, psychological well-being, and physical activity among girls at ages 11 and 13. Soc Sci Med. 2007;64(12):2391-404.
6. Mendle J, Turkheimer E, Emery RE. Detrimental psychological outcomes associated with early pubertal timing in adolescent girls. Dev Rev. 2007;27(2):151-71.

7. Weir K (2016). The risks of earlier puberty. [online] Available from: https://www.apa.org/monitor/2016/03/puberty [Last accessed October, 2020].
8. Waldhauser F, Boepple PA, Schemper M, Mansfield MJ, Crowley WF. Serum melatonin in central precocious puberty is lower than in age-matched prepubertal children. J Clin Endocrinol Metab. 1991;73(4):793-6.
9. Harinath K, Malhotra AS, Pal K, Prasad R, Kumar R, Kain TC, et al. Effects of Hatha yoga and Omkar meditation on cardiorespiratory performance, psychologic profile, and melatonin secretion. J Altern Complement Med. 2004;10(2):261-8.
10. Shannahoff-Khalsa DS, Kennedy B. The effects of unilateral forced nostril breathing on the heart. Int J Neurosci. 1993;73(1-2):47-60.
11. Malhotra V, Tandon OP, Patil R, Sen TK, Lobo SW, Nagamma T, et al. Suryanadi anuloma viloma pranayama modifies autonomic activity of heart. J Yoga. 2009;8:1-5.
12. Telles S, Nagarathna R, Nagendra HR. Breathing through a particular nostril can alter metabolism and autonomic activities. Indian J Physiol Pharmacol. 1994;38:133-7.
13. Gayathri V, Tl DA, Shivakumar DK. Effect of yoga on endocrine and nervous system in adolescent children: assessment using EPI parameters. J Ayu Herb Med. 2018;4(1):18-21.
14. Rangan R, Nagendra HR, Bhat GR. Effect of yogic education system and modern education system on memory. Int J Yoga. 2009;2(2):55-61.
15. Stewart M, Phillips K. Yoga for Children [Internet]. New York: Simon and Schuster; 1992 [Cited 2020. Oct 21]. Available from: https://books.google.com.cu/books?id=BDSHUWGMbgQC [Last accessed October, 2020].
16. Fontana D, Slack I. Teaching Meditation to Children: The Practical Guide to the Use and Benefits of Meditation Techniques. London: Watkins Publishing; 2012.
17. Mendelson T, Greenberg MT, Dariotis JK, Gould LF, Rhoades BL, Leaf PJ. Feasibility and preliminary outcomes of a school-based mindfulness intervention for urban youth. J Abnorm Child Psychol. 2010;38(7):985-94.
18. Noggle JJ, Steiner NJ, Minami T, Khalsa SB. Benefits of yoga for psychological well-being in a US high school curriculum: a preliminary randomized controlled trial. J Dev Behav Pediatr. 2012;33(3):193-201.
19. Conboy LA, Noggle JJ, Frey JL, Kudesia RS, Khalsa SB. Qualitative evaluation of a high school yoga program: feasibility and perceived benefits. Explore (NY). 2013;9(3):171-80.
20. Saxena K, Verrico CD, Saxena J, Kurian S, Alexander S, Kahlon RS, et al. An evaluation of yoga and meditation to improve attention, hyperactivity, and stress in high-school students. J Altern Complement Med. 2020;26(8):701-7.
21. Galantino ML, Galbavy R, Quinn L. Therapeutic effects of yoga for children: a systematic review of the literature. Pediatr Phys Ther. 2008;20(1):66-80.
22. Udupa K, Madanmohan, Bhavanani AB, Vijayalakshmi P, Krishnamurthy N. Effect of pranayam training on cardiac function in normal young volunteers. Indian J Physiol Pharmacol. 2003;47(1):27-33.
23. Telles S, Narendran S, Raghuraj P, Nagarathna R, Nagendra HR. Comparison of changes in autonomic and respiratory parameters of girls after yoga and games at a community home. Percept Mot Skills. 1997;84(1):251-7.
24. Manjunath NK, Telles S. Spatial and verbal memory test scores following yoga and fine arts camps for school children. Indian J Physiol Pharmacol. 2004;48(3):353-6.
25. Bhavanani AB, Madanmohan, Udupa K. Acute effect of Mukh bhastrika (a yogic bellows type breathing) on reaction time. Indian J Physiol Pharmacol. 2003;47(3):297-300.
26. Manjunath NK, Telles S. Improved performance in the Tower of London test following yoga. Indian J Physiol Pharmacol. 2001;45(3):351-4.
27. Madanmohan, Jatiya L, Udupa K, Bhavanani AB. Effect of yoga training on handgrip, respiratory pressures and pulmonary function. Indian J Physiol Pharmacol. 2003;47(4):387-92.
28. Slawta J, Bentley J, Smith J, Kelly J, Syman-Degler L. Promoting healthy lifestyles in children: a pilot program of be a fit kid. Health Promot Pract. 2008;9(3):305-12.
29. Donohue B, Miller A, Beisecker M, Houser D, Valdez R, Tiller S, et al. Effects of brief yoga exercises and motivational preparatory interventions in distance runners: results of a controlled trial. Br J Sports Med. 2006;40(1):60-3.
30. Sa'adah U, Kholisotin K, Munir Z, Fr H, Wahid AH. The effect of hatha yoga on dysmenorrhoea pain in adolescent principle. J Matern Care Reprod Health. 2019;2(2). [online] Available from: http://mcrhjournal.or.id/index.php/jmcrh/article/view/79 [Last accessed October, 2020].
31. Ulaa M, Lismidiati W, Hapsari ED. Differences use of yoga and self-tapping towards long pain of primary dysmenorrhea on adolescent. Indonesian J Nurs Pract. 2018;1(3):124-32.
32. Beets MW, Mitchell E. Effects of yoga on stress, depression, and health-related quality of life in

a nonclinical, bi-ethnic sample of adolescents: a pilot study. Hisp Health Care Int. 2010;8(1):47-53.
33. Gard T, Noggle JJ, Park CL, Vago DR, Wilson A. Potential self-regulatory mechanisms of yoga for psychological health. Front Hum Neurosci. 2014;8:770.
34. Kishida M, Mama SK, Larkey L, Elavsky S. "Yoga resets my inner peace barometer": A qualitative study illuminating the pathways of how yoga impacts one's relationship to oneself and to others. Complement Ther Med. 2017. [online] Available from: https://asu.pure.elsevier.com/en/publications/yoga-resets-my-inner-peace-barometer-a-qualitative-study-illumina [Last accessed October, 2020].
35. American Academy of Pediatrics. Diagnosing ADHD in Children: Guidelines and Information for Parents [Internet]. Itasca: American Academy of Pediatrics; 2017 [Cited 2020, Oct 21]. Available from: https://www.healthychildren.org/English/health-issues/conditions/adhd/Pages/Diagnosing-ADHD-in-Children-Guidelines-Information-for-Parents.aspx.
36. Jensen P, Kenny D. The effects of yoga on the attention and behavior of boys with attention-deficit/hyperactivity disorder (ADHD). J Atten Disord. 2004;7:205-16.
37. Mehta S, Shah D, Shah K, Mehta S, Mehta N, Mehta V, et al. Peer-mediated multimodal intervention program for the treatment of children with ADHD in India: one-year follow-up. ISRN Pediatr. 2012;2012:419168.
38. Hariprasad V, Arasappa R, Varambally S, Srinath S, Gangadhar BN. Feasibility and efficacy of yoga as an add-on intervention in attention deficit-hyperactivity disorder: an exploratory study. Indian J Psychiatry. 2013;55(Suppl 3):S379-84.
39. Farahani PV, Hekmatpou D, Khonsari AH, Gholami M. Effectiveness of super brain yoga for children with hyperactivity disorder. Perspect Psychiatr Care. 2019;55(2):140-6.
40. Cohen SC, Harvey DJ, Shields RH, Shields GS, Rashedi RN, Tancredi DJ, et al. The effects of yoga on attention, impulsivity and hyperactivity in pre-school age children with attention-deficit hyperactivity disorder symptoms. J Dev Behav Pediatr. 2018;39(3):200-9.
41. Barranco-Ruiz Y, Esturo Etxabe B, Ramírez-Vélez R, Villa-González E. Interventions based on mind-body therapies for the improvement of attention-deficit/hyperactivity disorder symptoms in youth: a systematic review. Medicina (Kaunas). 2019;55(7):325.
42. Artchoudane S, Bhavanani AB, Ramanathan M, Mariangela A. Yoga as a therapeutic tool in autism: a detailed review. Yoga Mimamsa. 2019;51(1):3-16.
43. Hewitson L. Scientific challenges in developing biological markers for autism. OA Autism. 2013;1(1):7.
44. Radhakrishna S, Nagarathna R, Nagendra HR. Integrated approach to yoga therapy and autism spectrum disorders. J Ayurveda Integr Med. 2010;1(2):120-4.
45. Koenig KP, Buckley-Reen A, Garg S. Efficacy of the get ready to learn yoga program among children with autism spectrum disorders: a pretest-posttest control group design. Am J Occup Ther. 2012;66(5):538-46.
46. Deorari M, Bhardwaj I. Effect of yogic intervention on autism spectrum disorder. Yoga Mimamsa. 2014;46(3):81-4.
47. Gwynette M, Warren N, Warthen J, Truleove J, Ross C, Snook C. Yoga as an intervention for patients with autism spectrum disorder: a review of the evidence and future directions. Autism Open Access. 2015;5(3):1000155.
48. Sotoodeh MS, Arabameri E, Panahibakhsh M, Kheiroddin F, Mirdoozandeh H, Ghanizadeh A. Effectiveness of yoga training program on the severity of autism. Complement Ther Clin Pract. 2017;28:47-53.
49. Litchke LG, Liu T, Castro S. Effects of multimodal mandala yoga on social and emotional skills for youth with autism spectrum disorder: an exploratory study. Int J Yoga. 2018;11(1):59-65.
50. Uma K, Nagendra HR, Nagarathna R, Vaidehi S, Seethalakshmi R. The integrated approach of yoga: a therapeutic tool for mentally retarded children: a one-year controlled study. J Ment Defic Res. 1989;33(Pt 5):415-21.
51. Bhavanani AB, Ramanathan M, Kt H. Immediate effect of mukha bhastrika (a bellows type pranayama) on reaction time in mentally challenged adolescents. Indian J Physiol Pharmacol. 2012;56(2):174-80.
52. Reina AM, Adams EV, Allison CK, Mueller KE, Crowe BM, van Puymbroeck M, et al. Yoga for functional fitness in adults with intellectual and developmental disabilities. Int J Yoga. 2020;13(2):156-9.
53. James-Palmer A, Anderson E, Zucker L, Kofman Y, Daneault JF. Yoga as an intervention for the reduction of symptoms of anxiety and depression in children and adolescents: a systematic review. Front Pediatr. 2020;8:78.
54. Miller R. Yoga Therapy: Definition, Perspective and Principles [Internet]. Little Rock: International Association of Yoga Therapists (IAYT); 2019 [Cited 2020, Oct 21]. Available

from: https://www.iayt.org/general/custom.asp?page=YogaTherapyDefinition.
55. Bhavanani AB. Health-and-well-being-a-yogic-perspective [Internet]. New Delhi: Ministry of Ayush; 2016 [Cited 2020, Oct 21]. Available from: https://moayush.wordpress.com/2016/06/20.
56. Rodefer E. Tips for Teaching Yoga to Teenagers [Internet]. California: Yoga Journal; 2007 [Cited 2020, Oct 21]. Available from: https://www.yogajournal.com/teach/teaching-yoga-to-teenagers.
57. Rimland B., Edelson M. Autism Treatment Evaluation Checklist [Internet]. California: Autism Research Institute; 1999 [Cited 2020, Oct 21]. Available from: https://www.autism.org/autism-treatment-evaluation-checklist/?sg_sessionid=1603356629_5f9147d5911ab2.67738581&__sgtarget=-1&__sgbrwsrid=56 b59f 46b8ed55 9a37840a7565 fb7a2e#sgbody-1329619.
58. Mehta S, Mehta V, Mehta S, Shah D, Motiwala A, Vardhan J, et al. Multimodal behavior program for ADHD incorporating yoga and implemented by high school volunteers: a pilot study. ISRN Pediatrics. 2011;2011:780745.
59. Muktibodhananda S. Hatha Yoga Pradipika. Bihar: Yoga Publications Trust; 2000. p. 50.

CHAPTER 16

Yoga for Substance Use Disorders

Venkata Lakshmi Narasimha, Sumana Venugopal, Bharath Holla, Hemant Bhargav

INTRODUCTION TO SUBSTANCE USE DISORDERS

Substance use disorder (SUD) refers to the consumption of psychoactive substances in harmful, hazardous or dependence pattern.[1] It contributes to a major share of illness-related morbidity and mortality. Both licit (alcohol and tobacco) and illicit substances are associated with harms starting from recreational use to a dependent pattern.[2] According to the World Drug Report 2019, 35 million people worldwide suffer from drug use disorders, while only one in seven of those receive treatment.[3]

According to the International Classification of Diseases, 10th Revision (ICD-10), dependence has been defined as the presence of three out of the six criteria for significant period in the last 12 months;[4] these six criteria include two physiological (tolerance and withdrawal), two psychological (craving and loss of control), and two psychosocial (use despite harm and salience) criteria. It also defines harmful use as usage of the psychoactive substance despite having psychological and physical harm not amounting to dependence. The prevalence of substance use varies across drugs and countries and it depends on multiple factors. For example, the UN Office on Drugs and Crime estimates that between 26 and 36 million people worldwide abuse opioids (use them without a prescription, in a way other than prescribed).

There are multiple theories, from neurobiological to social, which have tried to explain addiction to substances. Current understanding is that addiction is a brain disease resulting from neurobiological changes that happen in the brain. Koob and Volkow described three stages of addiction, along with the predominant neurotransmitters and areas involved. These include: binge/intoxication (dopamine and opioid peptides; involving basal ganglia), withdrawal/negative affect state (corticotropin releasing hormone and dynorphin; involving extended amygdala) and preoccupation/anticipation (glutamate; involving prefrontal cortex).[5]

Treatment for patients suffering from addictions are primarily focused at promoting abstinence and preventing frequent relapses. Despite advances in understanding the neurobiology of addiction, there are not many pharmacological treatments available for SUD. For example, till date only three pharmacological agents have been the US Food and Drug Administration (US FDA)-approved for the treatment of alcohol dependence. Of these, Disulfiram is an example of a deterrent drug, which produces unpleasant hypersensitivity to alcohol by blocking its oxidation at acetaldehyde stage. The remaining two are examples of anticraving drugs, Naltrexone (μ-opioid antagonist) and Acamprosate (putative glutamate modulator). Nalmefene, an opioid with μ-antagonism and partial κ-agonism, was recently approved for use by the European Medicines Agency to reduce alcohol consumption. Methadone (long acting μ-agonist) and Buprenorphine (partial μ-agonist) are approved for opioid detoxification and maintenance therapy in opioid dependence. Bupropion (norepinephrine-dopamine reuptake inhibitor) and Varenicline (partial α4β2 nicotinic acetylcholine receptor agonist) are approved for smoking cessation.

Psychosocial interventions including cognitive, behavioral, and motivational treatments have been rigorously studied across a broad range of addictions. These interventions are aimed at enhancing motivation to stop or reduce substance use, improving coping skills, changing reinforcement contingencies, and enhancing social supports and interpersonal functioning. Psychosocial interventions form the mainstay of treatment for relapse-prevention in cannabis, stimulants, inhalants, sedatives-hypnotics, and behavioral addictions. However, therapeutic effect sizes are generally modest for relapse prevention, even with judicious combination of both psychosocial and pharmacotherapeutic interventions.[6] Thus, better or adjuvant approaches that may enhance or facilitate the treatment of addictions by targeting motivation and control systems in the brain would be very valuable. Furthermore, there is a need to identify culturally appropriate and effective interventions for SUDs. Hence, add-on interventions such as yoga, which has been effective in various mental health conditions,[7] need to be explored as a treatment option for addictive disorders.

INTRODUCTION TO YOGA

Yoga is a tradition of lifestyle and spiritual discipline that has evolved over a period of nearly 5,000 years. The main sources of ancient yoga philosophy and practice are available from *Vedas, Upanishads, Smritis and Puranas*. In recent times, Yoga has evolved as a holistic therapy to treat the mind, body, and soul.[8] It includes various practices such as yoga postures, breathing practices, meditation, relaxation techniques, and guided imagery to improve physical and mental health. Several studies have demonstrated the usefulness of yoga in reducing stress, anxiety, and depression. The practice of yoga has also been shown to enhance prefrontal activation, reduce impulsivity, and promote positive behavioral changes with better self-regulation.[9,10] Withdrawal symptoms are characterized by sympathetic arousal. This can be countered effectively by yoga practices which have been demonstrated to bring a state of parasympathetic dominance.[11] Thus, yoga therapy may serve as a useful low-cost and low-risk adjunct in management of SUDs.

UNDERSTANDING ADDICTION FROM A YOGA PERSPECTIVE

Patanjali's Yoga Sutras (PYS) have an interesting way of describing the mind and its problems pertaining to addictions and craving, using the concept of five afflictions called *"kleshas"*. These afflictions are: *"Avidya"* or ignorance (delay discounting deficits: preference for smaller, immediate rewards over larger, delayed rewards); *"Asmita"* or excessive "I" ness (externalizing behaviors: strong identification with mind-body complex and material possessions with a resulting disposition to act out); *"Raga"* or excessive attachment (high reward dependence: persisting repetition of actions that are associated with rewards); *"Dwesha"* or excessive repulsion (novelty seeking: repulsion from situations where desires are not gratified with impulsive decision-making, avoidance of frustration, quick loss of temper, and avoidance of moral responsibilities); and *"Abhinivesha"* (harm avoidance: fear of losing what one possesses including fear of death). Persons suffering from these afflictions may be at higher risk for addictions according to this understanding. Patanjali also described potential obstacles in the path of Yoga (*Antarayaha*). Among the obstacles he described is *"Avirati"*, which refers to excessive craving for sensual gratification. Patanjali further said that such obstacles/mental distractions could be overcome and externalizing traits could be reduced by dedicating oneself to a committed practice of yoga and focused-meditation which involve (1) chanting of the cosmic sound "*Om*" with awareness of its transcendental meaning and (2) being mindful that there is calmness in the mind during the stillness of the breath, after complete exhalation and before inhalation (*Pracchardana vidharanabhyam va pranasya*) (PYS: 1.29; 1.32; 1.34).

Bhagavad Gita also describes how a person gets attached to pleasures which ultimately lead to compromise in his intellectual abilities. It states that *"Raga"* originates from *"Rajas guna"* (an attribute of the mind which creates unrest). Rajasic personalities who are passionate, ambitious, goal-oriented, and impulsive are more prone to develop *"Raga* (craving for more pleasures)". When the *"Raga"* is not fulfilled, such personalities get frustrated and turn toward a self-destructive mindset of *"Tamas"* (mental attributes of avoidance, lack of sensitivity, lack of foresight and ruthlessness) which is dominated by *"Dwesha"* (hatred) and *"Krodha"* (anger). Such anger clouds one's judgment, compromises higher intellectual abilities and discrimination power of the mind, allowing it to succumb to lower (animal) instincts. Specific lifestyle guidelines are provided in yoga texts to reduce *"Rajas"* and *"Tamas" guna,* and to promote the *"Sattva" guna* (mental attribute of balance and goodness characterized by prosocial traits). These include guidelines for eating habits, sleep, and behaviors including specific yogic practices (postures, breathing, and meditation). So, Yoga helps in the development of correct knowledge and provides insight into one's own mind and behavior.

The *Panchakosha* theory, derived from the *Taittiriya Upanishad* gives a detailed description about dimensions of human personality and self. Details of *Panchakosha* model are provided in *Chapter 1*. The main aim of Yoga therapy in addictive disorders ought to be to strengthen the *Vijnanamaya kosha* (layer of knowledge and understanding; probably related to activation of higher brain centers such as prefrontal cortex and anterior cingulate cortex which send inhibitory signals) and correct imbalances in *Manomaya kosha* (layer of emotions; probably related to amygdala and limbic system which are excitatory in nature) (see *Fig. 2* in *Chapter 1*). Research has shown that fast yogic breathing practices such as *Kapalabhati* (bellows breathing) may cause activation of prefrontal cortices[10] whereas chanting of the sound "Om" may cause limbic deactivation.[12] Counseling based on ethical precepts of *"Yamas"* (social restraints) and *"Niyamas"* (self-disciplines) given by Patanjali (see *Chapter 1* for more details) may also play an important role in strengthening the *Vijnanamaya kosha*. Asanas, *Pranayamas, Kriyas, Mudras,* and *bandhas* may further strengthen and enhance physical, mental, and spiritual well-being.

YOGA THERAPY FOR SUBSTANCE USE DISORDER: CURRENT EVIDENCE

The following section provides a selective narrative review of yoga therapy for SUDs. A number of recent studies have demonstrated effectiveness of yoga as an adjunctive treatment for managing SUDs. Studies have shown that regular practice of yoga not only reduced psychological stress, anxiety, and depression but curtailed substance usage and relapse rates. In addition, yoga enhanced overall sense of well-being and quality of life in this population.

A recent randomized controlled trial (RCT) was conducted on opioid-dependent patients ($n = 32$). Subjects were divided into two groups: (1) mindfulness-based therapy, or (2) treatment as usual, for 4 weeks. This study found that there was a close correlation between inferior frontal cortex function and mindfulness meditation,[13] suggesting a neurobiological basis for meditation practices in opioid dependence. In another study of opioid-dependent patients, yogic meditation was offered with conventional treatment, while control group was given treatment as usual for 12 weeks. It was found that add-on Yoga had greater effect in reducing perceived stress as compared to treatment as usual.[14] Another RCT on subjects with human immunodeficiency virus (HIV) and SUD (n = 73) looked at either add-on *Hatha Yoga* practice or treatment as usual for 12 sessions (90 min every week for 12 weeks). It was found that participants in the yoga group reported lesser stress than participants in the treatment as usual group. Relapse rate was also significantly lower in the yoga group.[15] Similarly, several studies have demonstrated the beneficial role of yoga in reducing substance use and impulsivity, and in improving abstinence.[16,17] Studies on subjects with alcohol dependence have observed the benefits of yoga in reducing alcohol consumption,[18] and improving depression and stress levels.[19] In subjects with nicotine dependence, studies have reported reduced cigarette smoking rate,[20-22] and improved anxiety and overall well-being.[21] Another pilot study reported improvement in the quality of life of cocaine users after 2 months of yoga practice.[23] **Table 1** provides a brief summary of the current evidence for use of yoga in SUD.

■ PROBABLE MECHANISMS OF YOGA IN SUBSTANCE USE DISORDER

Although direct studies that have examined the mechanism of action of Yoga in SUD are lacking, there is indirect evidence such as the effects of yoga on impulse control and

TABLE 1: Summary of current evidence for effectiveness of yoga in substance use disorder.

S. No.	Title of the study (Author name, Journal, and Year)	Population and sample size	Intervention and control intervention	Results
1.	Mindfulness-based therapy (MBT) modulates default-mode network connectivity in patients with opioid dependence (Fahmy M, et al. Eur Neuropsychopharmacology. 2019)	Opiate-dependent patients (n = 32)	Mindfulness-based therapy for 4 weeks (n = 16) as intervention and treatment as usual (TAU) (n = 16) as control group	Within the anterior default mode network (DMN), decreased right inferior frontal cortical connectivity was detected in patients who received MBT compared to TAU. In addition, within the MBT-group, decreased right superior frontal cortex connectivity was detected after treatment. Inferior frontal cortex function was significantly associated with mindfulness measures
2.	Yoga as an adjunctive intervention to medication-assisted treatment with Buprenorphine + Naloxone (Lander L, et al. J Addict Res Ther. 2018)	Opiate-dependent patients (n = 26)	Adjunctive yoga intervention while remaining in TAU for 12 weeks (n = 13) as intervention and TAU (n = 13) as control group	The treatment by follow-up time interaction effect was significant for perceived stress (p = 0.026) indicating that the yoga intervention had a larger effect than TAU. Changes in perceived stress decreased significantly over time in both the yoga intervention group and the TAU-matched control group

Contd...

Contd...

S. No.	Title of the study (Author name, Journal, and Year)	Population and sample size	Intervention and control intervention	Results
3.	A randomized trial of yoga for stress and substance use among people living with HIV in re-entry (Wimberly AS, et al. J Subst Abuse Treat. 2018)	Subjects with HIV and substance use disorder ($n = 73$)	Hatha Yoga practice for 12 sessions, weekly 90 minutes ($n = 37$) as intervention and TAU ($n = 36$) as control group	At 3 months, yoga participants reported less stress than participants in TAU. Yoga participants reported less substance use than participants in TAU at 1, 2, and 3 months
4.	A preliminary study of spiritual self-schema (3-S+) therapy for reducing impulsivity in HIV-positive drug users (Margolin A, et al. J Clin Psychol. 2007)	Users of illicit drugs, i.e., either heroin or cocaine ($n = 38$)	The specific meditation technique "anapanasati" for 12 weeks, each week for 60 minutes ($n = 21$) as intervention and methadone maintenance program only ($n = 17$) as control group	Compared to the control Group, the meditation group showed a trend to decreased alcohol and drug use, and improved impulsivity, spirituality, and motivation for abstinence; attendance in meditation group correlated to decreased substance use, impulsivity, and increased influence of spirituality on abstinence and HIV prevention motivation
5.	Mindfulness meditation and substance use in an incarcerated population (Bowen S, et. al. Psychol Addict Behav. 2006)	Users of various substances ($n = 305$)	Vipassana meditation (VM) for 10 days ($n = 63$) as intervention group and TAU aftercare ($n = 242$) as control group	At 3 months, compared to controls, meditation reduced alcohol, cocaine and marijuana use, and alcohol-related consequences, and improved psychiatric symptoms, drinking-related locus of control and optimism; the changes were related to the VM participation; At 6 months, recidivism rates (the only results reported for 6 months) were low, and comparable between the groups
6.	Yoga as an adjunct treatment for alcohol dependence: a pilot study (Hallgren M, et al. Complement Ther Med. 2014)	Alcohol-dependent patients ($n = 18$)	Treatment as usual + Yoga for 10 weeks in intervention group and only TAU in control group	Yoga was found to be a feasible and well-accepted adjunct treatment for alcohol dependence. Alcohol consumption reduced more in the TAU plus yoga group compared to the TAU only group
7.	Antidepressant efficacy and hormonal effects of Sudarshana Kriya Yoga (SKY) in alcohol dependent individuals (Vedamurthachar A, et al. J Affect Disord. 2006)	Inpatients of alcohol dependence ($n = 60$)	SKY therapy for 2 weeks ($n = 30$) in intervention group and continued inpatient care only ($n = 30$) as control group	In both groups, reductions in the Beck Depression Inventory (BDI) scores occurred but significantly more so in SKY group. Likewise, in both groups plasma cortisol as well as ACTH fell after 2 weeks but significantly more so in the SKY group. Reduction in BDI scores correlated with that in cortisol in SKY but not in control group

Contd...

Contd...

S. No.	Title of the study (Author name, Journal, and Year)	Population and sample size	Intervention and control intervention	Results
8.	Mindfulness training for smoking cessation: results from a randomized controlled trial (Brewer JA, et al. Drug Alcohol Depend. 2011)	Nicotine-dependent adults ($n = 88$)	Mindfulness training for weekly twice for 4 weeks ($n = 41$) as intervention and freedom from smoking (FFS) treatment ($n = 47$) as control group	88% of individuals received mindfulness training (MT) and 84% of individuals received FFS completed treatment. Compared to those randomized to the FFS intervention, individuals who received MT showed a greater rate of reduction in cigarette use during treatment and maintained these gains during follow-up. They also exhibited a trend toward greater point prevalence abstinence rate at the end of treatment, which was significant at the 17-week follow-up
9.	Yoga as a complementary treatment for smoking cessation in women (Bock BC, et al. J Women's Health. 2012)	Women with smoking addiction ($n = 55$)	Group-based cognitive behavioral therapy (CBT) for smoking cessation + yoga program (yoga) for twice a week for 8 weeks ($n = 32$) as intervention and CBT for smoking cessation plus a group-based wellness program ($n = 23$) as control group	Women in the yoga group had a greater 7-day point-prevalence abstinence rate than controls. Abstinence remained higher among yoga participants through the 6th month assessment, but not statistically significant. Women participating in the yoga program also showed reduced anxiety and improvements in perceived health and well-being when compared with controls
10.	Randomized trial comparing mindfulness training for smokers to a matched control (Davis JM, et al. J Subst Abuse Treat. 2014)	Smoking individuals ($n = 135$)	Mindfulness training for smokers (MTS) for 7 weeks which comprised of 2½-hour MTS every week for 7 weeks and a week of 6½-hour Quit day Retreat ($n = 68$) as intervention and FFS technique ($n = 67$) as control group	A significant difference was not found in the primary outcome; intent-to-treat biochemically confirmed 6-month smoking abstinence rates were mindfulness. Differences favoring the mindfulness condition were found on measures of urges and changes in mindfulness, perceived stress, and experiential avoidance. While no significant differences were found in quit rates, the mindfulness intervention resulted in positive outcomes
11.	A pilot feasibility and acceptability study of yoga/meditation on the quality of life (QOL) and markers of stress in persons living with HIV who also use crack cocaine (Agarwal RP, et al. J Altern Complement Med. 2015)	Users of crack cocaine who is also having HIV ($n = 24$)	Yoga/Meditation (YM) for 1 hour twice a week for 2 months ($n = 12$) as intervention and no intervention for control group ($n = 12$)	YM participants showed modest improvements on QOL. The Perceived Stress Scale (PSS) total score and the Impact of Events Scale (IES) intrusion score improved significantly 2 months after the intervention, but cortisol and dehydroepiandrosterone sulfate (DHEA-S) did not change

emotion regulation which points to probable mechanisms of action of yoga.

Studies have found that subjects with practice of mindfulness meditation showed greater prefrontal cortex activation[24-26] and deactivation of amygdalae[27] during an emotion-labeling test. Studies have also found structural neuroplastic adaptation effects in the areas of amygdala which shrunk in size after 8 weeks of mindfulness meditation practice.[28] These findings point to the potential role of mindfulness on inducing neuroplastic changes in regions that regulate affect and emotions. It was observed that in long-term meditators, the gray matter thickness in various areas of cortex (such as areas associated with attention, introspection, and self-regulation) was higher.[26] Parts of prefrontal cortex, i.e., anterior cingulate cortex, orbitofrontal cortex and insula can be strengthened by practicing mindfulness meditation. This may help in reasoning and cognition enhancement, and better regulation of emotions.[24,29] Enhanced connectivity between prefrontal cortex and limbic areas is found in meditators, possibly suggesting desensitization of negative affect and emotions. Meditation has also been shown to enhance connectivity between prefrontal cortex and limbic areas, to inhibit amygdalae, and to increase the hippocampal volume. This may lead to reduction of pain, stress and also behavioral changes which may manifest as enhanced ability to recognize what is important, better control over impulsive acts.[27,30] **Figure 1**, given here, depicts probable mechanisms of action of Yoga in SUD. Another probable way in which yoga might work is the greater functional connectivity between default mode network and other brain networks; this is found to enhance somatosensory processing and reduce emotional reactivity in the limbic system.[31,32]

Studies have also found reduction in levels of plasma norepinephrine and lowered stress levels after transcendental meditation.[33] Similarly, increase in plasma serotonin,[34] increase in peripheral melatonin, and reduction in cortisol levels[35] are other mechanisms which point to the role of yoga practice in bringing parasympathetic

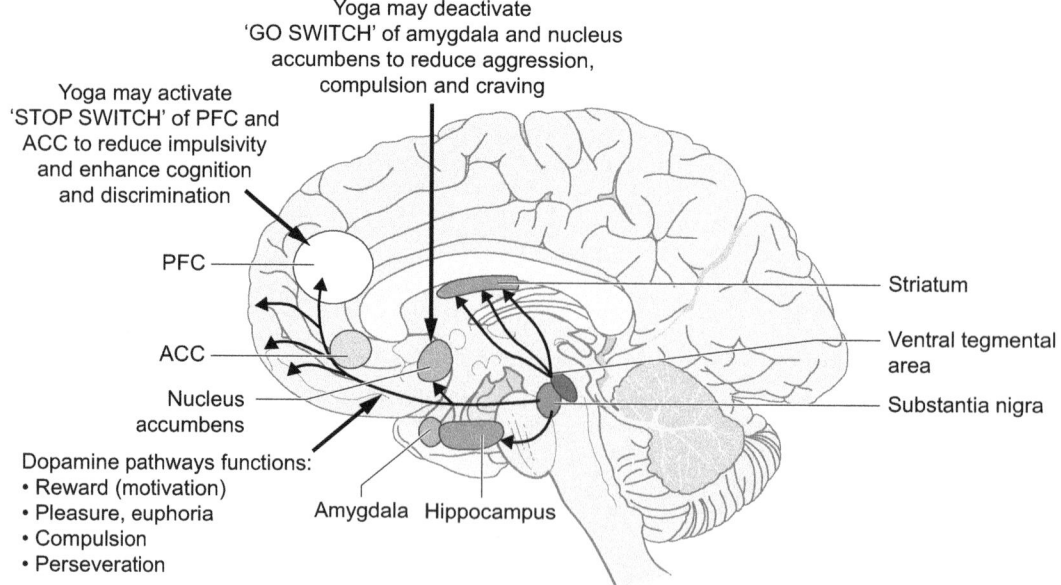

Fig. 1: Probable mechanisms of action of yoga in substance use disorder (SUD) (PFC: prefrontal cortex; ACC: anterior cingulate cortex).

dominance. Enhancement of GABA,[36] serum oxytocin[37] and plasma beta-endorphin levels[38] are other mechanisms which may be involved in the positive effects of yoga on improving mood, socialization, and well-being in those with SUD.

A YOGA MODULE FOR SUBSTANCE USE DISORDER

A Yoga module for opioid addiction has been developed and validated at the National Institute of Mental Health and Neuro Sciences (NIMHANS), Bengaluru. This module was developed by a thorough search of ancient and modern literatures with the objective of reducing opiate withdrawal symptoms (such as nausea, pain, running nose, fatigue, low mood, anxiety, and sleep disturbances) as well as craving associated with these drugs. This module also focuses on improving physical and mental strength of patients with opioid dependence. This yoga program was then validated by 13 experts who had more than 5 years of experience in treating psychiatric patients through yoga therapy.

Based on the suggestions given by experts, two Yoga modules were developed for patients with opioid dependence syndrome (ODS): (1) yoga module during the acute phase of withdrawal and (2) yoga module during the maintenance phase. After validation, four practices were deleted from the module as they did not reach the cutoff scores: (1) *Vrikshasana* (tree pose), (2) *Ujjayi pranayama* (victorious breath), (3) *Sitali pranayama* (cooling breath), and (4) *Chandra anuloma viloma pranayama* (left nostril breathing). All experts felt that *pawanamuktasana* breathing was useful but 70% of the experts suggested practicing *pawanamuktasana kriya* rather than the breathing (though *kriya* was not recommended in the acute symptomatic phase). Similarly, the following practices were not recommended by the more than 50% of experts for use during the acute symptomatic phase of drug withdrawal: (1) Straight leg raise breathing using both legs together (practice using alternate legs was allowed); (2) *Bhujangasana* (cobra pose) breathing; (3) *Naukasana* (boat pose) breathing; (4) *Vyaghrasana* (tiger stretch) breathing; (5) *Bhunamanasana* (earth salutation) breathing; (6) *Trikonasana* (triangle pose); (7) *Surya Namaskar* (sun salutation); and (8) *Kapalabhati* (skull shining breath). Experts also suggested adding the following practices into the module for the maintenance phase: (1) *Patangasana* (butterfly) and (2) *Bhramari in shanmukhi mudra* (humming breath). Two further modifications were: (1) Reducing the intensity of *Bhastrika* practice from 30 strokes/cycle to 20 strokes/cycle and (2) Replacing practice of "Om" chanting by *bhramari* (humming breath) in case the subject is unwilling or uncomfortable owing to his/her sociocultural background. This module was subsequently tested for feasibility in eight opioid-dependent inpatients (6 males and 2 females). All subjects received 10 sessions of the yoga program (1 hour/day, 5 days a week). Assessments were done before and after 10 sessions testing the ability to learn and perform the yoga practices, clinical symptoms, buprenorphine dosage, sleep latency and duration, and adverse effects of the module. *Kapalabhati* practices were not found to be feasible as subjects complained of stomach cramps during the practice. Hence, it was removed and the module was finalized. The content validity index (CVI) for the whole module (average of all content validity ratios) was 0.66. The module was found to be feasible and potentially useful as an adjuvant in managing withdrawal symptoms, reducing craving and promoting overall well-being in patients with ODS. **Appendix 1.9** provides details of the yoga module to be used in acute withdrawal phase as well as maintenance phase.

PRECAUTIONS TO BE FOLLOWED

By the Patient

There are some precautions which a patient suffering from SUD should follow while practicing yoga. These are as follows: (1) After consuming any solid food, give a gap of 3 hours before the practice of yoga; (2) Clothing should be loose and comfortable; (3) The place where yoga is practiced should be adequately ventilated and free of pollution; (4) Yoga should be practiced as per the capacity and is only to be increased in intensity very gradually; (5) While doing asanas, attention should be on the body parts that are being moved; (6) While doing pranayama, attention should be on the touch of the air in the nostrils; (7) Women should avoid fast and intense practices during menstruation and pregnancy; and (8) One should always consult a trained yoga teacher, reveal all health problems that one has and should only practice under supervision in the initial phase.

By the Yoga Therapist

Yoga therapists should be careful about following points while teaching Yoga to patients with SUDs: (1) Observe patience: Yoga therapists should give sufficient amount of time and energy to build a good rapport with the patient as patients with SUD may be less compliant in the initial phases (due to withdrawal symptoms and restlessness); (2) Start with less intensity: Patients may have aches and pains, and they may also feel lethargic. Hence, it is important to start with slow, simple and useful practices that are safe such as whole body joint loosening, relaxation techniques and slow pranayama; (3) Avoid being too slow: Since the patient is in a state of mind where they cannot remain focused for long and slow practices may make them more restless, it is important to change practices frequently and do them for shorter duration in the beginning; (4) Do not leave the patient alone: Such patients may have strong suicidal tendencies or they may abscond from hospital. A hospital staff should preferably accompany the patient from hospital to the yoga center; (5) Avoid emotional involvement with patients: Maintain empathy without compromising the professional role; and (6) Motivate patients to practice yoga regularly and motivate caregivers to monitor yoga practices by the patient.

CONCLUSION

With all these evidences, yoga can be considered as a viable option in treating SUD and as a holistic adjunct therapy. Yoga may help reduce severity and improve quality of life in patients suffering from SUDs.

ACKNOWLEDGMENTS

We would like to acknowledge Department of Science and Technology (DST), Government of India for financial support vide Reference no. DST/005/504/2018/01112 under Science and Technology of Yoga and Meditation (SATYAM) scheme to carry out the research in yoga for opioid use disorder.

CASE VIGNETTE

A 32-year-old married male from Manipur, suffering from ODS (ICD-10 criteria) for 8 years, was admitted to the Centre for Addiction Medicine (CAM) at NIMHANS in August 2018. This patient had been injecting heroin (1 g/day) for 8 years and was addicted. He had relapsed four times in the past with a maximum duration of abstinence of 1.5 months. He was admitted to NIMHANS and his predominant withdrawal symptoms were body pain, stomach cramps, running nose, goose flesh, and headache with strong craving for heroin. He also complained of weight loss and constipation. He was started on Buprenorphine 2 mg/day which was gradually increased over a week to 18 mg/day. On the 3rd day of admission, he was referred to the NIMHANS Integrated Centre for Yoga. He practiced a validated yoga program for 1 month (1 hour/day) under the supervision of a trained Yoga therapist. At the time of discharge, he was asymptomatic and denied craving. His sleep quality was better, the joint pains and constipation had reduced. He specifically reported that his ability to concentrate improved with yoga (was able to read books which was not possible earlier).

There was also a marginal increase in his basal plasma beta-endorphin levels from 2.02 pmol/L to 2.21 pmol/L after 15 days of yoga practice. He felt more confident of abstaining from heroin, after the practice of yoga. At the time of discharge, he was on 6 mg of Buprenorphine. Patient was given a booklet for yoga practice

Clinical Insights: Yoga Therapy for Substance Use Disorder

Prior to the session	• Therapists must be aware of the diagnosis, comorbidities, the stage of withdrawal and the medications that the patient is on at the time of first consultation. • Any emergency situations that are common in acute withdrawal phase such as seizures, delirium should be anticipated and appropriate referrals to medical services should be done. In these situations, using yoga as sole treatment should be avoided as they can be life-threatening and immediate medical intervention is required. • Therapist should emphasize on establishing a good rapport with the patient as this may contribute to compliance of treatment in the long run. • Long-term rewards of the sustained yoga practice should be emphasized to keep the patient motivated. • Avoid practices which can cause sympathetic overactivity (e.g., rapid *kapalabhati* and *bhastrika*) in the acute withdrawal phase. • Deep relaxation with breath regulation and mild simulations should be emphasized during the acute withdrawal phase, but advanced meditations should be avoided as patients may not have the sustained attention to practice that. • Patients may have stomach cramps due to withdrawal symptoms—in such case *Kapalabhati* practice should be avoided.
During the session	• The therapist should be aware that these patients may be irritable and may have very poor motivation to engage in the session. This should be dealt with patience and a lot of encouragement from the therapist. • In the initial phases (after the withdrawal phase is over), focus on fast dynamic practices as this will keep the patient engaged and may help to manage their cravings. • *Have frequent changes in the practices and avoid very slow practice so the patient's attention can be engaged.* • Practices should be designed keeping in mind the biological effects of substance use and withdrawal (e.g., practices to reduce sympathetic activity in case of alcohol withdrawal, improve endorphins in case of opioid dependence). • *Surya namaskar*, breathing techniques (slow but forceful *kapalabhati* and *bhastrika*), and mantra chanting (a, u, m or *Om*) followed by part-by-part deep relaxation of the body should be emphasized to help them control cue-induced craving in the maintenance phase. • *Many patients have difficulty in sleeping*—you can add left nostril breathing, humming breath, deep abdominal breathing with prolonged exhalations (inhalation/exhalation = 1:3) and *Om* mantra chanting at bedtime just before going to sleep. • Depending on the patient's receptivity, yoga-based spiritual counseling can be tried as an add-on intervention. • Any comorbid illness like depression and anxiety must be adequately addressed with the appropriate practices subsequently, once the patient is out of withdrawal.
After the session	• Encourage patients to continue yoga as a part of his/her lifestyle. • Depending on the type of personality, use *Karma yoga*, *Bhakti yoga*, *Jnana yoga* or *Raja yoga* philosophies to guide the patient toward growth. Use yoga to enhance the sense of purpose in patients' lives. • Along with yoga, other lifestyle modifications and treatments as suggested by the treating consultants should be continued. Appropriate collaboration is needed for a multimodal treatment approach.

and a video to continue practicing at home after discharge. He was asked to follow-up every 3 months. Assessments were done using standardized rating scales at baseline, at 3 and 9 months of follow-up, his plasma beta-endorphin levels were also assessed at baseline and 15 days of practice.

The dose of Buprenorphine was reduced to 6 mg after 3 months and 2 mg after 5 months. He stopped Buprenorphine completely on his own 5 months after the discharge, but increased smoking to 5–6 cigarettes per day. He continued to practice Yoga on and off (was practicing only on Saturdays and Sundays as he had started a job. At his 9-month follow-up, he had been off Buprenorphine for 4 months. He specifically mentioned that fast yoga breathing practice of "Bhastrika" (bellows breathing) 20 counts, 3 sets, regulated breathing, mantra chanting (a, u, m) and surya namaskar helped him overcome craving, and reduce restlessness, pain, and lethargy. There was a significant reduction in craving, withdrawal symptoms, anxiety, depression, pain, and constipation at 3 months which continued to improve till 9 months. There was also an improvement in his sexual functioning, sleep quality and in Clinical Global Improvement scale scores. He was last followed up in March 2020 and reported that he is doing well without Buprenorphine, and continues to practice yoga twice a week. However, his nicotine addiction still persists. On a more positive note, he continues to hold his job. He visits NIMHANS Integrated Centre for Yoga once a month for a booster yoga session and reports no craving. His urine screening for opioids was negative at 3rd, 6th, and 9th month of follow-up. At the last follow-up he said "lots of my friends died due to heroin overdose and I was scared that this would happen to me as well, for the first time in the last 8 years, I am able to abstain from heroin for such a long time (9 months). I feel confident that I can come out of it. I attribute 50% of my success to change of my place of residence and 50% to my yoga practice and support from my yoga teacher, which improved my will power".

REFERENCES

1. World Health Organization. Substance abuse. [online] Available from: https://www.who.int/topics/substance_abuse/en/ [Last accessed October, 2020].
2. World Health Organization. Global status report on alcohol and health 2018. [online] Available from: https://www.who.int/gho/alcohol/en/ [Last accessed October, 2020].
3. United Nation Office on Drugs and Crime (UNODC). World Drug Report 2019: 35 million people worldwide suffer from drug use disorders while only 1 in 7 people receive treatment. [online] Available from: https://www.unodc.org/unodc/en/press/releases/2019/June/world-drug-report-2019_-35-million-people-worldwide-suffer-from-drug-use-disorders-while-only-1-in-7-people-receive-treatment.html [Last accessed October, 2020].
4. World Health Organization (1993). The ICD-10 classification of mental and behavioural disorders. [online] Available from: https://apps.who.int/iris/handle/10665/37958 [Last accessed October, 2020].
5. Koob GF, Volkow ND. Neurobiology of addiction: a neurocircuitry analysis. Lancet Psychiatry. 2016;3(8):760-73.
6. Luty J. Drug and alcohol addiction: do psychosocial treatments work? BJPsych Advances. 2015;21(2):132-43.
7. Cabral P, Meyer HB, Ames D. Effectiveness of yoga therapy as a complementary treatment for major psychiatric disorders: a meta-analysis. Prim Care Companion CNS Disord. 2011;13(4):PCC.10r01068.
8. Balasubramaniam M, Telles S, Doraiswamy PM. Yoga on our minds: a systematic review of yoga for neuropsychiatric disorders. Front Psychiatry. 2013;3:117.
9. Bilderbeck AC, Farias M, Brazil IA, Jakobowitz S, Wikholm C. Participation in a 10-week course of yoga improves behavioural control and decreases psychological distress in a prison population. J Psychiatric Res. 2013;47(10):1438-45.
10. Bhargav H, Nagendra HR, Gangadhar BN, Nagarathna R. Frontal hemodynamic responses to high frequency yoga breathing in schizophrenia: a functional near-infrared spectroscopy study. Front Psychiatry. 2014;5:29.

11. Streeter CC, Gerbarg PL, Saper RB, Ciraulo DA, Brown RP. Effects of yoga on the autonomic nervous system, gamma-aminobutyric acid, and allostasis in epilepsy, depression, and post-traumatic stress disorder. Med Hypotheses. 2012;78(5):571-9.
12. Kalyani BG, Venkatasubramanian G, Arasappa R, Rao NP, Kalmady SV, Behere RV, et al. Neurohemodynamic correlates of "OM" chanting: a pilot functional magnetic resonance imaging study. Int J Yoga. 2011;4(1):3-6.
13. Fahmy R, Wasfi M, Mamdouh R, Moussa K, Wahba A, Schmitgen MM, et al. Mindfulness-based therapy modulates default-mode network connectivity in patients with opioid dependence. Eur Neuropsychopharmacol. 2019;29(5):662-71.
14. Lander L, Chiasson-Downs K, Andrew M, Rader G, Dohar S, Waibogha K. Yoga as an adjunctive intervention to medication-assisted treatment with buprenorphine + naloxone. J Addict Res Ther. 2018;9(1):354.
15. Wimberly AS, Engstrom M, Layde M, McKay JR. A randomized trial of yoga for stress and substance use among people living with HIV in reentry. J Subst Abuse Treat. 2018;94:97-104.
16. Margolin A, Schuman-Olivier Z, Beitel M, Arnold RM, Fulwiler CE, Avants SK. A preliminary study of spiritual self-schema (3-S+) therapy for reducing impulsivity in HIV-positive drug users. J Clin Psychol. 2007;63(10):979-99.
17. Bowen S, Witkiewitz K, Dillworth TM, Chawla N, Simpson TL, Ostafin BD, et al. Mindfulness meditation and substance use in an incarcerated population. Psychol Addict Behav. 2006;20(3):343-7.
18. Hallgren M, Romberg K, Bakshi AS, Andréasson S. Yoga as an adjunct treatment for alcohol dependence: a pilot study. Complement Ther Med. 2014;22(3):441-5.
19. Vedamurthachar A, Janakiramaiah N, Hegde JM, Shetty TK, Subbakrishna DK, Sureshbabu SV, et al. Antidepressant efficacy and hormonal effects of Sudarshana Kriya Yoga (SKY) in alcohol dependent individuals. J Affect Disord. 2006;94(1-3):249-53.
20. Brewer JA, Mallik S, Babuscio TA, Nich C, Johnson HE, Deleone CM, et al. Mindfulness training for smoking cessation: results from a randomized controlled trial. Drug Alcohol Depend. 2011;119(1-2):72-80.
21. Bock BC, Fava JL, Gaskins R, Morrow KM, Williams DM, Jennings E, et al. Yoga as a complementary treatment for smoking cessation in women. J Women's Health. 2012;21(2):240-8.
22. Davis JM, Manley AR, Goldberg SB, Smith SS, Jorenby DE. Randomized trial comparing mindfulness training for smokers to a matched control. J Subst Abuse Treat. 2014;47(3):213-21.
23. Agarwal RP, Kumar A, Lewis JE. A pilot feasibility and acceptability study of yoga/meditation on the quality of life and markers of stress in persons living with HIV who also use crack cocaine. J Altern Complement Med. 2015;21(3):152-8.
24. Creswell JD, Way BM, Eisenberger NI, Lieberman MD. Neural correlates of dispositional mindfulness during affect labeling. Psychosom Med. 2007;69(6):560-5.
25. Hölzel BK, Ott U, Gard T, Hempel H, Weygandt M, Morgen K, et al. Investigation of mindfulness meditation practitioners with voxel-based morphometry. Soc Cogn Affect Neurosci. 2007;3(1):55-61.
26. Kang DH, Jo HJ, Jung WH, Kim SH, Jung YH, Choi CH, et al. The effect of meditation on brain structure: cortical thickness mapping and diffusion tensor imaging. Soc Cogn Affect Neurosci. 2012;8(1):27-33.
27. Desbordes G, Negi LT, Pace TW, Wallace BA, Raison CL, Schwartz EL. Effects of mindful-attention and compassion meditation training on amygdala response to emotional stimuli in an ordinary, non-meditative state. Front Hum Neurosci. 2012;6:292.
28. Hölzel BK, Carmody J, Evans KC, Hoge EA, Dusek JA, Morgan L, et al. Stress reduction correlates with structural changes in the amygdala. Soc Cogn Affect Neurosci. 2009;5(1):11-7.
29. Esch T, Stefano GB. The neurobiology of stress management. Neuroendocrinol Lett. 2010;31(1):19-39.
30. Hölzel BK, Carmody J, Vangel M, Congleton C, Yerramsetti SM, Gard T, et al. Mindfulness practice leads to increases in regional brain gray matter density. Psychiatry Res. 2011;191(1):36-43.
31. Brewer JA, Worhunsky PD, Gray JR, Tang YY, Weber J, Kober H. Meditation experience is associated with differences in default mode network activity and connectivity. Proc Natl Acad Sci USA. 2011;108(50):20254-9.
32. Hasenkamp W, Wilson-Mendenhall CD, Duncan E, Barsalou LW. Mind wandering and attention during focused meditation: a fine-grained temporal analysis of fluctuating cognitive states. Neuroimage. 2012;59(1):750-60.
33. Infante JR, Torres-Avisbal M, Pinel P, Vallejo JA, Peran F, Gonzalez F, et al. Catecholamine levels in practitioners of the transcendental meditation technique. Physiol Behav. 2001;72(1-2):141-6.

34. Bujatti M, Biederer P. Serotonin, noradrenaline, dopamine metabolites in transcendental meditation-technique. J Neural Transm. 1976;39(3):257-67.
35. Solberg EE, Holen A, Ekeberg Ø, Østerud B, Halvorsen R, Sandvik L. The effects of long meditation on plasma melatonin and blood serotonin. Med Sci Monit. 2004;10(3):CR96-101.
36. Streeter CC, Jensen JE, Perlmutter RM, Cabral HJ, Tian H, Terhune DB, et al. Yoga asana sessions increase brain GABA levels: a pilot study. J Altern Complement Med. 2007;13(4):419-26.
37. Jayaram N, Varambally S, Behere RV, Venkatasubramanian G, Arasappa R, Christopher R, et al. Effect of yoga therapy on plasma oxytocin and facial emotion recognition deficits in patients of schizophrenia. Indian J Psychiatry. 2013;55(Suppl 3):S409.
38. Yadav RK, Magan D, Mehta N, Sharma R, Mahapatra SC. Efficacy of a short-term yoga-based lifestyle intervention in reducing stress and inflammation: preliminary results. J Altern Complement Med. 2012;18(7):662-7.

CHAPTER 17

Yoga in Chronic Pain Syndromes

Sowjanya Dumbala, Kankan Gulati, Sundarnag Ganjekar, Geetha Desai

INTRODUCTION

The word "Pain" is derived from the Latin word "*Poena*" meaning "to pay the penalty".[1] According to IASP (The International Association for the Study of Pain), pain is described as "an unpleasant sensory and emotional experience associated with actual or potential tissue damage or described in terms of such damage".[2] This definition includes not only sensory experiences but also emotional responses.[3] Both components have different characteristics. The first, i.e., the sensory component is characterized by the type of pain and its intensity. The type of pain can be described as "burning", "sharp", "dull" or "aching". The magnitude of pain describes its intensity. The second component, i.e., the reactive component comprises the emotional response to pain. Various words that are used to denote emotions are used to describe the emotional component, depending on the intensity or magnitude of pain.[4] Pain has been classified as acute and chronic, based on the duration of the experience of pain. In acute pain, the underlying cause is often evident and in chronic pain, multiple factors might be associated without a clear cause for the experience of pain.

Pain has been considered as a symptom of an underlying disease and hence the focus has been on treatment of the underlying cause. With the development of research in the area of pain, "Chronic pain" is now considered a distinct diagnostic entity. Treatment of chronic pain is often challenging as the cause may not be evident. Chronic primary pain (CPP) is a new diagnosis that has been added to the ICD-11 classificatory system.[5] It is intended to encompass several poorly understood pain conditions, while avoiding uncertain and confusing terms such as "somatoform", "nonspecific", or "functional". A distinct CPP syndrome classification will help in avoiding problems associated with previous classifications of chronic pain when the etiology is unclear but the emotional distress and functional disability associated with such pain are very evident.[6] In this chapter, we will focus on chronic pain types such as neck pain, fibromyalgia, dysmenorrhea, arthritis, and somatoform pain disorders.

Chronic primary pain may show up in any body-site such as the face, lower back, neck, abdomen, pelvis, urogenital region or any bodily system namely nervous, musculoskeletal or gastrointestinal systems. It can also be widespread, i.e., involving a combination of body sites.[6]

YOGIC UNDERSTANDING OF PAIN

According to Yoga, *Vyadi* (known as the disease in modern medicine) are of two types: (1) *Adhija* and (2) *Anadhija*. *Adhija* ailments are caused due to *Adhi or* stress and originate in the mind. *Anadhija* disorders caused due to trauma, injury, toxins, nutritional deficiencies and infections and are not originated in the mind. Similarly, the cause of pain can also be classified as *Adhija* (Functional) or *Anadhija* (Organic). Negative emotional states and stress

(*Adhija*) influence responses to trauma, injury or any other diseases caused by environmental factors (*Anadhija*). Hence it appears that chronic pain is a combination of *Adhija* and *Anadhija*. Chronic pain may also be caused due to non-specific causes related to modern lifestyle—*Adhija vyadis* which begins at the mind (*manas*) level.

To understand the cause of pain we first need to understand how the existence of human body is explained by yoga.

According to *Taittireya Upanishad*, the human body exists in five layers described as the *Panchakoshas*. Concepts in *Upanishads* are explained in the form of stories. *Bhrigu*, a student who was in search of reality was guided by his teacher who was also his father, *Varuna*. While searching for the ultimate truth, the five-layered existence of the human being was revealed to *Bhrigu*, which was nothing but the *Panchakosha* model. The five layers or the five *koshas* are as follows:[7]

1. *Annamaya kosha* (the physical layer): *Annamaya kosha* is the physical layer, which is the grossest of the five layers and is nourished by the food we consume.
2. *Pranamaya kosha* (the layer of *Prana*): *Prana* in Sanskrit means "life energy". It is subtler than the electromagnetic energy spectrum (electricity, sound, light, X-rays, etc.) known to modern science. It forms the basic fabric of the universe both inside and outside our bodies. A uniform and harmonious flow of *Prana* to every cell of *Annamaya kosha* keeps it alive and healthy.
3. *Manomaya kosha* (the mental layer): It is our mental and emotional library. It is the main aspect of one's personality and it performs different functions such as *Pramana* (conception), *Viparyaya* (misconception), *Vikalpa* (imagination), *Nidra* (sleep), *Smrithi* (memory), and *Ahankara* (ego).
4. *Vijnanamaya kosha* (the layer of wisdom): It is the fourth aspect of our existence. It is the conscience that continuously guides *Manomaya kosha* to get mastery over one's basic instincts. It gives us the power to discriminate between what is right and what is wrong and acts as our knowledge base.
5. *Anandamaya kosha* (the layer of bliss): This layer is the subtlest aspect of our existence. It is devoid of all forms of emotions, and is the state of total silence, complete harmony and perfect health.

It is believed that the stress or the disturbances of the *Manomaya kosha* (the mental layer) percolate through *Pranamaya kosha* and start showing its effects on the physical layer which is the *Annamaya kosha*. Therefore, to treat psychosomatic diseases it is important to work on all these levels of existence and not just on the physical sheath (*Annamaya kosha*).[8]

Also, according to *Patanjali Yoga Sutras*, *Kleshas* a kind of agony, is the root cause of pain to living beings. Sage *Patanjali* in the third verse of the second chapter mentions the five *Kleshas* namely *avidya* (ignorance), *asmita* (I-feeling), *raga* (liking), *dvesha* (repulsion), and *abhinivesah* (fear of death) which form the basis of all pain. These are afflictions that keep distracting the human mind. He then provides a solution to these mental afflictions and advises that one should practise *Kriya yoga* in order to eliminate these *Kleshas*. Kriya yoga constitutes of *tapas* (austerity), *swadhyaya* (self-study) and *Ishwara pranidhana* (surrender to god). By *tapas* he means self-discipline and austerity, i.e., a person practising *Kriya yoga* should lead a disciplined life. *Swadhyaya* or developing a perception about one's own self, will help one see their own consciousness and *Ishwara pranidhana* is merging with the inner awareness. Therefore, *Kriya yoga* is a combination of discipline, purification, observation and developing awareness about the self and helps in getting rid of the aforementioned afflictions.[9]

POSSIBLE MECHANISMS OF ACTION OF YOGA IN CHRONIC PAIN

Pain can be caused by any of the reasons described above. According to yoga, chronic pain is the result of long standing *Adhi* or stress, which begins in the *Manomaya kosha* and manifests initially as a psychological problem such as sleep disturbances, emotional instability, irritability and so on. After many years, this starts disturbing the *Pranamaya kosha* and slowly percolates to the *Annamaya kosha*. In the *Annamaya kosha*, it manifests as any one of the digestive problems such as constipation, indigestion or flatulence, which are known as common precursors of stress-induced diseases. When one is stressed, his/her mind is heavily loaded with a number of rushing thoughts. Such increased flow of thoughts in the mind is called *Adhi* or stress. The most efficient way to manage stress is to control the flow of the thoughts in our mind, which in turn can be controlled by manipulating one's breath rate. Depending on the degree of stress, there is an imbalance in the *Pranic* flow in the body. If this goes on for a few years, it manifests at the *Annamaya kosha* as unexplained pain in the form of sprain, strain, spasm, cramp, pain or inflammation. A combination of these imbalances settles down in one particular part of the body showing up as acute or chronic pain with no detectable physical or organic cause.

Practicing yoga and *pranayama* helps in controlling the mind by gaining control over breath, thereby removing blockages in the *Nadis* (energy channels). *Pranic* flow to the affected part is balanced, ultimately decreasing pain in the particular part of the body. Hence, yoga helps in eliminating stress-related disorders and reduces dependence on drugs in many pain-related disorders with no underlying physical cause. Also, musculoskeletal pain disorders can be treated by improving the function and increasing the range of movement, strength, balance, and dexterity.

THE RATIONALE FOR THE USE OF YOGA FOR CHRONIC PAIN

Mind-body interventions such as meditation or yoga have shown to increase pain acceptance and satisfaction in patients with chronic pain.[10] As compared to other interventions including standard care, self-care, therapeutic exercises, relaxing yoga, touch, and manipulation or no intervention, yoga significantly reduces the perception of chronic pain. Yoga is effective in chronic pain syndromes when used as a supplementary approach with moderate effect sizes.[11] Studies have reported that yoga significantly improved measures of function and pain which persisted even after 3 months.[12-14] Another study found that 6 weeks of *Vinyasa* yoga therapy was slightly better than exercise, moderately better than a self-care education book at 12 weeks follow-up of patients with chronic low back pain, and was superior to the self-care education book at 24 weeks.[12] Use of *Iyengar Yoga* therapy has reported a decline in the intake of the pain killer medications among self-referred patients with mild chronic low back pain and hence reduces the cost of treatment.[13] Yoga is also useful in musculoskeletal disorders as it involves slow movements and results in calming effects induced by breathing exercises and meditation.[15]

STUDIES ON YOGA FOR CHRONIC PAIN

There have been several studies evaluating the effectiveness of yoga in management of chronic pain, and many of these studies have focused on a particular type of pain such as chronic low backache, arthritis, migraine, fibromyalgia, dysmenorrhea, neck pain, etc. In this chapter, we have excluded lower back pain and migraine as these are dealt with in separate chapters in this book. Research articles were published in different languages (Chinese, German, and French) and include systematic reviews, meta-analyses, pilot studies, case reports, case studies, short communications, randomized controlled trials (RCTs) and others. Given below are some recent systematic reviews on yoga-based interventions in chronic pain conditions.

Li et al.[16] conducted the first meta-analysis and systematic review to evaluate the effects of yoga in patients with chronic nonspecific neck pain which included only RCTs and q-RCTs (10 trials, n = 686) measuring intensity of neck pain and disability associated with the neck, cervical range of motion (CROM), quality of life (QoL), and emotional state. The yoga intervention used was required to include any type of yoga, irrespective of physical postures, breathing techniques, meditation, or combination of one or more of them. Results showed that yoga had a positive effect on neck pain intensity ($Z = 4.75$, $p < 0.00001$), neck pain-related functional disability ($Z = 3.95$, $p < 0.0001$), CROM ($Z = 6.83$, $p < 0.00001$) and mood ($Z = 3.53$, $p = 0.0004$). Yoga can relieve neck pain intensity, improve pain-related functional disability, increase CROM, improve QoL and boost mood.[16]

Russell et al.[17] conducted a systematic review and meta-analysis to evaluate the effects of yoga on QoL and in women with chronic pelvic pain. This included three trials (single trial study, RCT and randomized case-controlled study) with intervention of *Iyengar* yoga for 90 minutes, 2 days/week for 6 weeks, yoga 2 hours, 2 days/week for 8 weeks, 1 hour of yoga, 5 days/week for 8 weeks for the three trials respectively. Outcome measures used for pain included: Endometriosis Health Profile-30 (EHP-30) pain domain; Numeric Pain Rating Scale (NPRS); Visual Analog Scale (VAS), Quality of Life: Impact of Pelvic Pain (IPP) Questionnaire, EHP-30 emotional well-being, and World Health Organization Quality of Life (WHOQoL-BREF) brief version. Results showed a statistically significant improvement following the yoga intervention for within-group analysis of QoL (ES = –1.4) pain (ES= –2.2) and the between-group analysis found statistically significant differences in QoL (ES = –1.5) pain (ES = –1.4), favoring the yoga group. Authors concluded that this systematic review provides moderate evidence to support the use of yoga to improve pain, and psychological and emotional QoL domains in women with CPP.[17]

Wang et al.[18] conducted a PRISMA (Preferred Reporting Items for Systematic Reviews and Meta-Analyses) compliant meta-analysis to evaluate the integrative effect of yoga practice in patients with arthritis of the knee using VAS and Short Form-36 Health Survey (SF-36), WOMAC (Western Ontario and McMaster Universities Osteoarthritis Index), HAQ (Health Assessment Questionnaire). This included 13 clinical trials (RCTs) and 1,557 individuals suffering from knee osteoarthritis or rheumatoid arthritis. Of these 13 clinical trials, five trials with 454 participants were further analyzed and provided clear evidence of yoga being more effective in lowering knee pain scores, assessed using VAS as compared to control group. The same study,[18] also describes that four trials with a total of 423 participants using SF-36 survey which is used to measure eight domains including Physical Function (PF), Role Physical (RP), Bodily Pain (BP), General Health (GH), Vitality (VI), Social Function (SF), Role Emotional (RE), and Mental Health (MH)[19] also established that yoga practice helps in reducing pain. Significant changes in scores of pain, functional disability, SF-36, SF-36 GH, SF-36 MH, and HAQ with $p < 0.05$ were reported. From the above findings, it was concluded that regular yoga training helps to reduce knee arthritis symptoms, promotes physical function and enhances general well-being in arthritic patients.

Hyun-Nam et al.[20] conducted a systematic review of RCTs to evaluate the effects of yoga on dysmenorrhea. This review included two RCTs of which one RCT used three poses (cobra, cat, and fish) for 20 min/day for 14 days and another RCT used *Yoga Nidra* for 35–40 min/day, 5 days/week for 6 months. They measured VAS to rate pain relief. Results showed a significant difference between experimental and control groups in pain intensity and pain duration ($p < 0.05$). Thyroid stimulating hormone ($p < 0.002$), follicle-stimulating hormone ($p < 0.02$), luteinizing hormone ($p < 0.001$) and prolactin ($p < 0.02$) decreased significantly in the intervention group, compared with the control group. Authors concluded that there was an overall improvement in symptoms and improvement in pathophysiological parameters.[20]

■ SOMATOFORM PAIN DISORDERS

Somatoform disorders are characterized by persistent, distressing bodily symptoms (e.g., burning, pain, tingling sensations, etc.) for which no underlying or organic cause has been established. This can lead to significant dysfunction and increased health-seeking behavior. Individuals may also experience symptoms of anxiety and depression along with bodily symptoms. In somatoform pain disorder, pain symptoms are persistent with no underlying cause found. Yoga helps in reducing stress levels and thereby helps in managing and preventing pain by giving stability at physical, mental and energy levels. A specific yoga module has been developed and validated for somatoform pain disorders[21] and the details of this module are provided in **Appendix 1.10.**

Practical tips to be kept in mind while practicing yoga for somatoform pain disorders:

a. *Precautions:*
   - Yoga should be learnt in the presence of an expert yoga instructor or under the guidance of a yoga teacher.
   - Each practice should be carried out with breath awareness along with body movement as suggested by the instructor.
   - Each practice should be done with specific awareness of the physical movement or breath or while concentrating on some specific *Chakra*.
   - Relaxation and sequence of practices should be kept in mind while practicing the module as they play a very important role.
   - Time and place of practice are very important factors. Yoga should be practiced on an empty stomach in a well-ventilated place.
   - Do not drink water immediately before and after the yoga session or even while practicing yoga as it may cause discomfort.
   - Clothes worn during yoga may also play an important role. Many people do not prefer to wear a yoga-specific clothes while practicing yoga, but most of the practices will be restricted without appropriate clothes or comfortable loose clothes.
   - Do not strain your body for the perfect *asana*, try to listen to your body while practicing yoga.

b. *Contraindications:*
   - Patients with headache should not practice *Ardhachakrasana, Padahasthasana* and *Ushtrasana*.
   - Patients with stomach pain should not practice *Navasana*.
   - Patients with neck or back pain should not practice *Uttanapadasana* or *Vipareetakarani*.

c. *Special instructions:*
   - The above-mentioned yoga module is for patients suffering from somatoform pain disorders. People suffering from back pain, neck pain and headache with specific medical reasons/conditions such as musculoskeletal disorders should follow the back pain or migraine module respectively, which will be discussed in subsequent chapters of this book.

– Anyone suffering from pain should first consult their doctor and an expert yoga instructor before attempting the above-mentioned yoga module, to confirm whether it can be practiced by them or not.

HOW DOES YOGA HELP IN REDUCING CHRONIC PAIN?

Biological Mechanisms

The mechanism of chronic pain is very complex as all the levels of the nervous system are involved. Chronic pain pathway becomes embedded in the spinal cord and it acts as a relay station where using local and distant networks incoming nociceptive signals are modified and further propagated to the brain. Repeated pain signals, as in chronic pain makes neural pathways hypersensitive. This happens due the alteration of plasticity and physiochemical changes in the neural pathways of the spinal cord and also due to development of resistance to antinociceptive (which help in reducing pain) inputs. Breaking these processes is what an effective mode of treatment should actually do.[22,23]

Normally the activation of innate immune system leads to activation of brain cytokine system. But the over sensitization brain cytokine system may outwardly manifest as somatization disorders.[24] Previous studies have reported increased blood levels of the inflammatory markers including interleukin-6 (IL-6)[25] tumor necrosis factor-alpha (TNF-α) and neopterin are increased in somatization syndromes[26] while a negative correlation was found with serum levels of sIL-2R.[25] Recent research establishes the fact that yoga has the ability to decrease the levels of proinflammatory markers such as IL-6, interleukin-2 (IL-2) and C-reactive protein by activating the vagus nerve.[27] In a RCT, 12 weeks of yoga training has shown to significantly decrease the levels of proinflammatory cytokines IL-1β and significantly increases anti-inflammatory cytokines IL-10 in healthy male volunteers.[28] Other research studies also show similar results, reporting lower levels of pro-inflammatory cytokines including TNF-α, IL-6,[29] high-sensitivity-C-reactive protein (hs-CRP)[30] and Interleukin-12[31] in yoga practitioners **(Fig. 1)**.

Brain-derived neurotrophic factor (BDNF) is a neurotrophin in the brain which plays an important role in pain sensation and serves as a pain modulator. Serotonin neurotransmitters play an important role in somatoform disorders are also influenced by BDNF. Previous studies have reported low levels of plasma BDNF in patients diagnosed with somatization disorder which increases post treatment with antidepressants.[32] Participants taking part in three months of yoga and meditation retreat have shown an increase in plasma BDNF levels with a decrease in self-reported anxiety and depression.[31]

Gamma-aminobutyric acid (GABA) neurons and receptors help in coordinating perception and response to pain at supra-spinal sites.[33] GABA binding with projection neurons help in decreasing pain transmission.[34] Chronic pain which is aggravated by stress is described to have low GABAergic activity, which improves when treated with pharmacologic agents. Yoga helps in stimulating the vagus nerve which increases the parasympathetic activity of the nervous system which further leads to correction of GABA underactivity.[35] Endorphins a part of endogenous opioid system are known to play an important role in modulation of chronic pain. Yoga a mind-body medicine is emerging as a potential alternative therapy to manage chronic painful conditions.[36]

Asanas include abdominal muscular stretches and contraction combined with spinal movements which have compressive/de-compressive effects on the blood flow of the underlying tissues.[37] Overall, yoga enhances blood flow to various parts of the body as it induces vasodilation while decreasing vascular

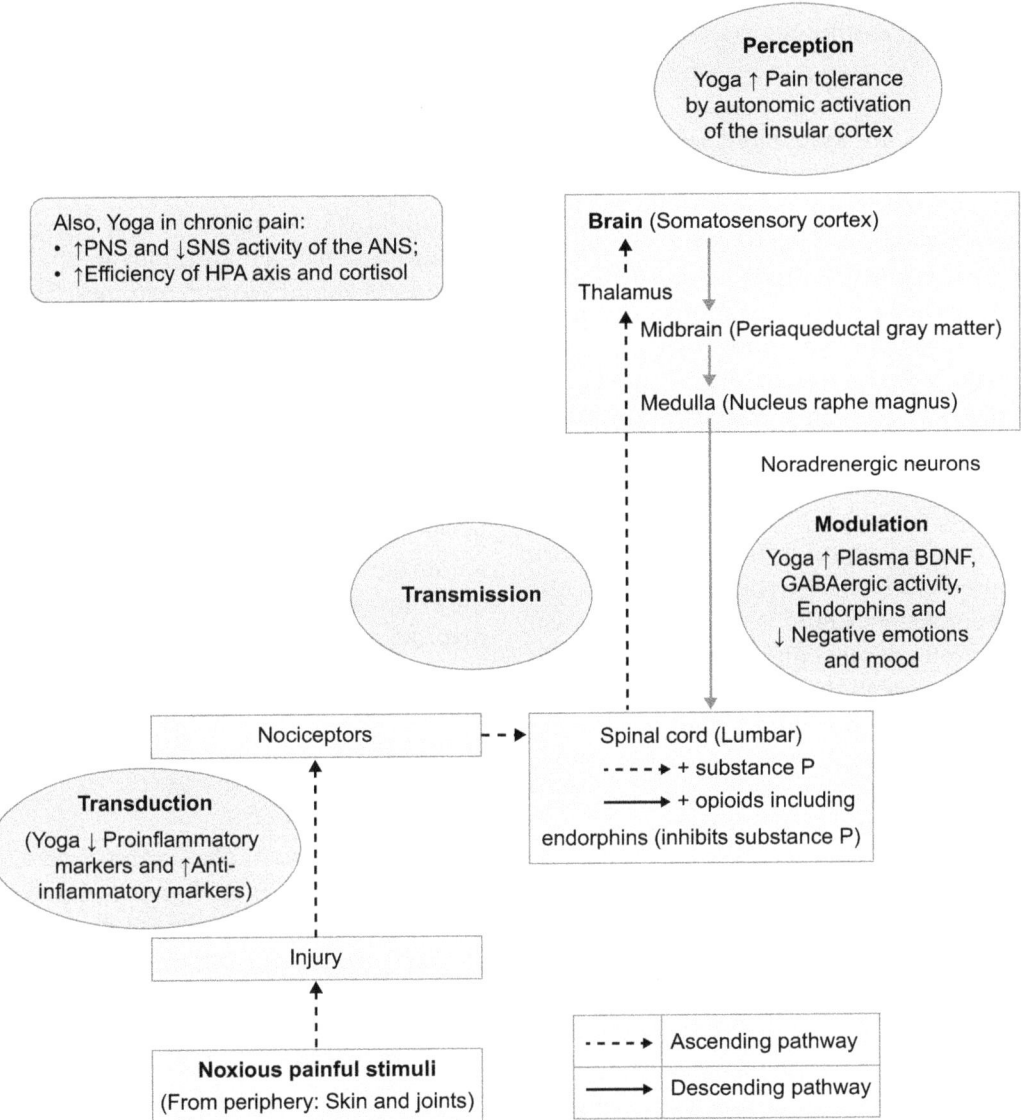

Fig. 1: Schematic diagram of the effects of yoga on pain pathway.

resistance.[38] As compared to healthy controls, a decrease in heart rate activity ("recovery response") during the resting period post performance of attention task has been seen in patients with somatization syndrome.[39] Evidences suggestive of autonomic imbalance, with higher sympathetic activity and lower parasympathetic activity have been established in patients diagnosed with somatoform disorders.[40] Yoga aids stimulation of the vagal nerve which shifts the autonomic balance toward parasympathetic dominance, decreasing sympathetic activity of the nervous system which is evident by lowering breath rate, heart rate, blood pressure and increasing heart rate variability (HRV),[41] thus inducing relaxation.[42]

The involvement of hypothalamic-pituitary-adrenal axis (HPA) in chronic pain is well established[43] and it influences the perception of pain.[44] HPA axis which is activated by stress and leads to hyperalgesia (abnormally heightened sensitivity to pain) following chronic states of distress.[45] Dysregulation of the HPA axis has been reported in many disease states involving chronic pain.[46] Somatoform syndromes are associated with blunted or varied activation pattern of HPA axis and reveal hypocortisolism, i.e., decreased cortisol levels in such patients.[47] A complex mechanism comprising of HPA-axis exhaustion along with reduced cortisol response forms the basis of somatic symptoms.[48] Yoga is known to have a positive effect on the functioning of the HPA axis[49] by influencing the level of cortisol. Healthy long-term yoga practitioners have displayed higher levels of cortisol, a sign of efficiency within the HPA axis, which may prove to be helpful if used for somatoform syndromes which report hypocortisolism. Also, higher efficiency of HPA axis correlates with improved adaptive physiological responses, QoL and psychological well-being.[50] Yoga improves sleep quality[51] and good sleep quality has been linked with higher cortisol reactivity.[52]

Yoga training equips practitioners with the ability to tolerate more pain or higher pain tolerance which can be attributed to the autonomic activation of the insular cortex. The increased pain tolerance of a yoga practitioner can be explained by an increase in the parasympathetic activity of the nervous system and interoceptive awareness, which leads to hypertrophy and connectional strengthening of the insular cortex.[53]

Psychological factors such as attentional and emotional factors activate the descending pathway and have the ability to influence pain perception in different ways. Focusing too much on the pain increases the perceived pain intensity whereas negative emotional states and mood increase the unpleasantness associated with the pain.[54,55] One week of yoga practice has the ability to reduce negative emotions and moods as well as increase positive emotions and moods.[49,56] Also, meditation helps in decreasing pain and also has a powerful effect on connectivity within pain modulatory circuit.[55]

CONCLUSION

Chronic pain syndromes are multi-factorial and complex in origin, manifestation and treatment responses. Yoga practice adopts a multidimensional and holistic approach to address chronic pain syndromes. There is growing evidence to show that yoga can be an effective adjunct therapy in various chronic pain syndromes. Some of the yoga practices can be tailored and customized according to the patient's condition, e.g., somatoform pain disorder, chronic headache, chronic lower backache and so on. Specific modules are designed for different pain disorders as the contraindicated practices for each pain disorder may be different. Future research should focus on RCTs and also on analyzing the efficacy of individual yoga practices on chronic pain.

CASE VIGNETTE

A 41-year-old female suffering from generalized body ache, knee pain, back pain and headache for 3 years was referred for further evaluation. She had undergone multiple consultations with minimal improvement. She was diagnosed with somatoform pain disorder and was prescribed an antidepressant and an anxiolytic with which there was no improvement. Initially, her headache was severe, back pain was moderate and whole-body aches were mild. She had severe hot and cold sensations, and also reported burning sensation (sensory somatic symptoms) with severe weakness of body, tiredness and moderate weakness in mind. The Pain score on the VAS was 6. Climbing stairs would exacerbate her pain. She was referred to the Integrated Centre of Yoga at NIMHANS for yoga-based therapy for her pain.

The treatment objectives included:
1. *Appreciate the importance of screening for the cause of pain.*

2. Understand the symptoms of somatoform disorder associated with pain.
3. Appreciate the role of yoga in somatoform pain disorder.

She underwent yoga therapy based on the yoga module for somatoform disorders for a period of 2 weeks. After 2 weeks, her pain score on VAS reduced from 6 to 2. Pain became mild and after 6 months her depression levels decreased and she was able to achieve normalcy.

Yoga helped in distributing Prana throughout the body and removed the energy blockages especially in the Manomaya Kosha (which can manifest as psychological problems like emotional instability); and yoga helped in increasing Pranic flow to Pranamaya Kosha and Annamaya Kosha thereby removing the energy blockages settled as pain. In summary, through regular practice of yoga (as is described in the module given below), her psychological

	Clinical Insights: Yoga Therapy for Somatoform Disorders
Prior to the session	• Realistic expectations regarding the benefits and limitations of yoga must be set by discussion with the patient and family members. • Patient's symptoms should never be undermined and should rather be duly acknowledged. Psychoeducation is to be done regarding the neurobiological and yogic concepts of origin of the illness and treatment (e.g., Neurobiological-Somatoform pain disorder is a problem where the pain pathways and chemicals in our brain are dysregulated creating excessive pain sensation. Yogic-Pranic energy is accumulated in a certain part of the body causing increased unpleasant sensations like pain in that part. *Focus of yoga will be to dissipate the prana to other parts of the body and develop equal body awareness*). • Collaboration is to be made with other treating consultants (psychiatrist/ psychotherapist/ physician) to ensure an integrated approach in treatment. • Individual or group sessions may be conducted as per the feasibility and symptom profile.
During the session	• *Practices should be designed to improve the mind-body awareness* (e.g., using instruction for equal body surface awareness and expansion of awareness beyond the body while delivering yoga sessions). • Practices may be of mild to moderate intensity. Forceful teaching of exercises may be counterproductive. Gradually build up the practice levels to enable the patient to get adjusted. • A balance should be maintained while dealing with the symptoms. There should be acknowledgement but not reinforcement of any symptom. (e.g., "I understand, Mr X, that you have this pain. It must be very difficult for you. But as we have already discussed, these exercises will help you overcome a lot of the pain in the long run. It may appear difficult in the beginning. But do not worry, it will be alright. And I must emphasize that to be better in the future, it is very important to do this exercise. I am afraid we cannot skip it. Now let us try again. Do not force yourself but please try. We will start slowly with fewer steps keeping in mind your comfort level.") • *Self-efficacy should be encouraged all throughout the practice to minimize therapist-dependence.* • Any positive or negative counter-transference in part of the therapist should be managed accordingly so that it does not come in the way of the professional therapist-patient relationship. • Old age, side effects of medicines should be taken care of as in most of the illnesses. Practices should be developed accordingly. • Positive reinforcements and reassurances must be given optimally so as to keep the patient motivated.
After the session	• Termination of sessions should be discussed appropriately to prepare the patient. • *The patient should be educated adequately about do's and don'ts of yoga at home (extreme bends should be avoided)*. The plan of further management including follow-ups should be discussed. • Follow-ups to be scheduled according to the clinical status and feasibility. • Every follow-up should contain repeat assessments. Supervised booster sessions may be conducted if required.

symptoms diminished, along with reduction in her joint pain and generalized body pain.

REFERENCES

1. Bastian B, Jetten J, Fasoli F. Cleansing the soul by hurting the flesh: the guilt-reducing effect of pain. Psychol Sci. 2011;22(3):334-5.
2. Flor H, Turk DC. Chronic Pain: An Integrated Biobehavioral Approach. Philadelphia: Lippincott Williams and Wilkins; 2015.
3. Beecher HK. Measurement of Subjective Responses: Quantitative Effects of Drugs. New York: Oxford University Press; 1959.
4. Johnson JE, Rice VH. Sensory and distress components of pain: implications for the study of clinical pain. Nurs Res. 1974;23(3):203-9.
5. World Health Organization. International classification of diseases for mortality and morbidity statistics, 11th Revision, Reference Guide (ICD-11). Geneva: World Health Organization; 2019.
6. Nicholas M, Vlaeyen JW, Rief W, Barke A, Aziz Q, Benoliel R, et al. The IASP classification of chronic pain for ICD-11: chronic primary pain. Pain. 2019;160(1):28-37.
7. Nagarathna R, Nagendra HR. Integrated Approach of Yoga Therapy for Positive Health. Bengaluru: Swami Vivekananda Yoga Prakashana; 2008.
8. Nagarathna R, Nagendra HR. Yoga for Back Pain. Bengaluru: Swami Vivekananda Yoga Prakashana; 2010.
9. Saraswati SS. Four Chapters on Freedom: Commentary on Yoga Sutras of Sage Patanjali. Bihar: Yoga Publications Trust; 2006. p. 139.
10. Saha FJ, Brüning A, Barcelona C, Büssing A, Langhorst J, Dobos G, et al. Integrative medicine for chronic pain: a cohort study using a process-outcome design in the context of a department for internal and integrative medicine. Medicine. 2016;95(27):e4152.
11. Hassed C. Mind-body therapies: use in chronic pain management. Aust Fam Physician. 2013;42(3):112-7.
12. Sherman KJ, Cherkin DC, Erro J, Miglioretti DL, Deyo RA. Comparing yoga, exercise, and a self-care book for chronic low back pain: a randomized, controlled trial. Ann Intern Med. 2005;143(12):849-56.
13. Williams KA, Petronis J, Smith D, Goodrich D, Wu J, Ravi N, et al. Effect of Iyengar yoga therapy for chronic low back pain. Pain. 2005;115(1-2):107-17.
14. Gatantino ML, Bzdewka TM, Eissler-Rnsso JL, Holbrook ML, Mogck EP, Geigle P, et al. The impact of modified Hatha yoga on chronic low back pain: a pilot study. Altern Ther Health Med. 2004;10(2):56-9.
15. Dillard JN, Knapp S. Complementary and alternative pain therapy in the emergency department. Emerg Med Clin North Am. 2005;23(2):529-49.
16. Li Y, Li S, Jiang J, Yuan S. Effects of yoga on patients with chronic nonspecific neck pain: a Prisma systematic review and meta-analysis. Medicine. 2019;98(8):e14649.
17. Russell N, Daniels B, Smoot B, Allen DD. Effects of yoga on quality of life and pain in women with chronic pelvic pain: systematic review and meta-analysis. J Women's Health Phys Ther. 2019;43(3):144-54.
18. Wang Y, Lu S, Wang R, Jiang P, Rao F, Wang B, et al. Integrative effect of yoga practice in patients with knee arthritis: a PRISMA-compliant meta-analysis. Medicine. 2018;97(31):e11742.
19. Guilfoyle MR, Seeley HM, Corteen E, Harkin C, Richards H, Menon DK, et al. Assessing quality of life after traumatic brain injury: examination of the short form 36 health survey. J Neurotrauma. 2010;27(12):2173-81.
20. Hyun-Nam K, Sam-Sun L, Sang-Dol K. Effects of yoga on dysmenorrhea: a systematic review of randomized controlled trials. Altern Integr Med. 2016;5(4).
21. Jha M, Dumbala S, Bhargav H, Arasappa R, Varambally S, Desai G. Yoga for Persons with Somatoform Pain Disorders: Practice Booklet. Bengaluru: NIMHANS Publication; 2018. p. 68.
22. Brookoff D. Chronic pain: 1. A new disease? Hosp Pract. 2000;35(7):45-59.
23. Cheng HT. Spinal cord mechanisms of chronic pain and clinical implications. Curr Pain Headache Rep. 2010;14(3):213-20.
24. Dantzer R. Somatization: a psychoneuroimmune perspective. Psychoneuroendocrinology. 2005;30(10):947-52.
25. Gil FP, Nickel M, Ridout N, Schwarz MJ, Schoechlin C, Schmidmaier R. Alexithymia and interleukin variations in somatoform disorder. Neuroimmunomodulation. 2007;14(5):235-42.
26. Euteneuer F, Schwarz MJ, Hennings A, Riemer S, Stapf T, Selberdinger V, et al. Psychobiological aspects of somatization syndromes: contributions of inflammatory cytokines and neopterin. Psychiatry Res. 2012;195(1-2):60-5.
27. McCall MC. How might yoga work? An overview of potential underlying mechanisms. J Yoga Phys Ther. 2013;3(1):1.
28. Rajbhoj PH, Shete SU, Verma A, Bhogal RS. Effect of yoga module on pro-inflammatory and anti-inflammatory cytokines in industrial workers of Lonavla: a randomized controlled trial. J Clin Diagn Res. 2015;9(2):CC01-5.

29. Vijayaraghava A, Doreswamy V, Narasipur OS, Kunnavil R, Srinivasamurthy N. Effect of yoga practice on levels of inflammatory markers after moderate and strenuous exercise. J Clin Diagn Res. 2015;9(6):CC08-12.
30. Shete SU, Verma A, Kulkarni DD, Bhogal RS. Effect of yoga training on inflammatory cytokines and C-reactive protein in employees of small-scale industries. J Educ Health Promot. 2017;6:76.
31. Cahn BR, Goodman MS, Peterson CT, Maturi R, Mills PJ. Yoga, meditation and mind-body health: increased BDNF, cortisol awakening response, and altered inflammatory marker expression after a 3-month yoga and meditation retreat. Front Hum Neurosci. 2017;11:315.
32. Kang NI, Park JI, Kim YK, Yang JC. Decreased plasma BDNF levels of patients with somatization disorder. Psychiatry Investig. 2016;13(5):526.
33. Enna SJ, McCarson KE. The role of GABA in the mediation and perception of pain. Adv Pharmacol. 2006;54:1-27.
34. Zhuo M. Cortical excitation and chronic pain. Trends Neurosci. 2008;31(4):199-207.
35. Streeter CC, Gerbarg PL, Saper RB, Ciraulo DA, Brown RP. Effects of yoga on the autonomic nervous system, gamma-aminobutyric acid, and allostasis in epilepsy, depression, and post-traumatic stress disorder. Med Hypotheses. 2012;78(5):571-9.
36. Suri M, Sharma R, Saini N. Neuro-physiological correlation between yoga, pain and endorphins. IJAPEY. 2017;2(9).
37. Vallath N. Perspectives on yoga inputs in the management of chronic pain. Indian J Palliat Care. 2010;16(1):1-7.
38. Oswal P, Nagarathna R, Ebnezar J, Nagendra HR. The effect of add-on yogic prana energization technique (YPET) on healing of fresh fractures: a randomized control study. J Altern Complement Med. 2011;17(3):253-8.
39. Rief W, Auer C. Cortisol and somatization. Biol Psychol. 2000;53(1):13-23.
40. Pollatos O, Dietel A, Herbert BM, Wankner S, Wachsmuth C, Henningsen P, et al. Blunted autonomic reactivity and increased pain tolerance in somatoform patients. Pain. 2011;152(9):2157-64.
41. Tyagi A, Cohen M. Yoga and heart rate variability: a comprehensive review of the literature. Int J Yoga. 2016;9(2):97.
42. Malhotra V, Tandon OP. A study of the effect of individual asanas on blood pressure. Indian J Tradit Knowl. 2005;4(4):367-72.
43. Clauw DJ, Chrousos GP. Chronic pain and fatigue syndromes: overlapping clinical and neuro-endocrine features and potential pathogenic mechanisms. Neuroimmunomodulation. 1997;4(3):134-53.
44. Rief W, Barsky AJ. Psychobiological perspectives on somatoform disorders. Psychoneuro-endocrinology. 2005;30(10):996-1002.
45. Pruessner JC, Hellhammer DH, Kirschbaum C. Burnout, perceived stress, and cortisol responses to awakening. Psychosom Med. 1999;61(2):197-204.
46. Aloisi AM, Buonocore M, Merlo L, Galandra C, Sotgiu A, Bacchella L, et al. Chronic pain therapy and hypothalamic-pituitary-adrenal axis impairment. Psychoneuroendocrinology. 2011;36(7):1032-9.
47. Rief W, Hennings A, Riemer S, Euteneuer F. Psychobiological differences between depression and somatization. J Psychosom Res. 2010;68(5):495-502.
48. Pukhalsky AL, Shmarina GV, Alioshkin VA, Sabelnikov A. HPA axis exhaustion and regulatory T cell accumulation in patients with a functional somatic syndrome: recent view on the problem of Gulf War veterans. J Neuroimmunol. 2008;196(1-2):133-8.
49. Ross A, Thomas S. The health benefits of yoga and exercise: a review of comparison studies. J Altern Complement Med. 2010;16(1):3-12.
50. Vera FM, Manzaneque JM, Maldonado EF, Carranque GA, Rodriguez FM, Blanca MJ, et al. Subjective sleep quality and hormonal modulation in long-term yoga practitioners. Biol Psychol. 2009;81(3):164-8.
51. Khalsa SB. Treatment of chronic insomnia with yoga: a preliminary study with sleep-wake diaries. Appl Psychophysiol Biofeedback. 2004;29(4):269-78.
52. Wright CE, Valdimarsdottir HB, Erblich J, Bovbjerg DH. Poor sleep the night before an experimental stress task is associated with reduced cortisol reactivity in healthy women. Biol Psychol. 2007;74(3):319-27.
53. Villemure C, Čeko M, Cotton VA, Bushnell MC. Insular cortex mediates increased pain tolerance in yoga practitioners. Cereb Cortex. 2014;24(10):2732-40.
54. Montoya P, Larbig W, Braun C, Preissl H, Birbaumer N. Influence of social support and emotional context on pain processing and magnetic brain responses in fibromyalgia. Arthritis Rheum. 2004;50(12):4035-44.
55. Bushnell MC, Čeko M, Low LA. Cognitive and emotional control of pain and its disruption in chronic pain. Nat Rev Neurosci. 2013;14(7):502-11.
56. Narasimhan L, Nagarathna R, Nagendra HR. Effect of integrated yogic practices on positive and negative emotions in healthy adults. Int J Yoga. 2011;4(1):13-9.

CHAPTER 18

Yoga for Low Back Pain

Ameya Patwardhan, Vinod Kumar, Tarachand Joshi, Suman Bista

INTRODUCTION

Low back pain (LBP) is a symptom rather than a disease and is defined by the location of pain, typically between the lower rib margin and the buttock creases. In both developed and developing countries, LBP is the leading cause of years lived with disability, with a mean point prevalence of 18.3%, and a 1-month prevalence of 30.8%.[1] LBP is more common in females and in those aged 40–69 years than in other age groups.[2] Prevalence of LBP rises steadily with age and up to 84% of adults will experience LBP during their lives with 50% of them having more than one episode.[1,3] LBP that is accompanied by activity limitation increases with age. If the LBP lasts for longer than 12 weeks that is generally considered as chronic LBP (CLBP). CLBP is 2.5 times more prevalent in the working population than in nonworking populations for reasons that are not clear.[1] About 90% of the time, LBP is short-lived (acute) and goes away within a few days or weeks without much inconvenience or trouble. A minority of patients, though, go on to have subacute back pain (lasting between 4 and 12 weeks) or chronic back pain (lasting 12 or more weeks). Recurrences are common and a few people end up with persistent disabling pain accompanied by a range of biophysical, psychological, and social factors.

Like most other ailments, LBP has a clear association with genetic as well as environmental factors. Genetic factors have been found to be more closely associated with chronic and disabling type of LBP than mild cases. People who have had previous episodes of LBP are at increased risk of a new episode. Likewise, people with other chronic conditions such as asthma, headache, diabetes, and poor mental health are more likely to report LBP than people in good health. Lifestyle factors such as smoking, obesity, and low levels of physical activity that relate to poorer general health, are also associated with episodes of LBP or development of persistent LBP.[1] Awkward postures, lifting, bending, and physically demanding tasks are associated with increased risk of developing LBP.

Low back pain is increasingly understood as a long-lasting condition with a variable course. Its severity of symptoms varies widely. Associated symptoms of LBP may include radicular pain characterized by leg pain, leg pain worse than back pain, and worsening of leg pain during coughing, sneezing or straining and while lifting the leg straight up. This may indicate associated radiculopathy (presence of weakness, loss of sensation, or loss of reflexes associated with a particular nerve root, or a combination of these) in the lower limbs.[1] People with LBP and radicular pain or radiculopathy are reported to be more severely affected and have poorer outcomes compared with those only with LBP. Lumbar spinal stenosis, confirmed by the presence of both symptoms and imaging findings, is clinically characterized by pain or other discomfort with walking or extended standing that radiates into one or both lower limbs and is typically relieved by rest or lumbar flexion (neurogenic claudication).

Most of the time (90%), LBP is nonspecific. In other cases, it may arise from either problems beyond the lumbar spine (e.g., leaking aortic aneurysm); specific disorders affecting the lumbar spine (e.g., epidural abscess, compression fracture, *spondyloarthropathy*, malignancy, cauda equina syndrome); or radicular pain, radiculopathy, or spinal canal stenosis. Diagnostic investigations such as imaging [X-ray of the spine, computed tomography (CT) scan and magnetic resonance imaging (MRI)] are ordered when the clinician suspects a specific disease process that has different management implications from nonspecific LBP. According to the American College of Physicians' guidelines for diagnostic imaging, immediate imaging is recommended when there are major risk factors for cancer, spinal infection, cauda equina syndrome, or severe neurological deficits.[2]

Magnetic resonance imaging findings that have a reasonably strong association with LBP include disk bulge, disk extrusion, and spondylolysis. Disc herniation in conjunction with local inflammation is the most common cause of radicular pain and radiculopathy. Besides, there are some serious causes of persistent LBP (malignancy, vertebral fracture, infection, or inflammatory disorders such as axial spondyloarthritis, tuberculosis, and intra-abdominal causes) that require identification and specific management targeting the cause, but these account for a very small proportion of cases.[1] In such cases, collaboration with back pain specialists is essential for diagnostic clarification and management.

Chronic LBP is the number one cause of disability globally.[1] The overall increase in the global burden of LBP is almost entirely due to population increase and aging, as opposed to increased prevalence. Most people with LBP have low levels of disability, although disability is highest in working age groups. In older people, LBP is associated with increased limitation of activity.

Costs associated with health care and work disability attributed to LBP are enormous, vary between countries, and are affected by multiple factors such as social norms, healthcare approaches and legislation. Despite the existing initiatives to address the global burden of LBP as a public health problem, there is a need to identify cost-effective and context-specific strategies for managing LBP to take care of the consequences of the current and projected future burden.[1]

■ YOGA FOR LOW BACK PAIN: EVIDENCE-BASED

Medical managements for LBP in many cases are intrusive, addictive, and expensive and they often fail. Surgical interventions are reserved for severe cases or cases with progressive neurological deficits. This approach for the management of back pain is common but contrary to the existing evidence. Commonly followed dictum of not returning to work until symptom free does not hold true for patients with LBP. About 63% of Indians believe that bed rest is the mainstay of therapy.[4] Research evidence suggests that exercise alone, or in combination with education, is the most effective for prevention of LBP. To be more specific, current guidelines (Denmark, UK, and USA) recommend the use of exercise and a range of other nonpharmacological therapies alone or in combinations such as massage, acupuncture, spinal manipulation, Tai chi, and Yoga.[4] Since there is no evidence that one form of exercise is better than other forms, guidelines recommend exercise programs that take individual needs, preferences, and capabilities into account in deciding the type of exercise. Factors such as cultural acceptability of treatments, patient attitudes toward and adherence to treatment, and treatment providers vary between countries and cultures, and influence treatment outcomes.[4] This makes yoga even more relevant due to its basic idea of individualized approach.

Yoga is an ancient mind-body discipline which has become popular for its role in yoga therapy. Back pain is one such condition where yoga is beneficial. It is difficult to be precise about the onset of use of yoga in patients with LBP, but it is one disorder where yoga has been found to be beneficial in the short term and long term. Over a period of time, experts in this field have identified Yoga practices which are considered to be relevant, useful and feasible for this patient population.

Keeping in mind the need for a nonpharmacological intervention which is culturally acceptable, feasible, with minimal adverse effects and which takes care of the individual requirements, preferences, and capabilities, yoga emerges as a relevant choice for patients with LBP, especially in the Indian population.

LITERATURE REVIEW OF YOGA FOR LOW BACK PAIN

Yoga is being increasingly studied as a treatment strategy for patients with LBP. There are a limited number of trials available for role of yoga for acute or subacute cases of LBP. Majority of the evidence is for CLBP. It has been found that yoga can be safely accomplished, is feasible, lacks any serious adverse effects, is cost-effective and overall received positively by patients with CLBP. Potential advantages of yoga over other therapies are that it is usually group-based and delivered in a community rather than a hospital setting and it has been also shown to have other health benefits. Apart from efficacy studies of various schools of yoga such as *viniyoga, hatha yoga, Iyengar yoga*, a scientific generic *yoga* module to take care of the needs of patients with LBP has also been proposed.[5]

Most yoga studies do demonstrate beneficial effects for adults suffering from CLBP and it has also been shown that the beneficial effect is comparable to exercise. In a systematic review, of 14 randomized controlled trials (RCTs), Chang et al. found that yoga can reduce pain and disability, can be practiced safely, and is well received by participants.[6] In another systematic review and meta-analysis of eight RCTs, Cramer et al., reported that there is strong evidence for short-term effects of yoga on pain, back-specific disability, and global improvement. In addition, there is strong evidence for a long-term effect on pain and moderate evidence for a long-term effect on back-specific disability. The reviewers found no evidence for either short-term or long-term effects on health-related quality of life. This review suggested that yoga can be recommended as an additional therapy to CLBP patients.[7] Holtzman et al., in a meta-analysis of eight RCTs, found strong and consistent evidence for the short-term benefits of yoga on functional disability.[8] In a systematic review of seven RCTs, Posadzki et al. suggested that yoga leads to a significantly greater reduction in LBP than usual care, education or conventional therapeutic exercises.[9] Hill, in another systematic review which included four RCTs, concluded that yoga led to a significant improvement in back function and back pain when compared with certain other care modalities.[10] In another systematic review on efficacy of Iyengar yoga for CLBP, strong evidence for effectiveness was established.[11] In one recent review published in 2017, small-to-moderate improvements were reported for back-related function.[12] Overall, the benefits reported after yoga practice are improved mobility, reduced pain and disability, and reduced use of pain medication.

Thus, it may be safely said that yoga therapy for patients with LBP has the potential to be considered in clinical settings. However, there are practical limitations in its use due to lack of clear clinical guidelines, dose-response relationships, information on specificity and sensitivity of practices, overall number of sessions for optimum results, strategies to prevent relapses, and lack of availability of adequate number of yoga therapists.

The summary of evidence for use of yoga in back pain has been shown in **Table 1**.

TABLE 1: Yoga for back pain—summary of evidence.

S. No.	Authors (Year)	Design	Number of studies	Participants	Conclusion
1.	Cramer et al. (2013)	Systematic review and meta-analysis	Ten randomized controlled trials (RCTs)	967 patients with chronic low back pain	• Strong evidence for short-term effects on pain, back-specific disability, and global improvement • Strong evidence for a long-term effect on pain and moderate evidence for a long-term effect on back-specific disability • No evidence for either short-term or long-term effects on health-related quality of life • Yoga was not associated with serious adverse events[7]
2.	Posadzki et al. (2011)	Systematic review	Seven RCTs	403 patients with low back pain	• Five studies suggested that yoga leads to a significantly greater reduction in low back pain than usual care, education or conventional therapeutic exercises • Two studies showed no between-group differences. Yoga has the potential to alleviate low back pain[9]
3.	Chang et al. (2016)	Systematic review	14 RCTs	1,277 patients with low back pain	• As effective as other nonpharmacologic treatments in reducing the functional disability of back pain • More effective in reducing pain severity of chronic low back pain when compared to usual care or no care • Positive impact on depression and other psychological comorbidities • An effective and safe intervention for chronic low back pain[6]
4.	Hill (2013)	Systematic review	Four RCTs	711 patients with chronic low back pain	• All four papers found that yoga lead to a significant improvement in back function • Three demonstrated a significant improvement in back pain when compared with certain care modalities • Further well-designed RCTs are warranted, with multiple, specified comparator care modalities before firm conclusions can be gained[10]
5.	Crow et al. (2015)	Systematic review	Six RCTs	570 patients with back or neck pain	• Yoga can decrease pain and increase functional ability in patients with spinal pain

Contd...

Contd...

S. No.	Authors (Year)	Design	Number of studies	Participants	Conclusions
					• Evidence of *Iyengar Yoga* interventions being useful in treating spinal pain and having other therapeutic effects[11]
6.	Sawyer et al. (2012)	Systematic review and meta-analysis	Six RCTs	373 patients with low back pain	• Medium beneficial effect on chronic low back pain significantly less functional disability after the intervention • The improvements in pain and function for yoga subjects remained statistically significant 12–24 weeks after the end of the intervention[13]
7.	Diaz et al. (2013)	Systematic review	Ten RCTs	1,024 patients with low back pain	• Yoga significantly improve quality of life and reduce disability, stress, depression, and medication usage associated with chronic low back pain in eight of the ten trials when compared with usual care, self-care book, or exercises • More research is necessary before recommendations can be made[14]
8.	Goode et al. (2016)	Systematic review	Ten RCTs	956 patients with chronic low back pain	• Benefit of yoga in midlife adults with nonspecific chronic low back pain for short- and long-term pain and back-specific disability • The effects of yoga for health-related quality of life, well-being and acute low back pain are uncertain[15]
9.	Holtzman et al. (2013)	Meta-analysis	Eight RCTs	743 patients with chronic low back pain	• Medium-to-large effect on functional disability and pain • Follow-up effect sizes for functional disability and pain were smaller, but remained significant • Moderate-to-high level of variability in effect sizes[8]
10.	Kelly (2009)	Systematic review	Five RCTs and two case series	344 patients with low back pain	• Positive impact on low back pain and function, with effects comparable to education combined with aerobic and strengthening exercise and more effective than education alone or no treatment • Yoga may provide an inexpensive and easily accessible way for patients with low back pain to manage their symptoms[16]

Contd...

Contd...

S. No.	Authors (Year)	Design	Number of studies	Participants	Conclusions
11.	Whitehead (2018)	Systematic review	12 RCTs	1,080 patients with low back pain	• More effective than nonexercise interventions and either as effective as or slightly more effective than non-yoga exercise interventions • Yoga results in more adverse events than psychological or educational interventions but has the same number of adverse events as non-yoga exercise[17]

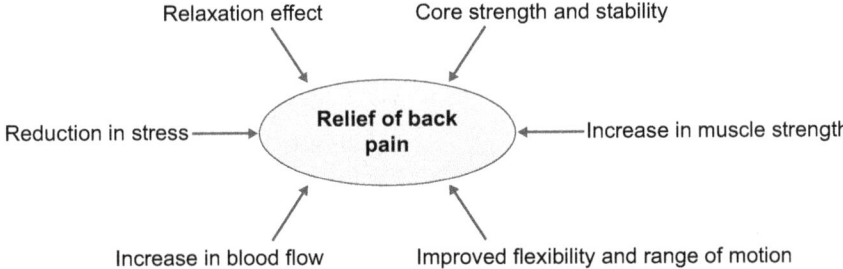

Fig. 1: Possible mechanisms of action of yoga in relieving back pain.

POSSIBLE MECHANISMS OF ACTION OF YOGA

There is no single clearly established mechanism to explain the action of yoga for CLBP. It is likely to be a complex interaction of physiological, psychological, and emotional pathways through which yoga provides relief to patients with LBP. Due to similarities in the basic nature of the physical components of yoga and exercises, it is easy to understand that there is overlap in the possible mechanisms of action of yoga for patients with LBP. Yoga practices can be hypothesized to have beneficial effects for a number of reasons which are depicted in **Figure 1**.

1. *Core strength and stability*: Yoga provides benefits for core strength and overall stability which could possibly explain benefits for patients with LBP.
2. *Increase in muscle strength*: Yoga postures help in improvement in muscle strength which can help support the spine.
3. *Improved flexibility and range of motion*: Yoga practices improve flexibility in the back, which can help people's functional movement and get them back to their normal living.
4. *Increase in blood flow*: Yoga practices might increase blood flow to the soft tissues in the back, which results in healing and reduces stiffness.
5. *Relaxation effect*: Pranayama, meditation, and relaxation techniques after practice of yogasana helps to relax joints and muscles and calms the mind.
6. *Reduction in stress*: Reduction in stress is another possibility which helps in reduction of associated psychological symptoms along with improvement in quality of life.

YOGA MODULE INCLUDING RECOMMENDATIONS FOR PRACTICE

There is a lack of literature about specificity and sensitivity of yoga practices for patients with CLBP. Patil et al. attempted development and validation of yoga module to cater to the needs of patients with CLBP.[5] This was based on the inputs from experts in the field of yoga therapy and can be considered as most scientific set of yoga practices. We hereby are providing a set of yoga practices which can be useful for patients with CLBP of varied etiology. Although yoga is considered as safe, the practices listed here are to be initiated under supervision only. We have provided a validated yoga module for LBP in **Appendix 1.11** at the end of this book.[5]

Practical Tips for Yoga including Precautions, Contraindications, and Special Instructions

- *Simplification*: Start with simple yoga practices. Consider simplification of difficult practices. Example: *Saral bhujangasana* is a simplified version of *bhujangasana*.
- *Moderation*: Ensure that yoga practices are done in moderation followed by brief relaxation at the end. A yoga therapy session should be rejuvenating and energizing. Any yoga therapy session resulting in tiredness/fatigue is likely to be counterproductive.
- *Stepping-up*: Difficulty level for practices is to be gradually increased. *Yoga* postures can initially be taken in the breathing practices. These can later be followed by shorter holds before longer holds. Examples: *Ardha salabhasana breathing, ardha salabhasana, salabhasana breathing,* and *salabhasana* are in the increasing order of difficulty levels.
- *Slowness and stability*: These are the core concepts of yogic practices. It is to be ensured that there are no jerky movements while entering or coming out of the postures.
- *Individual practices*: Efforts should be made to identify specific yoga practices based on individual needs.
- *Fast and dynamic practices*: All fast and dynamic practices are to be avoided in patients with CLBP. Examples include *Surya namaskar,* dog breathing, *mukha dhouti, kapalabhati, bhastrika,* and *agnisara kriya*.
- *Order of practices*: Examples: For patients bedridden due to severe back pain, start with supine and prone postures, followed by sitting and then standing postures.

CONCLUSION

Chronic pain can affect an individual in multiple dimensions. Beyond the physical level, the hyperaroused state can negatively affect the muscle tension, breathing patterns, energy levels, and mindset, all of which can affect the quality of life of the individual and family.[18] Yoga in its entirety is a practice that influences an individual at the physical, emotional, and spiritual level and hence gains importance in this context of chronic back pain. Number of systematic reviews and meta-analyses point toward beneficial effect of yoga in terms of pain reduction, improved functionality and sense of well-being in back pain, thus providing a strong evidence for its clinical utility.[13-17]

CASE VIGNETTE

A 38-year-old lady (Ms UL) was referred from the Department of Physiotherapy to the NIMHANS Integrated Centre for Yoga (NICY), NIMHANS in July 2019 with complaints of LBP for the last 3 years. She was apparently fine 3 years back when she started having mild LBP radiating to the left leg and toe. The severity of pain gradually increased over a period of 1 week and the patient started having disturbed sleep. Pain was associated with numbness/tingling sensation in the left lower extremity. She had used several medications including anti-inflammatory drugs, topical gels, multivitamins and sedatives over the past few months. An MRI of the lumbosacral spine was done in 2017 which suggested L4-5 posterior and paracentral disk protrusion impinging the thecal sac and L5 traversing nerve roots. Hence, she was advised certain exercises and surgical intervention. Ms UL continued Pregabalin and Methylcobalamin medication for the prescribed duration of 15 days and stopped thereafter. During this time, she reported 90% improvement although she also observed drowsiness as a side effect of the medication. The severity of pain increased again after stopping medication and the patient received Ayurveda treatment for 1-hour daily for 15 days. Specific dietary restrictions were also advised. By the 15th day severity of pain reduced but 30–40% of symptoms still persisted.

She restarted her routine teaching job, although the pain persisted. Pain used to worsen while lifting heavy weights, while suddenly bending forward and while driving. While at work, she used a lumbar belt on a regular basis to support her back. She used topical analgesics as and when required. Back pain and mild disturbance in sleep became a part of her routine with occasional episodes of heavy headedness and headache. With this continuous pain, the patient visited the physiotherapy department at the NIMHANS in July 2019. During one of her visits to NIMHANS, she consulted the NICY, after which yoga therapy sessions were planned.

The first yoga session offered to her was an orientation session and she was introduced to yoga therapy. She was made to understand the panchakosha concept of existence and further details about adhija vyadhi were elaborated. With the premise that yoga therapy should be able to influence all levels of existence, yoga therapy was initiated. Some preliminary practices were taught in the first session. From the second day onward she started attending our regular group yoga session for patients with LBP. The first 5 days of yoga sessions were difficult for her due to an increase in severity of symptoms. Yoga practices were mellowed down to adjust to her needs. Patient was made to do only supine and prone postures for the first 2 weeks. Practices included were saral bhujangasana breathing, setu bandhasana breathing, folded legs lumbar stretches (with feet together), single leg lumbar stretches, and single leg pawanamuktasana breathing. As pain was acute, postures were done in the form of slow continuous movement with awareness and none of the final postures were maintained for more than 5 seconds in the first week, 10 seconds in the second week, and so on. Besides to ensure engagement of back muscles patient was asked to keep folded towel to support the back in supine position and then press and release was advocated.

By the 10th day, the patient reported improvement in her symptoms. She stopped regular use of the lumbar belt by the 25th day. Sleep quality improved and headache also decreased. Once the acute pain subsided, a long-term management plan with yoga therapy was discussed with the patient. For the long-term management, standing and sitting postures were also introduced gradually. Duration of maintenance of posture was also increased. Practices for long-term management included hands-in-and-out breathing, hands-stretch-breathing, tadasana stretch, ardhakati chakrasana, ardha chakrasana, bhujangasana, setu bandhasana, lumbar stretches (folded legs, feet together and separate), crossed legs lumbar stretches, and ekapada uttanasana for strengthening of muscles were kept in mind while planning yoga therapy for long-term management.

Motivated with the results, Ms UL continued supervised yoga sessions till December 2019 at NICY and thereafter started practicing at home. By that time, she reported 95% improvement in back pain. According to the patient, practices which benefited her most were setu bandhasana, lumbar stretches, pawanamuktasana and bhujangasana. She especially appreciated the component of synchronized breath and body movements which helped her to have a connection of body-breath-mind. Apart from these, she also considered pranayama (particularly nadi shuddhi and bhramari) and chanting (nadanusandhana and pranavajapa) as an important part of practice. Currently she practices yoga at home for 90 minutes daily for at least 20 days a month. She reports experiencing no pain during her day-to-day activities. She uses the lumbar belt only occasionally. She has also not had any analgesic in the past 12 months. She subsequently also started attending Tele-yoga programs initiated by the Department of Integrative Medicine at NIMHANS.

Low back pain can be a chronic debilitating illness as depicted in the above case vignette. However, in patients like Ms UL, yoga therapy when practiced consistently can bring about significant improvement in symptoms as well as quality of life.

Clinical Insights: Yoga for Low Back Pain

Prior to the session	• Most patients would be having a chronic history of pain and disability, so the therapist should always exercise a calm and empathetic attitude toward the patient. • It is absolutely necessary to be aware of the patient's medical and surgical history. The cause of LBP should be in mind while deciding the yoga module for the patient. • The rationale for yoga and the expectations of the patient should be discussed prior to starting the session. • Appropriate props such as pillows, bolsters, cushions, straps, meditation chair for back support can be used as and when necessary.
During the session	• Start with easy exercises in the position the patient is most comfortable with. For example, a therapist can consider starting the sessions with practices performed while the patient is in supine or prone condition. • Gradual gradation of exercises can be considered depending on the patient's response and ability to follow the exercises. • Give clear instructions to patients on how to sit during yoga practices, how to use support to comfortably change posture from sitting to supine and vice versa without strain on their back are important. • Avoid any fast pacing yoga practices and asanas that require acute forward bends (e.g., *surya namaskar, padahastasana, shashankasana*, tiger breathing). • Avoid fast repetitions of physical practices and fast breathing practices which may produce a jerk to the back (e.g., *kapalabhati*). • Do not push the patients beyond their limit, instead encourage patients to be aware of their body limitations and gradually perform the practices within those limits. • Patients may use the concept of diffusing the excessively accumulated "*prana*" or "*vayu*" in the most painful region through mindfulness. • *If the patient develops acute exacerbation of pain during any of the practices, they should be advised to stop the practices immediately and rest in shavasana position or most comfortable position*. Gentle *pawanamuktasana* breathing with "press" and "release" practices (with breath synchronization) should be taught. Practices should be gradually initiated again as the pain intensity comes down. • *Good relaxation of muscles in shavasana (or the most comfortable posture) and gentle rhythmic breathing at the end of practices is the key*, at least 15 minutes of relaxation is a must after 40–45 minutes of asana and breathing practices. No yoga session should end abruptly without relaxation, this may aggravate the pain. • If a patient has associated neuropathy, necessary precautions need to be taken while doing the exercises (e.g., a patient with sensory or motor neuropathy may require help with standing postures and hand support). • In some cases of CLBP, there may be chances of misuse atrophy of muscles, so therapists must be aware of this and can target the individual muscles for strengthening.
After the session	• Encourage a caretaker to be with the patient while they perform the exercises back at home. • Caretaker should be educated on necessary precautions. • Regular practice should be encouraged for prolonged benefits. • Aim at improving the quality of life rather than a complete cure.

REFERENCES

1. Hartvigsen J, Hancock MJ, Kongsted A, Louw Q, Ferreira ML, Genevay S, et al. What low back pain is and why we need to pay attention? Lancet. 2018;391(10137):2356-67.
2. Maher C, Underwood M, Buchbinder R. Non-specific low back pain. Lancet. 2017;389(10070):736-47.
3. Shemshaki H, Nourian SM, Fereidan-Esfahani M, Mokhtari M, Etemadifar MR. What is the source of low back pain? J Craniovertebr Junction Spine. 2013;4(1):21-4.
4. Foster NE, Anema JR, Cherkin D, Chou R, Cohen SP, Gross DP, et al. Prevention and treatment of low back pain: evidence, challenges, and promising directions. Lancet. 2018;391:2368-83.
5. Patil NJ, Nagarathna R, Tekur P, Patil DN, Nagendra HR, Subramanya P. Designing, validation, and feasibility of integrated yoga therapy module for chronic low back pain. Int J Yoga. 2015;8(2):103-8.
6. Chang DG, Holt JA, Sklar M, Groessl EJ, Diego S, Diego S, et al. Yoga as a treatment for chronic low back pain: a systematic review of the literature. J Orthop Rheumatol. 2016;3(1):1-8.
7. Cramer H, Lauche R, Haller H, Dobos G. A systematic review and meta-analysis of yoga for low back pain. Clin J Pain. 2013;29(5):450-60.
8. Holtzman S, Beggs RT. Yoga for chronic low back pain: analysis of randomized controlled trials. Pain Res Manag. 2013;18(5):267-72.
9. Posadzki P, Ernst E. Yoga for low back pain: a systematic review of randomized clinical trials. Clin Rheumatol. 2011;30(9):1257-62.
10. Hill C. Is yoga an effective treatment in the management of patients with chronic low back pain compared with other care modalities—a systematic review? J Complement Integr Med. 2013;10(1):1-9.
11. Crow EM, Jeannot E, Trewhela A. Effectiveness of Iyengar yoga in treating spinal (back and neck) pain: a systematic review. Int J Yoga. 2015;8(1):3-14.
12. Wieland LS, Skoetz N, Pilkington K, Vempati R, D'Adamo CR, Berman BM. Yoga treatment for chronic non-specific low back pain. Cochrane Database Syst Rev. 2017;1(1):CD010671.
13. Sawyer A. Impact of yoga on low back pain and function: a systematic review and meta-analysis. J Yoga Phys Ther. 2012;02(04):2-4.
14. Diaz AM, Kolber MJ, Patel CK, Pabian PS, Rothschild CE, Hanney WJ. The efficacy of yoga as an intervention for chronic low back pain: a systematic review of randomized controlled trials. Am J Lifestyle Med. 2013;7(6):418-30.
15. Goode AP, Coeytaux RR, McDuffie J, Duan-Porter W, Sharma P, Mennella H, et al. An evidence map of yoga for low back pain. Complement Ther Med. 2016;25:170-7.
16. Kelly Z. Is yoga an effective treatment for low back pain: a research review? Int J Yoga Ther. 2009;19(1):103-12.
17. Whitehead PB. The effect of yoga on chronic nonspecific low back pain. Am J Nurs. 2018;118(2):64.
18. Vallath N. Perspectives on yoga inputs in the management of chronic pain. Indian J Palliat Care. 2010;16(1):1-7.

CHAPTER 19

Yoga for Migraine

Usha Rani MR, Sujan MU, Kaviraja Udupa, Sathyaprabha TN

INTRODUCTION

Headache is one of the most common disorders of the nervous system worldwide. Headache is defined as pain or discomfort felt in the head or face. Headaches can differ in terms of their location, intensity of the pain, and how often they occur. Some of the pain sensitive regions include the scalp, nerves in the face, mouth and throat, muscles around the head, neck and shoulders, and blood vessels at the base of the brain.

Headaches are divided into primary (benign, recurrent headaches not caused by underlying disease or structural problems) and secondary headaches (caused by an underlying disease such as an infection, head injury, vascular disorders, brain bleed or tumors). Migraine is considered to be the 3rd most common and the 6th most disabling disorder among primary headache disorders. Symptoms of migraine include unilateral or bilateral, moderate to severe throbbing and pulsating head pain, associated with nausea, vomiting, and sensitivity to light (photophobia) and sound (phonophobia). Migraine headaches may occur with aura, i.e., disturbances such as flashes of light, blind spots, vision changes, or tingling sensation in the hand or face before the attack or simply without aura (without the above-mentioned disturbances).

FOUR PHASES OF MIGRAINE

1. *Premonitory (before the onset of headache)*: One may experience stiffness in the neck, craving for food, constipation, fatigue, depression/irritability, sensitivity to light and sound, yawning and increased frequency of urination.
2. *Aura*: One may see zigzag lights/feel numbness on the side of the face/trouble recollecting or understanding what people are saying.
3. *Headache*: One may experience one-sided or both-sided headache lasting 4–72 hours.
4. *Post-dromal (post-headache)*: One may experience low mood and feel fatigued with poor concentration.[1]

CONVENTIONAL MANAGEMENT

The pharmacological treatments for acute (acetaminophen, nonsteroidal anti-inflammatory drugs, triptans, antiemetics, ergot alkaloids, and combination analgesics)[2] and chronic migraine (beta-blockers, anticonvulsants, calcium-channel blockers, tricyclic antidepressants, serotonin antagonists, antihypertensives, and antidepressants, selective serotonin reuptake inhibitors, noradrenergic-specific serotonergic antidepressants)[3] have shown to be poorly tolerated by some of the patients. The unpleasant side effects of medicines and their inefficiency to meet an optimal control over migraine pain has led to low treatment compliance and other complications, such as prolongation (chronicity) of headache[4] and interference with patients' daily lives.[5] These constraints might have led patients chose complementary and alternative medicine (CAM) either alone or in combination with drugs.[6] The other treatment strategies for migraine include:

Noninvasive neuromodulation treatments (transcranial direct current stimulation, "repetitive or patterned" transcranial magnetic stimulation (TMS), percutaneous mastoid stimulation, transcutaneous cranial nerve stimulation, vagus nerve stimulation, handheld brachial and cervical electric stimulation such as gammaCore) and *invasive neuromodulation treatments* (occipital nerve stimulation, sphenopalatine ganglion stimulation, high cervical spinal cord stimulation); nutraceuticals [riboflavin (vitamin B_2) and magnesium]. They are limited in their usage due to nonavailability in most of the countries and side effects such as pain, infections, and lead migration, respectively.

Although *behavioral techniques* (relaxation, thermal and electromyographic biofeedback, and cognitive behavioral therapy) have been effective when used along with classic pharmacological therapies and allow a certain degree of self-management, these strategies may not target the migraine biology or the actual pain mechanisms.

While the strength of evidence is low for the use of *acupuncture, nutraceuticals* such as [riboflavin (vitamin B_2) and magnesium] have been found to be cost-effective, easily available and a good option for patients with comorbidities, those who are on concomitant medications, or in patients who are unable to tolerate the side effects of drugs.[4]

However, despite the incidence of migraine is high in India, most of these people often ignore or do not seek help for their headache as they feel it is manageable or due to cultural/social factors. Migraine is more common in women compared to men, affecting the age group between 15–49 years. This duration is the most crucial time for an individual to complete their education, career-building, start a family, raise children and plan the future progress in life. Therefore, it is critical to treat migraine on time.

■ YOGIC UNDERSTANDING OF MIGRAINE

Yoga is a spiritual and holistic science aimed at the development of one's physical, mental and moral-spiritual aspects of being. Yoga's philosophy and practical approaches are applicable in one's day-to-day life. Yoga's perspective about ailments is based on the classification of diseases into *adhija vyadhi* (psychosomatic and stress-related disorders) and *anadhija vyadhis* (infectious disease, toxins, accidents, etc., i.e. not born due to stress), as described in an ancient text called *Yoga Vāsiṣtha*.

Diseases that are thought to arise due to stress can be understood through the concept of *Panchakosha viveka* described in *Taittiriya Upanishad*. In modern times, it has been gaining traction in the field of Yoga, largely due to its applications in therapy.

The *Panchakosha* model divides the human personality into five sheaths, with each succeeding sheath being contained in the preceding one as explained here:

1. *Annamaya kosha (AMK)*: The first sheath is the "sheath of food"—the physical body made up of bones, flesh, blood, etc. It is also called the "*Sthula Sharira*" or gross body.
2. *Pranamaya kosha (PMK)*: The second sheath is the "sheath of vital life force", made up of the five vital airs—*Prana, Apana, Vyana, Udana,* and *Samana*. It is said to be possessed with *Kriya Shakti* (power of action), since it is the PMK which animates and sustains the AMK.
3. *Manomaya kosha (MMK)*: The third sheath is the "sheath of mind". It is endowed with Ichchha Shakti (power of desire) and serves as the receptacle of all sense inputs. But, it may not interpret or understand them and respond reflexively. It is also the part of the personality that is the cause of

diversity, i.e., "I" and "mine" with respect to one's body and possessions—the sense of ego.
4. *Vijnanamaya kosha*: The fourth sheath is the "sheath of intellect", the characteristic of which is determination. It is the sphere of knowledge, where one understands the meaning behind what the senses and the mind perceive and does all actions with volition. The *Pranamaya, Manomaya* and *Vijnanamaya koshas* together are said to be the "*Sukshma Sharira*" (subtle body), since they do not present themselves to the senses.
5. *Anandamaya kosha*: The fifth and last sheath is the "sheath of bliss". It is the sheath of ignorance, which one experiences during the deep sleep state. It is also called the "*Karana Sharira*" (causal body), since it is into it that all the other sheaths merge during deep sleep and it is from it that they all arise.[7,8]

The five sheaths are known to be pervaded by prana as it nourishes, sustains and maintains the relationship between the koshas. The prana acts as a neutral space to allow movement between the koshas and prana is required to carry out functions of the physical body.

UNDERSTANDING MIGRAINE IN TERMS OF ADHIJA VYADHI—PSYCHOSOMATIC DISEASE

Yoga emphasizes the importance of maintaining a healthy lifestyle. The components of a healthy lifestyle include ahara (healthy and nourishing diet), vihara (recreational activities to relax body and mind), achara (healthy activities such as yoga asanas), and vichara (right thoughts and right attitude).

Stress according to yoga is the uncontrolled persistent repetitive thought arising in the mind. The root cause of migraine is a wrong lifestyle that begins as stress at the level of MMK. This imbalance in the mind is transferred to the body via prana. On exposure to enormous stress, the disturbing thoughts pick up the intensity and there is an excess flow of prana to the head region. This extreme prana activity in the region of the head gets hostile leading to imbalance (endocrine/nervous) at the level of AMK and shows up as migraine. The excess flow of prana to the head region can lead to an inappropriate distribution of prana in other regions of the body. The associated complications of migraine such as nausea and vomiting can be a result of reduced flow of prana to the stomach region. Reducing the stress at MMK level helps to restore balance at all sheaths of an individual. Thus, yoga as a therapy is helpful in improving the quality of life by producing positive emotional and psychological effects in any situation that an individual is undergoing.[9,10]

It should also be noted that not all people undergoing stress will be prone to migraine. It depends on: (1) the type of personality, i.e., the way he/she reacts to the stressors,[11] (2) the genetic predisposition to a particular disease, and/or (3) an inherent weakness or vulnerability of the organ in that particular individual.[12]

RATIONALE FOR THE USE OF YOGA IN MIGRAINE

Migraine can be associated with physical issues (musculoskeletal disorders and fibromyalgia) and mental issues (anxiety, panic disorder, and depression). A combination of physical and mental distress may trigger the emotional component *(fear)* of pain. As a result, symptoms of migraine increase, leading to a disability affecting the quality of life of the affected individual.

Another important concern about migraine is the frequency of headache. It varies from one individual to another. This *"natural"* within-person variation makes it difficult to treat migraine successfully. Therefore, an intervention that is individualistic, reduces stress, and allays pain (or fear of pain) at all levels (physical, mental, and emotional) is of utmost importance in treating migraine. Furthermore, lifestyle measures such as regular sleep, regular meals, exercise, avoidance of stress and dietary triggers can also be helpful. Several nonpharmacological approaches such as yoga, biofeedback, relaxation training, and neck loosening exercises (neck tilt: side to side, up and down; neck turn and stretch)[13] are known to significantly reduce frequency and severity of episodes of headaches in these patients. About 40% of patients in America suffering from neurological and pain disorders seek nonpharmacological management, i.e., CAM. Yoga is a holistic mind-body intervention that encompasses a series of practices such as postures, breathing exercises, relaxation, and meditation. The core objective of all these practices is to cultivate awareness.

Self-awareness: Yoga asanas help to increase awareness of the physical body.[14] When an individual performs any posture and continues to maintain the posture with full attention for a while, an unpleasant internal sensation gradually gets transformed into a tolerable sensation. Since the mind is diverted, the stress due to fear about migraine attack/pain reduces and relaxation sets in. This transformative effect is due to the effect of self-awareness.

Breath awareness: Yogis often emphasize the "breathing to the affected part".[14] Observing the breath passively and mobilizing the affected part of the body through prolonged exhalation calms down the mind and reduces the pain respectively.

Mindfulness: Migraine attacks can be due to external (food, environment, etc.) or internal factors (stress perception and responses). It is not surprising that patients with migraine are stressed about the attacks in the past due to stress/food and anticipate similar attacks in the future. This anticipation is by itself a strong triggering factor for migraine. Practicing mindfulness helps to be in the present moment without being affected by the past or future.

Overall, yoga practice may help to recognize the signals of pain at an early stage and can then help control it through self-regulatory mechanism.[15]

LITERATURE REVIEW

Several studies have found yoga therapy to be effective in reducing the intensity, frequency, and duration of pain in migraine and these changes were noticeable even after 3–6 months of post-yoga practice. Meditation alone has shown to improve tolerance toward pain. Patients with migraine without aura are known to have endothelial dysfunction which increases the risk for several vascular disorders such as ischemic stroke and coronary artery disease. A study of yoga intervention for 3 months found a decrease in the vascular cell adhesion molecule thereby reducing the risk for vascular diseases.[16] The physiological changes that might have led to the improvement in patients with migraine as a result of yoga therapy was evident through changes in heart rate variability and surface electromyography. From the above studies, it can be concluded that yoga may be used as an adjunct in the management of migraine.

A summary of the studies conducted so far on yoga for migraine is listed here.
In summary, all these studies[5,16-20] **(Table 1)** have demonstrated that yoga when introduced as a complementary therapy reduced the clinical severity, subjective pain, and frequency of headache. Hence, yoga is recommended as a complementary therapy for patients with migraine.

YOGA MODULE INCLUDING RECOMMENDATIONS FOR PRACTICE

There are no studies on the validation of a specific yoga module for migraine and also safety issues with few practices.[21] In this context, the yoga practices beneficial for migraine were collated and validated through an expert's opinion. This testing was

TABLE 1: Yoga for migraine—evidence-based.

S. No.	Author	Methodology	Study intervention	Control intervention	Outcomes	Conclusion
1.	John[17]	• A randomized controlled trial • 72 patients with migraine without aura were randomized into two groups	Yoga therapy	Self-care	• Headache intensity and frequency • Pain rating index • Affective pain rating index • Total pain rating index	A significant reduction in migraine headache frequency and associated clinical features, in patients treated with yoga over a period of 3 months
					Anxiety and depression scores and symptomatic medication use was significantly lower in the yoga group compared to the self-care group	
2.	Sharma[18]	• A randomized controlled trial • 70 patients with migraine were randomized into two groups	• Individualized yoga treatment for 12 weeks with four consecutive therapeutic sessions a week • 6-month follow-up	Standard care	• Self-perceived pain intensity • Pain frequency • Duration of pain • Functional status • Depression • Prescription and nonprescription medication use	The yoga group experienced statistically significant change in frequency, intensity and duration of pain. Depression decreased and functional status improved in yoga group and these differences were retained at 6-month follow-up
3.	Kisan[19]	• A randomized controlled trial • 60 migraine patients were divided into two groups	• Yoga along with conventional care • Yoga sessions were given 5 days a week for 6 weeks	Conventional care	• Clinical assessment (frequency, intensity of headache, and headache impact) • Autonomic function tests were done at baseline and at the end of the intervention	• Both yoga and conventional care group showed significant improvement • Yoga therapy showed an additional beneficiary effect on patients with migraine by reducing frequency and intensity

Contd...

Contd...

S. No.	Author	Methodology	Study intervention	Control intervention	Outcomes	Conclusion
4.	Naji-Esfahani[16]	- *A randomized controlled trial* - 42 women patients with migraine were divided into two groups	- Hatha Yoga practices along with conventional care - Individualized yoga therapy at three sessions per week (each session 75 minutes) for 12 weeks	Conventional care	- Intercellular adhesion molecule (ICAM) - Vascular cell adhesion molecule (VCAM) levels	Integrated yoga therapy is an effective treatment for migraine and also improved vascular function
5.	Wachholtz[5]	- *Nonrandomized study* - 92 meditation naive participants were divided into four groups	Spiritual Meditation Group (SMG), Internally Focused Secular Meditation (IFSM) Externally Focused Secular Meditation (EFMG), Progressive Muscle Relaxation (PMR)	NIL	- Migraine frequency decreased in SMG compared to other groups - Migraine severity ratings did not differ across groups - Usage of migraine medication decreased and improved pain tolerance in SMG compared to other groups	Spiritual meditation may be more effective for pain tolerance and migraine coping than nonspiritual meditation alternatives
6.	Vasudha[20]	- *An open-labeled nonrandomized study* - 60 migraine patients were divided into two groups	- Ayurveda and Yoga (AY) group underwent traditional Panchakarma (biopurification) using therapeutic purgation followed by yoga therapy - Yoga sessions were started after 15–17 days of Ayurveda treatment - Individualized yoga therapy sessions for 40 minutes for 7 days and asked to do home practice for 5 days/week for 90 days	Conventional care	Migraine disability assessment score, perceived stress, heart rate variability (HRV), and surface electromyographies (EMGs) of frontalis muscle were measured on Day 1, 30, and 90	The AY group therapy reduced migraine-related disability, perceived stress, sympathetic arousal, and muscle tension

carried out at Central Council for Yoga and Naturopathy—National institute for Mental Health and Neuro Sciences (NIMHANS) Collaborative Center (see **Appendix 1.12** for the yoga module for migraine).

Neck pain and muscle tension are common symptoms of a migraine attack. In this view, the patient may incur benefits from the following practices: The stretching and relaxing exercises (neck exercises, shoulder rotation, finger clench) followed by breathing into the affected area (*Shashankasana* breathing and head rolling) may help to relax and ease tension in the head, neck, and shoulders and increase tolerance and control.[14,17,22] Similarly, the self-awareness induced by asanas (ardhakati chakrasana and pawanamuktasana) coupled with breath awareness and prolonged exhalation during pranayama (nadi shodhana and bhramari) may alter the perception of pain and reduce the stress, anxiety, and depression associated with pain respectively. The applied relaxation techniques (quick relaxation technique) may be helpful in recognizing the stimulus (external or internal) and induce relaxation whenever the painful symptoms appear.[14]

Practices that are fast, vigorous (*Kapalabhati*) and practices involving high concentration and light (*Trataka*) may be avoided as they have been found to increase headache and eye pain respectively.[23,24]

Practical Tips for Yoga

Following are a few basic things to be kept in mind before starting yoga:
- *Time*: Yoga can be done during morning or evening hours.
- *Place*: Yoga should be practiced on a level floor in a well-ventilated room.
- *Outfit*: Choose loose and light (preferably cotton) and comfortable clothing.
- *Accessories*: Remove jewelry, wristwatch, belt, spectacles, etc., that may interfere while practicing.
- *Diet:* Sattvic foods like fresh fruits and vegetables; freshly cooked vegetarian food that is nonspicy and light for digestion should be consumed.

Considerations before Practicing Yoga

Although yoga is assumed to be safe, the following concerns are important to note:
- The patient must undergo a clinical examination by the neurologist and yoga consultant before practicing the yoga module.
- Yoga must be learnt under the supervision of a certified yoga expert, preferably who has experience in dealing with neurological disorders.
- As there are numerous schools of yoga, it is suggested to follow any one school of yoga which is evidence-based to avoid confusion.
- The duration of yoga practice depends on the duration and severity of the illness. But, any sign of improvement does not mean it is time to stop practicing yoga. Consult the doctor and the yoga expert who will modify the yoga practices. Adding yoga as a part of the daily routine is always an advantage to maintain overall well-being.
- Further, any improvement in symptoms does not mean that the patient can stop taking medications or alter its dosage. It is better to consult the primary treating doctor to evaluate the status of the condition and follow his/her advice. Likewise, if the patient wishes to change medications or use any form of alternate medication along with conventional (allopathic) medications, they should keep their primary doctor informed about the same.

POSSIBLE MECHANISMS OF ACTION OF YOGA

There is limited empirical evidence to support the precise underlying mechanisms for the clinical effects of yoga for migraine. Hence some of the possible mechanisms that explain the benefits of yoga in pain management in general are explained here.

Endocrine system: There is evidence that yoga has a positive impact on the stress hormone regulation. Studies have shown decreases in salivary cortisol associated with decrease in perceived stress and anxiety levels leading to increased feelings of well-being and improvement in pain management.[25] Regular practice of yoga also increased melatonin levels owing to improvement in the quality of sleep and immunity.[26]

Another mechanism that has been proposed is that of improvement in cardiac autonomic balance (e.g., enhancement of vagal tone and reduction in the sympathetic drive) through yoga practice. Pranayama practices increase frequency and duration of inhibitory neural impulses by activating stretch receptors of the lungs after maximum inhalation (more than normal tidal volume) in accordance with the Hering–Breuer reflex. During lung inflation, slowly adapting receptors in the lungs initiate inhibitory impulses. This plays an important role in controlling the role of autonomic functions such as heart rate and systemic vascular resistance. Synchronization of electrical signals between hypothalamus and the brainstem is said to be responsible for inducing the parasympathetic response. Further, a decrease in sympathetic system drive through relaxation techniques enhances sleep. Yoga has been proved to enhance the vagal tone and reduce the frequency and severity of headaches, thus improving the quality of life. Thus, modulating the autonomic balance is one of the main pain-relieving factors that can be achieved through a regular practice of yoga by patients with migraine.[27]

Inflammation: Yoga is known to be effective in decreasing proinflammatory cytokines such as interleukin-6 (IL-6), IL-2. and C-reactive protein attributing to yoga's capacity to stimulate the vagus nerve.[28]

Nerve conduction: Sleep and pain perceptions are related and good sleep is known to improve the long-term prognosis of individuals with migraine. It is speculated that yoga therapy is similar to a massage therapy in inducing deep sleep by reducing "substance P" levels.[29]

Psychology and cognition: Studies have indicated that yoga practices increase the awareness of physical and mental states.[30] This improved self-satisfaction, self-confidence, self-control and self-care could lead to improved pain management.

Behavioral/social: Yoga treatment programs have been shown to be effective in bringing about a lifestyle change in terms of making the right choice of food, maintain sleep hygiene, and reinforce physical activity, self-care and socialization which is all healthy ways of responding to stress. This change of attitude is the first step toward pain management.[31]

CONCLUSION

Regular yoga practice has shown many benefits in patients with migraine. Although some of these yoga-related benefits could be linked to a reduction in stress, modulation of cardiac autonomic balance, regulation of inflammatory cytokines and behavioral changes in sleep and lifestyle changes, more comprehensive studies required to understand the bigger picture. Nevertheless, yoga (with some contraindications for specific practices) can be offered as add-on therapy in patients with migraine to provide improvement in management of pain as well as the quality of life.

CASE VIGNETTE

Given here is a first-person account of a patient (anonymized) with migraine who practiced yoga:

Clinical Insights: Yoga for Migraine

Prior to the session
- Make sure that yoga is practiced indoors.
- Make sure that the yoga room is free from noise and artificial lights.
- Subjects should either practice in the morning or evening, practicing yoga during meal times may be avoided.
- After an acute episode which may require medications to manage the pain, practices such as head rolling, slow alternate nostril breathing and deep relaxation techniques may be offered once the pain subsides.
- *"Pranic"* model of excessive accumulation of *"prana"* or *"vayu"* in the head region due to imbalances in lifestyle and dysregulated emotions should be explained.
- How yogic practices aim at equidistribution and balance of *"prana"* throughout the body should be emphasized.

During the session
- *Loud mantra chanting may aggravate or precipitate headaches* and should be avoided; it is better to focus on gentle humming chants. *Highly focused meditations can be avoided.*
- *Fast breathing practices such as Bhastrika and Kapalabhati should be avoided.* They cause hyperventilation which may lead to increase in headaches by vasodilation or metabolic acidosis.
- *Emphasis on* yoga practices that enhance quality of sleep such as *slow mindful breathing techniques alternate nostril breathing (nadi shuddhi pranayama), very gentle humming breath (bhramari pranayama) with grounding of the head, and deep relaxation technique (in reverse direction, i.e., from head to toes).*
- Include practices which enhance digestive fire such as sitting twisted pose (*vakrasana*).

After the session
- Caretaker should be educated on necessary precautions.
- Regular 10-minute practice of *nadi shuddhi pranayama* and gentle *bhramari* in moon (*shashankasana*) pose (with forehead touching the ground) for 5 minutes should be done every day in the morning. Regular practice may be useful in preventing headache episodes.
- *Diet plays a very important role*: Patient and caregivers should be educated on avoiding rajasic and tamasic diet and sattvic diet should be promoted.
- Aim at improving the quality of life rather than a complete cure.

"I (Mr X) was around 27 years of age when I got my first migraine attack. I was apparently fine till then. After completing my engineering, I found a job which offered only night shifts. For the initial 6 months, there were no issues. One fine day, as I stepped out of the house in the afternoon, I experienced a severe, headache especially on the left side. I also had intense pain in my left eye and was unable to open my eyes. I also felt stiffness in the neck and felt nauseated. The headache was quite severe and did not subside till I vomited whatever I had for lunch. I did not feel relaxed despite taking rest for 2 hours. I was feeling weak, fatigued, and low. I experienced similar episodes the following week as well. I met a physician who referred me to a neurologist who diagnosed with migraine. My job posed a lot of challenges for which I had to take out extra time to complete. The medications used to make me feel drowsy as the migraine attacks were not less than 3-4 times per week. I was unable to work continuously on computers as it was increasing the headache. It went on for 6 months and I could see my productivity at work decreasing. This had a huge impact on my career. I was both physically and mentally disturbed. I was also not sharing my difficulties with anyone and as a result, it reflected in my behavior which was not acceptable to me and made me feel guilty. I then decided to share my health concerns with a friend for which he suggested to try yoga. I informed my doctor about the same and I was encouraged to go ahead and also was directed to a therapist who had expertise in teaching yoga practices for migraine per se.

I started attending three sessions per week and continued to practice at home. After 25 *days, I began to notice subtle improvements but the pain was still persisting. I changed my job to one that only had day shifts. After 6 months of continuous yoga practice, I noticed a significant change in migraine attacks: they were mild and occurred hardly once or twice in a month. I was also able to get over the attack in a short while.*

REFERENCES

1. Neck exercises: Do's and don'ts. New Jersey: American Migraine Foundation; 2020 [online] Available from: https://americanmigraine foundation.org/living-with-migraine/ [Last accessed October, 2020].
2. Mayans L, Walling A. Acute migraine headache: treatment strategies. Am Fam Physician. 2018;97(4):243-51.
3. Agostoni EC, Barbanti P, Calabresi P, Colombo B, Cortelli P, Frediani F, et al. Current and emerging evidence-based treatment options in chronic migraine: a narrative review. J Headache Pain. 2019;20(1):1-9.
4. Puledda F, Goadsby PJ, Prabhakar P. Treatment of disabling headache with greater occipital nerve injections in a large population of childhood and adolescent patients: a service evaluation. J Headache Pain. 2018;19(1):5.
5. Wachholtz AB, Malone CD, Pargament KI. Effect of different meditation types on migraine headache medication use. Behav Med. 2017;43(1):1-8.
6. Wells RE, Smitherman TA, Seng EK, Houle TT, Loder EW. Behavioral and mind/body interventions in headache: unanswered questions and future research directions. Headache: J Head Face Pain. 2014;54(6):1107-13.
7. Carlson BM. Human Embryology and Developmental Biology, 4th edition. St. Louis: Mosby; 2009. p. 541.
8. Nikhilananda S. Vedantasara of Sadananda, 13th edition. Kolkata, India: Advaita Ashrama; 1931.
9. Swāhānanda S. Pañcadaśī of Śrī Vidyāraṇya Swāmī: With an Introduction by Dr TMP Mahādevan. Madras: Sri Ramakrishna Math; 1967.
10. Saraswati SS, Hiti JK. Asana Pranayama Mudra Bandha. Bihar, India: Yoga Publications Trust; 1996.
11. Bhavanani AB. Application of yogic concepts in the promotion of positive health. [online] Available from: http://icyer.com/documents/ APPLICATION%20OF%20YOGIC%20 CONCEPTS%20IN%20PROMOTION%20OF%20 POSITIVE%20HEALTH.pdf [Last accessed October, 2020].
12. Saraswati SN. Prana and Pranayama, 13th edition. Bihar, India: Yoga Publications Trust; 2013.
13. Nagarathna R, Nagendra HR. Integrated Approach of Yoga Therapy for Positive Health. Bengaluru: Swami Vivekananda Yoga Prakashana; 2003.
14. Nespor K. Pain management and yoga. Int J Psychosom. 1991;38(1-4):76-81.
15. Roche LT. Yoga: a self-regulation process. Yoga Mimamsa. 2018;50(1):16.
16. Naji-Esfahani H, Zamani M, Marandi SM, Shaygannejad V, Javanmard SH. Preventive effects of a three-month yoga intervention on endothelial function in patients with migraine. Int J Prev Med. 2014;5(4):424-9.
17. John PJ, Sharma N, Sharma CM, Kankane A. Effectiveness of yoga therapy in the treatment of migraine without aura: a randomized controlled trial. Headache: J Head Face Pain. 2007;47(5):654-61.
18. Sharma N, Singhal S, Singh AP, Sharma CM. Effectiveness of integrated yoga therapy in treatment of chronic migraine: randomized controlled trial. J Headache Pain. 2013;14(1):1.
19. Kisan R, Sujan MU, Adoor M, Rao R, Nalini A, Kutty BM, et al. Effect of yoga on migraine: a comprehensive study using clinical profile and cardiac autonomic functions. Int J Yoga. 2014;7(2):126-32.
20. Vasudha MS, Manjunath NK, Nagendra HR. Lifestyle—a common denominator for the onset and management of migraine headache: complementing traditional approaches with scientific evidence. Int J Yoga. 2019;12(2):146-52.
21. Anheyer D, Klose P, Lauche R, Saha FJ, Cramer H. Yoga for treating headaches: a systematic review and meta-analysis. J Gen Intern Med. 2020;35(3):846-54.
22. Kaniecki RG. Migraine and tension-type headache: an assessment of challenges in diagnosis. Neurology. 2002;58(9 suppl 6):S15-20.
23. Nivethitha L, Mooventhan A, Manjunath NK, Bathala L, Sharma VK. Cerebrovascular hemodynamics during the practice of Bhramari Pranayama, Kapalbhati and Bahir-Kumbhaka: an exploratory study. Appl Psychophysiol Biofeedback. 2018;43(1):87-92.
24. Goadsby PJ, Holland PR, Martins-Oliveira M, Hoffmann J, Schankin C, Akerman S. Pathophysiology of migraine: a disorder of sensory processing. Physiol Rev. 2017;97(2):553-622.
25. McCall MC. How might yoga work? An overview of potential underlying mechanisms. J Yoga Phys Ther. 2013;3(1):1.

26. Rao RM, Vadiraja HS, Nagaratna R, Gopinath KS, Patil S, Diwakar RB, et al. Effect of yoga on sleep quality and neuroendocrine immune response in metastatic breast cancer patients. Indian J Palliat Care. 2017;23(3):253-60.

27. Vasudha MS, Manjunath NK, Nagendra HR. Changes in MIDAS, perceived stress, frontalis muscle activity and non-steroidal anti-inflammatory drugs usage in patients with migraine headache without aura following ayurveda and yoga compared to controls: an open labeled non-randomized study. Ann Neurosci. 2018;25(4):250-60.

28. Kiecolt-Glaser JK, Christian L, Preston H, Houts CR, Malarkey WB, Emery CF, et al. Stress, inflammation, and yoga practice. Psychosom Med. 2010;72(2):113-21.

29. Lander L, Chiasson-Downs K, Andrew M, Rader G, Dohar S, Waibogha K. Yoga as an adjunctive intervention to medication-assisted treatment with buprenorphine + naloxone. J Addict Res Ther. 2018;9(1):354.

30. Büssing A, Michalsen A, Khalsa SB, Telles S, Sherman KJ. Effects of yoga on mental and physical health: a short summary of reviews. Evid Based Complement Alternat Med. 2012;2012:165410.

31. Wells RE, Baute V, Wahbeh H. Complementary and integrative medicine for neurological conditions. Med Clin North Am. 2017;101(5):881-93.

Yoga in Parkinson's Disease

Diya Chatterjee, Shantala Hegde, Arun Thejaus KP, Pooja Mailankody

INTRODUCTION

Parkinson's disease (PD) is a disease of the brain and its symptoms include tremors of the limbs, slowness of movements, stiffness of the body parts, and impairment of balance. In addition to problems affecting movement, patients can also have depression, anxiety, sleep, memory disturbances, pain, absent or decreased smell, and constipation. PD is understood to be caused due to decreased levels of dopamine in the brain.

Parkinson's disease is now recognized as one of the most common neurological disorders to affect people over the age of 55, with a prevalence rate of 0.5–1.0% among people aged 65–69 years, rising to 1–3% among those aged 80 years and over. Symptomatic therapy for PD can provide some benefit for many years. However, by the end of 5 years about half of these patients develop levodopa-related motor complications, such as worsening of symptoms and dyskinesias.[1] Moreover, the disease relentlessly progresses and patients experience additional motor and nonmotor problems such as "freezing", falls, speech disturbance, autonomic dysfunction, psychiatric disturbances (depression, anxiety, psychosis), sleep disturbances and impairment of cognition that do not adequately respond to dopamine replacement therapy.[2] These problems markedly impair the quality of life (QoL) and functional status of patients. Managing these patients is a challenge to physicians and caregivers.

TREATMENT

Treatment of PD is mainly with Dopa and dopamine agonists. Levodopa, commonly used in the treatment of PD, produces improvement in stiffness and slowness. Other features such as imbalance, falls, constipation, memory, and sleep disturbances do not respond to levodopa.[2] As the disease progresses, the response to levodopa also begins to decrease. The duration of beneficial effects of the drug decreases (wearing off) and some patients develop abnormal involuntary movements called dyskinesias after taking levodopa.

A surgical procedure called deep brain stimulation (DBS) of certain areas in the brain also helps in managing symptoms of PD, especially in advanced stages when patients have severe disease and intolerable side effects. Nevertheless, not all patients with PD (PwPD) are suitable candidates for surgery. DBS cannot be done in patients with psychosis or dementia. Tremor, rigidity, slowness of movements, dyskinesias, and motor fluctuations improve after DBS. It does not produce improvement in falls, depression, anxiety, memory disturbances or constipation.[3] The cost of DBS is prohibitive and majority of PwPD, in a resource-constrained setting like India, cannot afford this surgical intervention.

NONMOTOR SYMPTOMS IN PARKINSON'S DISEASE

At its core, although PD is a complex neurological motor disorder, its conceptualization continues to evolve. Apart from the well-cited motor symptoms, nonmotor symptoms (NMS) of PD are being increasingly discussed in recent times. Some of these NMS precede the motor dysfunction by more than a decade.[4] NMS of PD are a key determinant of health, QoL and societal cost for individuals with the disorder and is being discussed briefly in the following section.

Psychotic symptoms such as visual hallucinations, sense of "presence" or passage, visual illusions, paranoid delusions[5] or dopaminergic drug-induced psychosis are reported in PwPD. *Sleep disturbances*, sleep attacks, insomnia, sleep fragmentation and rapid eye movement sleep behavior disorder (characterized by increased violent dream content, yelling, kicking and other potentially injurious motor activities)[6] are also seen. *Sensory disturbances* such as hyposmia (reduced ability to smell), pain, paresthesia, akathisia, impaired visual acuity and visual processing, and *autonomic disturbances* in the form of nausea and loss of appetite, lower urinary tract symptoms and sexual dysfunctions have been reported in several studies.[5,7] *Emotional disturbances* including depression, anxiety, apathy[5] and impairments in expressing and recognizing emotions[8] can be very disabling.

Cognitive deficits in PwPD often develop before the onset of motor symptoms. An estimated 50% of individuals with PD have mild cognitive impairments (MCIs) in the absence of dementia[9] and 25–30% of individuals with PD meet criteria for dementia.[10] Patients with MCI in PD present with executive dysfunction, and attention and memory deficits. PwPD perform poorly on tasks of complex attention, divided attention, planning, response inhibition, working memory, mental flexibility, and abstract reasoning. Memory deficits include both verbal and nonverbal explicit memory, domains of immediate recall, delayed recall, and recognition. They also perform poorly on tasks of visuoperceptual/visuospatial components. Language impairments are seen on measures of phonemic verbal fluency, semantic verbal fluency and visual confrontation naming.[11] Cognitive impairments pose a life-time adjustment risk to PwPD, thus making it imperative to focus on its understanding and management.

COGNITIVE REMEDIATION

Cognitive deficits in PD can adversely affect activities of daily living, thereby lowering an individual's level of independence and well-being. Pharmacotherapy has shown limited benefit in the treatment of cognitive impairments.[12] Such individuals are more likely to benefit from specialized cognitive remediation (CR) programs. CR involves structured, theoretically-driven modules to teach strategies and guide practice to improve cognitive domains and areas of functioning.

Cognitive remediation involves structured, theoretically driven modules to teach strategies and guide practice for improving cognitive domains and areas of functioning. CR programs for executive functions in PD inpatients have focused upon working memory facilitation using search tasks, matrices, puzzles, speech production, picture completion, and storytelling along with occupational therapy, physiotherapy, and physical treatment.[13] CR in PD has shown significant improvements in measures of attention, processing speed, memory, visuospatial abilities, executive functions, and semantic and verbal fluency.[14] Findings from a randomized controlled study for the efficacy of a cognitive rehabilitation program in PD population showed significantly increased brain connectivity between the left inferior temporal lobe and the bilateral dorsolateral prefrontal cortex compared to the control group post-training thereby implying the role of cognitive training in enhancing brain connectivity and activation.[15]

Cognitive remediation in PD shows subjective and objective gains and presents itself as a vital adjunct to pharmacotherapy, successfully leading to improved functioning in cognitive domains as well as better QoL and overall functioning.

MUSIC AND NADA YOGA: RESEARCH DIRECTIONS FOR THE FUTURE

"With total attention, listen to the sound of a stringed instrument, or any other musical instrument. Be absorbed in the all-pervading stillness."

–Vijnana Bhairava Tantra

Another novel realm of treatment for nonmotor as well as motor symptoms in PD is the field of music and rhythm-based interventions. Music is ubiquitous; however, it is in the past three decades or so that music has been studied as a basic and distinctive cognitive faculty. Music is a specialized cognitive function, subserved by various neural networks. Research on how brain processes music is emerging as a rich and stimulating area of investigation in the field of neuropsychology and neurosciences. Music has the potential to be valuable in rehabilitation targeting motor and NMS in PD. Engaging in music (actively or passively) is known to facilitate neurogenesis leading to neural plasticity.[16] Rhythmic auditory stimulation (RAS) methods through metronome sounds or marching music have shown to improve motor functions, especially speed of gait and reduce freezing of gait in PD.[17] Today, music and rhythm-based interventions are studied and clinically applied as scientific methods of intervention to improve speech and language, cognition and emotion, in addition to motor functions. Indian Classical Music and its beneficial effects on health have been documented in literature and philosophy. *Nada Yoga* for instance, considers *"naada"* or sound and music to have the power to heal as well as to enhance psychological and spiritual health. Indian classical music has its origins in the *Samaveda* and is an ever-evolving art. This music has, over years, taken various forms and has branched out into different traditions. *Raga Chikitsa*—healing through various ragas of the classical tradition—has been an integral part of the ancient healing system, the *Ayurveda*. Music, combined with yogic practice, can bring about expanded consciousness involving deep relaxation and awareness of the internal bodily acoustics. It involves listening deeply to the internal sounds and the music of the natural world, where every element has its own vibration—from blossoms, trees and animals to the human mind. In a study exploring the effect of music learning as part of *Nada Yoga Sadhana* in a group of music practitioners, it was found that learning music as part of *Nada Yoga Sadhana* positively increased alpha rhythm on electroencephalography and also improved the general well-being of study participants.[18] This implicates that practice of Nada yoga can instill a deep sense of relaxation and can also be effective in reducing stress. Music and yoga incorporated into therapeutic techniques for the motor and NMS of PD is yet to be examined systematically. It is imperative that systematic research in this area is carried out in coming years to establish the scientific evidence for therapeutic benefits.

YOGA FOR THE TREATMENT OF PARKINSON'S DISEASE

Dopamine deficiency in PD has been well established. Yoga restores the production of dopamine. In addition, the ability of the brain to change or neuroplasticity is stimulated through yoga.[19-21]

Studies have shown that symptoms of slowness of movements and stiffness of the limbs improve with yoga. Other features of PD such as anxiety, depression and balance problems, which do not respond to Levodopa, also improve with yoga.[22-26] Some of the *asanas* can decrease the shortening of the certain muscles that lead to the abnormally flexed posture in PD.[27] In a study by Sharma et al. (2015), 8 PwPD who underwent yoga for 12 weeks were compared with five patients who did not and they found significant improvement in Unified Parkinson Disease Rating Scale (UPDRS) motor scores. Positive trends of improvement were also noted in depression scores. It was also shown that falls decreased by 25% as a result of yoga.[23] Boulgarides et al. (2014) found that there was significant improvement in depression as well as balance after 8 weeks of yoga in 10 PwPD.[24] A study of 14 older adults by Schmid et al. (2010) found significant reduction in fear of falling and improvement in static balance after 12 weeks of yoga.[25] Yoga helps to improve the mobility and activities of daily living in PwPD. Yoga is a safe and effective complementary method for managing motor symptoms and improves the motor function in PD. Yoga can be an effective tool to prevent functional deterioration in PD.[26] Metri et al. developed and validated a module of yoga for PwPD with a detailed review of classical textbooks of Yoga and inputs from 20 experts in the field[28] (see **Appendix 1.13** for the yoga module for PD).

MECHANISMS OF YOGA IN PARKINSON'S DISEASE

The concept of yoga comes from textbooks of ancient Indian philosophy. The application of yoga as a therapeutic intervention to mitigate the severity of certain diseases began in the early 20th century.[29] There are multiple elements in yoga that provide benefits for specific disease conditions that demand further research and exploration. Some elements of yoga include *asanas* postures; *pranayama* voluntary regulated breathing techniques, relaxation techniques, and *dhyana* meditation, mindfulness, and self-reflection. In yoga, these elements could either be practiced as a standalone technique or as a combination based on the application and intended result.[30] In recent years, yoga has been used as an adjunct therapy for several neurological conditions.[31]

Even though the role of oxidative stress in the pathogenesis of neurodegenerative disease is well established, the exact etiology of heterogeneous and slowly progressing disorders such as Alzheimer's disease (AD) and PD is yet to be clearly understood. Cumulative oxidative stress can induce cellular damage, impairment of the DNA repair system and also cause mitochondrial dysfunction. These have been shown to play a key role in acceleration of the aging process and the development of neurodegenerative disorders.[32] Studies have found that the level of systemic oxidative stress is lower in yoga practitioners but the specific yoga technique, which brings about this change, has not been identified. Another component of yoga, namely "relaxation technique", has also been shown to reduce oxidative stress during short as well as long-term sessions. This reduces oxidative stress by inducing upregulation of biological oxidative genes, buffering against cellular reaction with over expenditure of mitochondrial energy and downregulation of nuclear factor kappa-light-chain-enhancer of activated B-cells (NF-κB) inflammatory gene.[33]

Yoga Nidra is a voluntarily-induced suppression of the executive system via relaxed meditation. A study conducted in healthy volunteers with 7–26 years of experience in practicing meditation showed an increase of dopamine levels in the ventral striatal region of the brain during *Yoga Nidra*. Other than *Yoga Nidra*, 3-month practice of other yoga techniques also demonstrated significant improvement in the level of dopamine in healthy individuals.[19] This directly correlated with metrics for assessment of mental relaxation and parasympathetic dominance. Such techniques to enhance dopamine levels in ventral striatum are yet to be explored in PD.[19]

Brain-derived neurotrophic factor (BDNF) is a protein encoded by the *BDNF* gene, that plays an important role in differentiation, regeneration, and plasticity mechanisms in the human brain. PwPD have lower BDNF compared with healthy people and this has a role in the pathophysiology of PD. It also affects motor cortex plasticity and motor learning in

PD. It has been shown that endurance exercises can influence the up regulation of BDNF in PD and improve motor cortex plasticity.[20,21] Yoga and meditation practices increase the plasma BDNF significantly, mostly due to the decrease in stress level in healthy individuals. This is associated with decrease in the cortisol level and improved heart rate variability (HRV) variables. Such techniques could be used to treat comorbidities of PD such as depression and anxiety.

The precise mechanisms to explain the effects of yoga are yet to be fully understood but yoga can be used as biopsychosocial model for a better understanding of the physiological and psychological factors, which influence the individual during the state of illness. The positive effects of yoga are facilitated by changes in the central nervous system (CNS) and peripheral nervous system (PNS), along with the action of endocrine and immune system. Yogic practices that focus on breathing techniques and attention could influence a downregulation of hypothalamic-pituitary-adrenal (HPA) axis and sympathetic nervous system (SNS). This in turn leads to dominance of parasympathetic over SNS mediated by the stimulation of the vagus nerve. There are numerous studies that support the action of yogic practices such as breathing and awareness-based techniques on enhanced autonomic control resulting in reduction of blood pressure and heart rate.[34]

Yogic concept of health is different from the Western concept, which considers the absence of disease as health. According to the Yogic terms, when you are really your "Self", you are truly at "ease". So, the loss of "self" creates disease[30] and this is well explained with the *Panchakosha* concept. The internal imbalance due to long-standing stressful and demanding situations of life is the start of any disease. And in the context of PD, intense surges of uncontrolled excessive speed of responses to the demanding situations at an emotional level (*Manomaya kosha*), conflicts between value systems (*Vijnanamaya kosha*), depression, dislikes, etc. (*Manomaya kosha*) are seen in the initial stages of PD and then later the cardinal symptoms manifest in *Pranamaya* and *Annamaya koshas*. The practice of yoga by "mastery over the mind" helps to correct this imbalance, harmonize the disturbances at each of the five levels (*Panchakosha*).[35]

CONCLUSION

Stretching a muscle improves its control; thus, *asana* practice could enhance better muscle activity. *Pranayama* could improve even distribution of oxygen to cells of the body, providing reduction in pain and better utilization of nutrients through better blood supply. Relaxation procedures such as *Yoga Nidra* could decrease stress related effects in the body thus improving overall well-being and better sleep for improved repair mechanisms to the body. The effects of the practice of yoga on the nervous system and the HPA axis substantiate the application of yoga for the management of PD. In addition to problems associated with movement, yoga helps in management of anxiety, depression and balance issues in PD.

CASE VIGNETTE

A 63-year-old college professor presented with tremulousness of the left upper limb and slowness of activities performed with left hand of 4 years' duration. On clarifying, he revealed that he had been suffering from constipation since many years. His wife also reported that he had decreased perception of smell for the past 5-6 years. There was no family history of similar illness. He was on treatment with Levodopa 6 times a day. When this medication was started 2 years ago, his symptom response was good with benefits lasting for around 4 hours after taking the medication. The slowness would improve and he would perform all his activities of daily living with ease. However, for the past 2 years, the beneficial effects of medication had

Clinical Insights: Yoga for Parkinson's Disease

Prior to the session	• Clinical symptoms of the patient have to be assessed. Patients who have problems with balance, gait and exhibit intense tremors may require one-to-one sessions. • Caregiver assistance to the patient during the session is advisable for cases with severity of stage 3 and above on Hoehn and Yahr scale. • Caregivers also must be given instructions on how to provide passive assistance to the patients with severe morbidity. • It is important to be aware of the medications and other modes of therapy the patient is undergoing. • The yoga therapist should be aware of the ON-state and OFF-state conditions of the anti-parkinsonian medications. The therapist should not intensify the yoga practices mistaking the ON-state conditions with the improvement in symptoms. • Educate the patient on how yoga may help him/her. Also, highlight about the necessities and precautions to be taken during the yoga session.
During the session	• Special emphasis on practices such as *Sithilikarana vyayama* (whole body joint loosening), *Kapalabhati*, *Nadanusandhana* (mantra chants) and relaxation techniques should be given. • Whole body joint loosening should be performed 2–3 times a day apart from regular yoga sessions to reduce stiffness. • Chronically ill patients should be appreciated for any slight advancement in their yoga practice. This will motivate and encourage the patient. • Use of a chair is strongly recommended, especially in the cases with severity of stage 3 and above on the Hoehn and Yahr scale, i.e., for those with postural instability or severe disability due to tremors or those who are wheelchair-bound. • Patient may need support from therapist while changing the postures from sitting to supine, prone to supine, etc., and vice versa. This must be done under the observation of caregiver. • If the patient is unable to attain the final posture, the therapist should advise modifications in the posture to make the patient comfortable. If required supportive props such as pillows, bolsters, meditation chair with back support may be used. • Make sure that the patient is not extremely fatigued with the pace and intensity of the practices. The patient may experience bodyaches and may get discouraged to continue the yoga practices. Start with simple low-intensity practices such as joint loosening and mantra chantings and gradually build up. • Voice culture yoga practices of tongue rotation, tongue massage, *simha mudra*, matching the voice to sound "*Om*" by whispering and gentle chantings, *ujjayi* breathing should be used in patients with speech difficulties. • If patient displays easy fatigability, it is better to schedule two yoga sessions of shorter duration (30 min) in a day rather than teaching the entire yoga module in one session.
After the session	• Inquire about the subjective difficulties in the yoga practices after each class and address them. • Schedule follow-up assessments in coordination with the neurologist treating the patient. • Educate the patient and caregiver on the small modules of practices such as joint loosening followed by relaxation that can be practiced multiple times by the patient at home.

only been lasting for 1–2 hours (wearing off). At the time of presentation, he also reported low mood and loss of interest in his routine activities.

Psychiatric opinion was sought for his mood problems. The option of DBS was discussed with the patient and his relatives but was deemed to be unaffordable. He attended yoga sessions for 3 days a week for 4 weeks. A validated yoga module for PD developed by Metri et al.[28] was administered by the yoga therapist (**Appendix 1.13**). Assessment after 1 month of supervised yoga sessions revealed improvement in both motor symptoms and mood leading to improved QoL.

REFERENCES

1. Nussbaum RL, Ellis CE. Alzheimer's disease and Parkinson's disease. N Engl J Med. 2003; 348(14):1356-64.
2. Olanow CW, Watts RL, Koller WC. An algorithm (decision tree) for the management of Parkinson's disease (2001): treatment guidelines. Neurology. 2001;56(Suppl 5):S1-88.
3. Malek N. Deep brain stimulation in Parkinson's disease. Neurol India. 2019;67(4):968-78.
4. Kalia LV, Lang AE. Parkinson disease in 2015: evolving basic, pathological and clinical concepts in PD. Nat Rev Neurol. 2016;12(2):65-6.
5. Chaudhuri KR, Healy DG. Schapira AH, National Institute for Clinical Excellence. Non-motor symptoms of Parkinson's disease: diagnosis and management. Lancet Neurol. 2006;5(3):235-45.
6. Menza M, Dobkin RD, Marin H, Bienfait K. Sleep disturbances in Parkinson's disease. Mov Disord. 2010;25(Suppl 1):S117-22.
7. Biousse V, Skibell BC, Watts RL, Loupe DN, Drews-Botsch C, Newman NJ. Ophthalmologic features of Parkinson's disease. Neurology. 2004;62: 177-80.
8. Sotgiu I, Rusconi ML. Investigating emotions in Parkinson's disease: what we know and what we still don't know. Front Psychol. 2013;4:336.
9. Goldman JG, Litvan I. Mild cognitive impairment in Parkinson's disease. Minerva Med. 2011;102(6): 441-59.
10. Aarsland D, Zaccai J, Brayne C. A systematic review of prevalence studies of dementia in Parkinson's disease. Mov Disord. 2005;20(10):1255-63.
11. Watson GS, Leverenz JB. Profile of cognitive impairment in Parkinson's disease. Brain Pathol. 2010;20(3):640-5.
12. Seppi K, Weintraub D, Coelho M, Perez-Lloret S, Fox SH, Katzenschlager R, et al. The movement disorder society evidence-based medicine review update: treatments for the non-motor symptoms of Parkinson's disease. Mov Disord. 2011;26(Suppl 3): S42-80.
13. Biundo R, Weis L, Fiorenzato E, Antonini A. Cognitive rehabilitation in Parkinson's disease: is it feasible? Arch Clin Neuropsychol. 2017;32(7): 840-60.
14. Diez-Cirarda M, Ibarretxe-Bilbao N, Peña J, Ojeda N. Efficacy of cognitive rehabilitation in Parkinson's disease. Neural Regen Res. 2018;13(2):226-7.
15. Díez-Cirarda M, Ojeda N, Peña J, Cabrera-Zubizarreta A, Lucas-Jiménez O, Gómez-Esteban JC, et al. Increased brain connectivity and activation after cognitive rehabilitation in Parkinson's disease: a randomized controlled trial. Brain Imaging Behav. 2017;11(6):1640-51.
16. Reybrouck M, Vuust P, Brattico E. Music and brain plasticity: how sounds trigger neurogenerative adaptations. In: Chaban V (Ed). Neuroplasticity: Insights of Neural Reorganization. Croatia: IntechOpen; 2018. pp. 85-103.
17. Thaut MH, McIntosh GC, Rice RR, Miller RA, Rathbun J, Brault JM. Rhythmic auditory stimulation in gait training for Parkinson's disease patients. Mov Disord. 1996;11(2):193-200.
18. Kumar K. Effect of learning music as a practice of Nada yoga on EEG alpha and general well-being. Yoga Mimamsa. 2011;43:215-20.
19. Kjaer TW, Bertelsen C, Piccini P, Brooks D, Alving J, Lou HC. Increased dopamine tone during meditation-induced change of consciousness. Cogn Brain Res. 2002;13(2):255-9.
20. Pal R, Singh SN, Chatterjee A, Saha M. Age-related changes in cardiovascular system, autonomic functions, and levels of BDNF of healthy active males: role of yogic practice. Age (Dordr). 2014;36(4):9683.
21. Foster PP. Role of physical and mental training in brain network configuration. Front Aging Neurosci. 2015;7:117.
22. Kwok JY, Kwan JC, Auyeung M, Mok VC, Lau CK, Choi KC, et al. Effects of mindfulness yoga vs stretching and resistance training exercises on anxiety and depression for people with parkinson disease: a randomized clinical trial. JAMA Neurol. 2019;76(7):755-63.
23. Sharma NK, Robbins K, Wagner K, Colgrove YM. A randomized controlled pilot study of the therapeutic effects of yoga in people with Parkinson's disease. Int J Yoga. 2015;8(1):74-9.
24. Boulgarides LK, Barakatt E, Coleman-Salgado B. Measuring the effect of an eight-week adaptive yoga program on the physical and psychological status of individuals with Parkinson's disease. A pilot study. Int J Yoga Therap. 2014;24:31-41.
25. Schmid AA, Van Puymbroeck M, Koceja DM. Effect of a 12-week yoga intervention on fear of falling and balance in older adults: a pilot study. Arch Phys Med Rehabil. 2010;91(4):576-83.
26. Cheung C, Bhimani R, Wyman JF, Konczak J, Zhang L, Mishra U, et al. Effects of yoga on oxidative stress, motor function, and non-motor symptoms in Parkinson's disease: a pilot randomized controlled trial. Pilot Feasibility Stud. 2018;4:162.
27. Corcos DM, Robichaud JA, David FJ, Leurgans SE, Vaillancourt DE, Poon C, et al. A two-year randomized controlled trial of progressive resistance exercise for Parkinson's disease. Mov Disord. 2013;28(9):1230-40.

28. Kakde N, Metri KG, Varambally S, Nagaratna R, Nagendra HR. Development and validation of a yoga module for Parkinson disease. J Complement Integr Med. 2017;14(3).
29. Büssing A, Michalsen A, Khalsa SB, Telles S, Sherman KJ. Effects of yoga on mental and physical health: a short summary of reviews. Evid Based Complement Alternat Med. 2012;2012:165410.
30. Stephens I. Medical yoga therapy. Children (Basel). 2017;4(2):12.
31. Mishra SK, Singh P, Bunch S, Zhang R. The therapeutic value of yoga in neurological disorders. Ann Indian Acad Neurol. 2012;15(4):247-54.
32. Kandlur A, Satyamoorthy K, Gangadharan G. Oxidative stress in cognitive and epigenetic aging: a retrospective glance. Front Mol Neurosci. 2020;13:41.
33. Bhasin MK, Dusek JA, Chang BH, Joseph MG, Denninger JW, Fricchione GL, et al. Relaxation response induces temporal transcriptome changes in energy metabolism, insulin secretion and inflammatory pathways. PLoS One. 2013;8(5):e62817.
34. Lawrence M, Celestino FT, Matozinho HH, Govan L, Booth J, Beecher J. Yoga for stroke rehabilitation. Cochrane Database Syst Rev. 2017;12:CD011483.
35. Villacres MD, Jagannathan A, Nagarathna R, Ramakrsihna J. Decoding the integrated approach to yoga therapy: qualitative evidence based conceptual framework. Int J Yoga. 2014;7(1):22-31.

CHAPTER 21

Yoga for Epilepsy

Praveen Angadi, Nivedha Mohan Raj, Malla Bhaskara Rao

INTRODUCTION

India carries an enormous burden of epilepsy. By conservative estimates, there are over 10 million people/patients with epilepsy (PWE) in India.[1,2] Antiepileptic drugs (AEDs) can stop the seizures in about 60–70% of PWE and 10–20% of PWE can be benefited by surgery. Reports show that methods including lifestyle changes, yoga, and meditation may play a significant role in achieving the cure or control of epilepsy and improvement in the quality of life. However, these methods are currently underutilized. In a Science and Technology of Yoga and Meditation-Department of Science and Technology (SATYAM-DST), Government of India funded project, the authors are investigating the role of yoga and meditation in the management of people with chronic drug-resistant epilepsy (DRE). Based upon the literature review as well as the ongoing research, an overview on the role of yoga for epilepsy is presented in this chapter. Along with physicians, yoga therapists can play an important role in the management of PWE and reducing the disease burden in India.[3]

Epilepsy

Seizures are the result of synchronized hyperexcitation in neuronal networks. Epilepsy is a chronic condition of the brain characterized by the generation of recurrent unprovoked seizures and by the neurobiological, cognitive, psychological, and social consequences of this condition. DRE may be defined as the condition in which two-approved AEDs (independently or in combination) fail to provide freedom from seizures. Epileptogenesis is defined as the development of tissue capable of generating spontaneous seizures, including development of an epileptic condition and progression. Epilepsy surgery is the removal or functional manipulation of part of the brain with the aim to reduce seizures, improve the cognitive function and the quality of life. Lesion is a volume of altered cerebral tissue detected by neuroimaging techniques or during surgery. Focus is a volume of brain tissue that contains the epileptogenic area or the epileptogenic zone.[4-6] Gamma-aminobutyric acid (GABA), the principal inhibitory neurotransmitter in the cerebral cortex, maintains the inhibitory tone that counterbalances neuronal excitation. When this balance is perturbed, seizures may ensue. Experimental and clinical study evidence indicates that GABA has an important role in the mechanism and treatment of epilepsy. Poor seizure control was associated with low brain GABA concentration. GABA concentration, remote from the seizure focus, is a risk factor for seizure recurrence.[7] Medical conditions including depression, epilepsy, and post-traumatic stress disorder (PTSD) tend to have low heart rate variability (HRV) and low GABAergic activities and reduced GABA system activity.[8]

Yoga

The ancient practice and philosophy of yoga is increasingly becoming a point of therapy and research in epilepsy for seizure treatment.

In the *Ayurveda* tradition, epilepsy is called *apasmara*, meaning loss of consciousness of the body. The ancient Indian texts, the *Vedas*, describe four types of epilepsy and nine disorders causing convulsions in children. For the treatment of epilepsy, the physical discipline of yoga seeks to re-establish a balance (union) between those aspects of a person's health that cause seizures. Yoga is one of the oldest formal practices known whose purpose is to restore this balance.

Pranayama causes changes in metabolism, blood flow, and oxygen levels in the blood. The practice of *pranayama*, i.e., controlled deep diaphragmatic breathing, helps restore normal respiration; this can reduce the chances of going into a seizure or stop the seizure before it becomes full blown. The *yogasanas* aid in restoring balance to the body and its metabolic systems. Practicing *asanas* increases physical stamina and calms the nervous system. *Asanas*, used as a physical exercise alone, improve circulation, respiration, and concentration, while decreasing the chances of having a seizure. These exercises also help to improve the health-related quality of life (HRQOL).[3]

Stress is a well-recognized trigger of seizure activity. *Dhyana* or meditation soothes the mind even as it heals the body. Meditation improves blood flow to the brain and slows the production of stress hormones. Meditation also increases the levels of neurotransmitters, like serotonin, which keep the body's nervous system calm. Practicing relaxation techniques such as yoga meditation is well known as a definitive aid in seizure control.[9]

In 1996, The Indian Journal of Medical Research published the results of a study on the effects of *Sahaja Yoga* practice on seizure control. In this study, a group of PWE who practiced *Sahaja Yoga* for 6 months experienced 86% decrease in their seizure frequency. The practice of yoga regulates body physiology through control of posture, breathing, and meditation. The effects of yoga on the autonomic functions of patients with refractory epilepsy, as quantified by standardized autonomic function tests, were determined in another study. The yoga group showed significant improvement in parasympathetic parameters and a decrease in seizure frequency scores.[10]

EFFECT OF YOGA ON EPILEPSY

Rajesh *et al.* performed a prospective, nonrandomized clinical trial, in which patients with DRE adhered to a twice-daily yoga meditation protocol. 19/20 subjects reported a decreased frequency of seizures within 3 months, and 6 of those 19 demonstrated significant reductions (<50% reduction in seizure frequency). Additionally, patients usually report stress as a factor that increases the likelihood of auras or a seizure episode.[11] Panjwani demonstrated that PWE responded to *Sahaja Yoga* in reducing stress, in a randomized controlled study. This provides hope to patients with refractory epilepsy that nonpharmaceutical techniques may be successful in reducing seizure frequency.[12]

Furthermore, Sirven surveyed the use of complementary and alternative medicine (CAM) treatments including yoga among the Epilepsy Foundation of Arizona (EFAZ) members. The survey questioned the type of therapy used, level of seizure control, and their perceptions on the various CAM treatments for seizures. Results showed that 42% of all respondents had tried CAM for nonseizure conditions, and 44% had used CAM for their seizures. Yoga was reported as effective in seizure control in 57% of participants. All CAM modalities were partly perceived to be beneficial; however, botanicals, stress reduction, and yoga were reported as being the most helpful.[13]

In a randomized controlled trial, involving 18 patients with electroencephalography (EEG)-diagnosed epilepsy, yoga showed therapeutic effects of decreasing seizure index along with an improvement in quality of life.

Subjects participated in professional and group yoga sessions including booster sessions 6- and 12-month post-treatment. Results of yoga therapy demonstrated a significant reduction in seizure index and a significant increase in quality of life over time. Augmenting yoga to help PWE presents an inexpensive, noninvasive, enjoyable, and potentially cross-cultural, supplementation to epilepsy control and quality of life improvement.[14]

A Cochrane review of yoga in adults with refractory epilepsy found only two unblinded, controlled trials[15] and was unable to draw reliable conclusions about the efficacy of such treatment due to the limited number of studies, small number of participants, and lack of blinding. Nevertheless, there was a beneficial effect in control of seizures, with better efficacy of yoga when compared to no intervention or *"sham yoga"* (e.g., postural exercises mimicking yoga or muscle relaxation). The meta-analysis recommended that yoga should only be used as an adjunct to AEDs.

Sathyaprabha et al. conducted a short-term, unblinded, controlled study of the impact of yoga, which included postures, meditation, and breathing exercises, on autonomic function in epilepsy. The yoga group had a decrease in seizure frequency after 10 weeks of daily sessions, not seen in a simple routine exercise control group.[16] The mechanism by which relaxation and yoga may reduce seizure frequency is unclear, but may relate to direct physiochemical or electrographic changes, changes in the autonomic nervous system (ANS) and vascular tone, alterations of CO_2 and O_2 concentrations, or indirect effects on the limbic system.[17]

Overall, the studies of yoga are small and bound by certain limitations. The nature of these interventions, e.g., makes double-blinding largely impossible. In addition, the studies often fail to meet the standards of high-level evidence due to small sample sizes, inadequate randomization methods, or uncontrolled designs. Unlike drug studies in which blood levels or pill bottle opening may be tracked, protocols are based on home practice for which adherence cannot be verified. Some studies were also potentially confounded by changes in AEDs and differing baseline characteristics across groups. Despite these constraints, yoga has been associated with multiple health benefits and poses little risk; we would consider its use in medically refractory patients whose seizures may be exacerbated by stress and who are not candidates for, or do not desire, further medication trials, surgery, or implantable devices, with the understanding that current empirical support is limited.

Deepak[18] conducted a study on 11 adult patients of refractory epilepsy who were taught meditation. They practiced for 1 year. The control group was matched for age and duration of epilepsy. The results of the trial showed that the meditation group showed decrease in frequency and duration of seizures (as compared to the baseline) after 6 months of yoga practice. No changes were seen in the control group. The practitioner of yoga combines physical posture, breathing exercises, relaxation, and meditation to attain optimal physical fitness. In a study of 32 PWE, randomized to group 1 ($n = 10$ receiving yoga therapy), group 2 ($n = 10$, receiving sham yoga) and group 3 ($n = 12$, control group), 40% of group 1 became seizure-free after 6 months.[19]

It has been reported that brain GABA levels increase by 27% after a 1-hour yoga asana practice in experienced practitioners and suggests that the practice of yoga should be explored and compared to other exercise modalities as a treatment or adjunctive treatment for disorders associated with low GABA states.[20] The development of an inexpensive, widely available intervention, with few side effects, that is effective in alleviating the symptoms of disorders associated with low GABA states has clear public health advantages.

MECHANISM OF ACTION

Yoga may induce relaxation, stress reduction, and influence the electroencephalogram and the ANS, thereby controlling seizures. Meditation induces ketosis, which may increase brain GABA, and hence would be expected to inhibit epileptiform activity. In epilepsy, homeostasis can be restored through yoga practices by reducing allostatic load in stress systems. Hypothetically, it can be said that stress induces imbalance of the ANS with decreased parasympathetic nervous system (PNS) and increased sympathetic nervous system (SNS) activities, underactivity of the GABA system (the primary inhibitory neurotransmitter system) and increased allostatic load. It is further hypothesized that yoga-based lifestyle intervention (YBLI) practices correct underactivity of the PNS and GABA systems partially through stimulation of the vagus nerves, which are main peripheral pathway of the PNS and reduce allostatic load.[8]

Several studies have shown that yoga can have demonstrable physiologic effects. For instance, *Sahaja Yoga* has been shown to produce alterations in galvanic skin resistance (GSR), blood lactate level, and urinary vanillylmandelic acid (VMA). These alterations may collectively indicate reduced stress following yoga practice. Additionally, *Sahaja Yoga* has been observed to produce EEG changes in PWE, with power spectral analysis showing a shift in frequencies from 0–8 Hz to 8–20 Hz. Such EEG changes may be because of the modulation of hypothalamic and endocrine effects on the limbic system and SNSs.[10]

In such conditions, YBLIs show improvement in symptoms. The possible mechanism of action suggested is that yoga increases brain desynchronization. Yoga also reduces stress, increases central inhibitory GABA levels, and alters blood flow of the central nervous system and leads to a shift in autonomic balance toward relative parasympathetic dominance.[8,16] Yoga practices stimulate the activation of alpha, beta and theta waves of the brain and these waves are associated in improving cognition, memory, mood, and anxiety.[21]

METHODS

Patients with DRE may benefit from alternative/adjunctive treatment modalities. One such alternative treatment modality is yoga, which is widely accepted and practiced all over the world. A nonrandomized study offering yoga meditation two times a day with weekly yoga program demonstrated significant reductions in seizure frequency in 19 out of 20 patients after 3 months of yoga practice and six patients were seizure-free for 6 months. According to the yogic understanding, it is believed that pranic imbalance is evident in PWE and yogic practices create balance in breath, mind, and pranic flow to the head region. As yoga practices can increase awareness and mindfulness in the brain, epilepsy associated conditions such as stress, depression, suicidal ideations, anxiety, reduced quality of life, sleep disturbance, irritability, mood swings, and loss of memory can be effectively addressed.[8,22] A suggested yoga schedule for PWE can be found in **Appendix 1.14** at the end of the book. PWE must be aware that lack of sleep, photic stimulation as well as hyperventilation can precipitate seizures. Hence these provoking factors have to be avoided while practicing yoga and meditation.

PRACTICAL CONSIDERATIONS DURING YOGA THERAPY

The yoga therapy practices have to be chosen wisely based upon scientific evidence and modulated as per the individual requirement. Patients belong to various socioeconomic and educational back grounds. Keeping their need, motivation, intelligence quotient (IQ), memory, cognition, and understanding capacity the module has to be taught in such a way they understand the concepts underlying the yoga practices. Language is strongest tool as well as barrier to convey the information from one to another. The *yoga* therapy practices have to be delivered in a language understood by the patient to get to know the concepts. One has to start practicing slowly and moderation plays a very important role. The practices should not be done beyond one's capacity. Daily increase as per the capacity and to withstand practice effects helps participants a lot.

During supervised yoga sessions, it is good to have a better understanding between yoga therapist and the participant. Yoga therapist is advised to assess patient's physical strength, limitations, comorbidities, sleep duration, daily activities, recent surgeries if any and willing to undergo yogic practices. Patients to be asked to come in loose, comfortable clothes. One has to clear the bowel and bladder before the session commencement. One has to avoid strong perfumes and solid food for 2–3 hours and liquids 45–60 minutes before the session. After 30 minutes of the session, patient can have liquid/solid food. To learn the practice properly, patients are advised to observe instructor carefully and follow the practices one by one. Patients should also observe their physical, mental, emotional, and breathing status before and after the session. Once they become familiar with the practices, they can practice as per own phase and speed. Oneness with mind body complex and tracing the effect of gross and subtle impact of the practices makes huge difference in the yoga therapy outcome. It is advised to practice Yoga at home/therapy center in a calm and quiet room without external disturbance. Yoga can be practiced in a comfortable way in the morning or evening or both times with or without yoga video guidance. It is advised to observe silence and relaxation after each practice of the module and keeping breath flow slow, deep, spontaneous, rhythmic and regulated. Instructor's assurances and clarifications of the yoga practices often make patients relaxed and motivated.

INDICATIONS

Yoga and meditation can be added during the early course of the disease for better efficacy for many DREs. During the later course of the disease, once drug resistance develops, all forms of therapeutic interventions, both pharmacological as well as nonpharmacological, will be less effective. Yoga and meditation need willingness and cooperation of the patients, and children and elderly may require alteration in the modules to make it easier for them to practice. Similarly, pregnant women may find it difficult to practice yoga and meditation especially during the late stages of pregnancy. People with not only primary epilepsy, but also secondary epilepsy due to traumatic brain injury, stroke as well as tumors can practice yoga and meditation and derive the benefits.

The prevalence of psychological distress, especially depressive and anxiety disorders, is higher in epilepsy than in other chronic health conditions. These comorbid conditions contribute even more than epileptic seizures themselves to impaired quality of life in PWE. The link between these comorbidities and epilepsy appears to have a neurobiological basis, which is at least partly mediated by stress through psychological and pathophysiological pathways. It is therefore crucial for clinicians to take stress-related conditions and psychiatric comorbidities into account when managing PWE and to propose clinical support to enhance self-control of stress, as stress is a major seizure trigger. Management includes both pharmacological treatment and nonpharmacological methods for enhancing self-management of stress (e.g., mindfulness-based therapies, yoga, cognitive-behavioral therapies, biofeedback), which may not only protect against psychiatric comorbidities but also reduce seizure frequency.

SATYAM-DST PROJECTS

In a DST-SATYAM funded project at the National Institute of Mental Health and Neuro

Sciences (NIMHANS), we have been studying the effect of yoga on people with chronic DRE awaiting epilepsy surgery in a randomized controlled study. In a cohort of 90 subjects, 72 people with mesial temporal lobe epilepsy (MTLE) with mesial temporal sclerosis (MTS) were recruited so far. In the ongoing project, it was hypothesized that yoga and meditation would increase the hippocampal volume and improve memory. People of both gender with in age range of 18–50 were recruited in the project. For people with MTLE and MTS, unilateral anterior temporal lobectomy with amygdalohippocampectomy is the standard of care for cure/control of the seizures. The surgical candidates are identified based upon clinical, multimodality neuroimaging [magnetic resonance imaging (MRI), positron emission tomography (PET)-MRI, and magnetoencephalography (MEG)], video-EEG telemetry, and neuropsychology assessments methods. In this project, clinical, EEG, MRI of the brain, neuropsychology, biochemical as well as autonomic functional evaluation is being carried out 3 months prior to surgery, at the time of surgery, as well as 6 months after the surgery. The following assessments would be carried out as part of the research program and all three time-points' assessments will be compared and studied. Of 72, 36 subjects were randomized to yoga group and 36 in Waitlist group. Of 36, 32 patients underwent 12 supervised yoga therapy sessions and were asked to continue home-based practice for 3 months prior to surgery. A video-guided yoga module DVD was given for home practice. After 3 months of Yoga practice, they were subjected to surgery and postsurgery, 6 days of booster Yoga sessions were carried out and they were asked to continue home-based yoga practice for 6 months. Waitlisted group had treatment as usual. Till date 72 baseline, 60 presurgery and 47 post-6 months of surgery assessments have been completed. Fifty-two people have undergone surgery. Most of the patients practiced yoga one time (preferably in the morning) and some two times (morning and evening) a day. The yoga at home was practiced on an average of 30–90 minutes in their own phase and interest. Out of the 32, 15 people expressed that *Surya namaskar* (sun salutations) was their favorite practice, 14 people liked each and every component of yoga module, four people liked *Pranayama* (regulated breathing practice), *Yoga Nidra* (guided deep relaxation technique), and meditation and the rest did not specify. The reported benefits on practicing the yoga module are alleviation of stress, reduced anger, mental calmness, improvement in memory and gait, reduced seizure episodes, reduced body weight and increased physical activity, energy levels and better quality of sleep. Majority of these subjects are positive about continuing their Yoga sessions at home for long time. In this ongoing research proposal, reduction in seizure frequency and reduction in the duration of episodes have been observed in 25 among the 32 subjects who practiced yoga and meditation regularly (Rao et al., unpublished data). Out of the 32 patients, only three experienced epileptic episodes during the yoga practice. Keeping this in the mind, it is advised to avoid breathing practices such as Kapalabhati, Bhastrika, breath holding, fast breathing practices, and Trataka in flickering light which mimics photic stimulation.

Though an interim analysis showed no statistically significant change in imaging, autonomic, biochemical, and neuropsychological parameters, majority of the patients subjectively felt that surgical outcome and yoga practice helped to improve their education level, job opportunities, quality of life and sleep, family relationships, and connectivity with social life. Five female patients in the project were immensely happy with yoga practice and delivered children uneventfully.

In the second project, as a follow-up, the resected hippocampus from the patients is being utilized for research in neurogenesis by immunohistochemical and electrophysiological studies. To test the impact of yoga and meditation on adult neurogenesis in the hippocampus, in our work at the NIMHANS we are studying the membrane property and excitability of dentate gyrus (DG) neurons by patch-clamp electrophysiology. The electrophysiological characteristics of neurons obtained from newly regenerated and mature DG neurons from MTS individuals with and without yoga are being compared. Research outcomes of both these projects will be available in due course.

BENEFITS OF YOGA IN EPILEPSY

- Complementary treatments help those with epilepsy, both by enhancing quality of life and by decreasing seizure activity.
- Interventions can be integrated into an outpatient clinic, even across cultures, with good results.
- Treatment of epilepsy can be noninvasive and low cost and can be conducted even in the presence of language barriers and cultural differences.

HIGHLIGHTS AND LIMITATIONS

Yoga is considered as one of the "mind-body" approaches. It appears to be an effective method to cope with chronic stress by inducing relaxation. Successful yoga interventions have been reported in stress reduction and depression care. It is hypothesized that yoga practice reduces stress responses through inducing increased PNS and GABA system activity and decreased HPA-axis activity, so that optimal homeostasis is restored. This mechanism could be an explanation of the potential efficacy of yoga practice in seizure frequency and quality of life in the management of refractory epilepsy. Indeed, in one study, yoga practice was associated with reduction of about 50% in seizure frequency and improvement in quality of life.[11] Only a few studies have investigated the effects of yoga in the management of refractory epilepsy and its associated comorbidities. Its practice can be encouraged but with the present lack of outcome research its effectiveness remains to be fully evaluated.

PATIENTS' PERSPECTIVE OF YOGA PRACTICES

Appendix 1.14 *provides a yoga module for epilepsy that we found useful in our clinical practice.* Most of the patients felt practices are easy to learn and follow. Regular and long-term practice helped them to understand the effect of each practice on their mind-body complex. Most of the people liked *Surya namaskar* as it involves all systems of the body and mind. They felt that *Bhramari* is immediately relieving their stress. Relaxation techniques and meditation helped them to overcome their over thinking about the disease. Overall, yoga practice brought the difference in their quality of life and sleep apart from the conventional treatment.

Of all our patients, only three experienced epileptic episodes during the yoga practice. Keeping this in the mind, it is advised to avoid practices which cause hyperventilation and photic stimulation such as *Kapalabhati*, *Bhastrika*, breath holding, fast breathing practices, and *Trataka* in flickering light (which mimic photic stimulation).

PRACTICAL IMPLICATIONS AND LIFESTYLE ADVICE

Irrespective of patients' education levels, yoga has to be taught in a way that patients understand. They have to memorize the name of the practice, how to practice and how not to practice. They should take help from the experienced practitioners. They should know their body limitation well during the practice. Patients are advised home-based practice 1–2 times in a day in own pace. In addition to yoga, lifestyle advice was given such as (1) early to bed and adequate sleep hours; (2) avoid overthinking and stressful conditions; (3) avoid prolonged fasting, overeating and skipping of antiseizure drugs (ASDs); (4) only by practicing yoga regularly in moderate way can bring changes in their health and disease; and (5) encouragement in pursuing education, job, marriage and having children and leading a happy and healthy life.

CONCLUSION

As a result of the COVID-19 pandemic, management of PWE has become more difficult. Anxiety and stress are known factors to precipitate and aggravate epilepsy. Along with antiseizure medication, surgery in selected candidates, lifestyle modifications, PWE will immensely benefit with physical exercise, cognitive stimulation, caloric restriction, intermittent fasting, yoga, and meditation. Physicians and yoga therapists can play a significant role in improving the quality of life of PWE.

CASE VIGNETTE

Ms Kavitha (name changed) experienced first episode of seizure at the age of 3 years. For the first time in her life, it was a big shock and she did not know what to do about it. Her family members took her to a local doctor. She started taking medications without knowing what they were or how they worked. Later on, the seizure episodes continued to occur. She consulted many doctors over the subsequent years. Although various medications were tried, there was no improvement. She was left thinking that there was no solution. That is when she decided to go to a specialist hospital for treatment. She consulted doctors at the NIMHANS and her medicines were adjusted. She continued to have 7–8 seizure episodes in a month in spite of ASDs. She used to get episodes irrespective of place and time of the day and worried about loss of memory, behavioral issues, delayed recalling capacity and understanding capacity. On further tests (MRI and EEG), it was noted that there were minor changes in her brain. Doctors at the NIMHANS advised her to take ASDs and undergo yoga and meditation therapy. She voluntarily agreed and received 3 months of yoga training under the supervision of Yoga experts at the NIMHANS. Initially she was not very hopeful if yoga would help but continued with the practice. After 12 weeks of supervised sessions (1 hour/day 5 days a week), she felt relaxed and calm. Physically, she was energetic, enthusiastic to practice yoga. She continued practicing yoga at home subsequently with the help of a recorded video. At 6 month follow-up, she experienced reduction in the frequency and duration of seizure episodes. She has practicing yoga regularly for last 1.5 years now. Her current seizure frequency has decreased to once in a month. After the yoga practice, she has been more confident of facing any situation and issues in her life. She also felt that her memory has improved. She prefers to continue with her yoga practice as it has immensely benefited her life according to her. She shared her positive experiences with others so that they too may get motivated and derive similar benefits.

	Clinical Insights: Yoga for Epilepsy
Prior to the session	• Be more careful with the patients with higher risk of a possible emergency (such as uncontrolled seizure, status epilepticus or continuous seizure episode, etc.). Assessment of clinical history and diagnosis is mandatory. Appropriate referral must be made in that case. • History of the last seizure episode, frequency of episodes, details of the type of episode (whether generalized tonic-clonic or absence or partial seizures), triggering factors, medications and patient's current cognitive status are to be obtained to avoid any untoward happenings. • Therapists should be careful about the settings for the yoga session. Yoga should not be practiced at a place where safety may be compromised like close to a staircase or a swimming pool, or places containing hard or sharp objects where patients may get hurt. • Expectations from yoga must be discussed with patient and caregivers and realistic goals set.

Contd...

Contd...

Clinical Insights: Yoga for Epilepsy

During the session	• Sleep deprivation and stress are well-known triggers for seizure. Yoga practices should be designed to alleviate those problems. Practices for enhancing sleep quality such as left nostril breathing, humming breath, and "*Om*" chanting should be advised at bedtime. • Practice intensity should be moderate to high based on the capacity of the patient. Better to split yoga sessions into shorter capsules to be practiced two or three times a day rather than a single session lasting an hour or more. • Practices such as Kapalabhati and Bhastrika which involve hyperventilation should be avoided. • Slow breathing practices such as alternate nostril breathing (*nadi shuddhi*) and humming breath (*bhramari*) should be advised with adequate time for relaxation and breath normalization. • Any sudden severe sensory stimulus (e.g., bright light) may precipitate seizure and thus should be avoided. Precaution to be observed while practicing Trataka procedure. • Patients with chronic epilepsy may have cognitive deficits. Instructions should be clear, concise, repeated and unhurried. Patience and empathy are important on the therapist's part. • Patients should be encouraged to memorize the sequence of the practices. The therapist may encourage the patient in doing so, by asking "next steps" after initial supervised training for 10–12 sessions. • Antiepileptics may have different side effects (e.g., sodium valproate causing nausea/sedation). A knowledge of the side effects may enable design practices according to the need of the patient. Specific practices for the alleviation of side effects may be advised if required. • Weight gain is an important side effect of some antiepileptic medications (such as sodium valproate), yoga practices should also thus focus on weight loss (without using above-mentioned contraindicated practices). • Cognitive improvement can be another important goal for yoga intervention. • Assess clinical condition at every session to detect any worsening at the earliest and practices should be modified accordingly. • Group or individual sessions may be conducted as per the therapist's discretion and patient's suitability. • If any acute seizure episode occurs during the yoga session, the therapist should not panic. The patient should be put in a lateral recumbent position in an area where patient's safety is ensured (away from any anticipated danger) and referral to the nearest emergency medical facility should be done at once.
After the session	• The patient and the caregiver should be educated adequately about do's and don'ts of yoga while practicing at home. The plan of further management including follow-ups should be discussed. • Even if the patient has had no seizures in last many years, the therapist should refrain from advising discontinuation of medication. Suggest them to meet the treating neurologist. • Caregivers should be made aware of the possible yoga practice-related triggers so that adequate precautions can be taken at home. • Every follow-up should contain repeat assessments. Supervised sessions may be conducted if required.

REFERENCES

1. Rao M. Addressing the burden of epilepsy in India. Neurol India. 2017;65:S4-5.
2. Rao M. Epilepsy in India: Bridging the treatment gap. Neurol India. 2018;66:1060-1.
3. Saxena VS, Nadkarni VV. Nonpharmacological treatment of epilepsy. Ann Indian Acad Neurol. 2011;14(3):148-52.
4. Santhosh NS, Sinha S, Satishchandra P. Epilepsy: Indian perspective. Ann Indian Acad Neurol. 2014;17(Suppl 1):S3-S11.
5. Gourie-Devi M. Epidemiology of neurological disorders in India: Review of background, prevalence and incidence of epilepsy, stroke, Parkinson's disease and tremors. Neurol India. 2014;62(6):588-98.
6. Rathore C, Rao MB, Radhakrishnan K. National epilepsy surgery program: realistic goals and pragmatic solutions. Neurol India. 2014;62(2):124-9.
7. Petroff OA, Rothman DL, Behar KL, Mattson RH. Low brain GABA level is associated with poor seizure control. Ann Neurol. 1996;40(6):908-11.

8. Streeter CC, Gerbarg PL, Saper RB, Ciraulo DA, Brown RP. Effects of yoga on the autonomic nervous system, gamma-aminobutyric-acid, and allostasis in epilepsy, depression, and post-traumatic stress disorder. Med Hypotheses. 2012;78(5):571-9.
9. Kanhere S, Bagadia D, Phadke V, Mukherjee P. Yoga in children with epilepsy: a randomized controlled trial. J Pediatr Neurosci. 2018;13(4):410-5.
10. Panjwani U, Selvamurthy W, Singh SH, Gupta HL, Thakur L, Rai UC. Effect of Sahaja yoga practice on seizure control and EEG changes in patients of epilepsy. Indian J Med Res. 1996;103:165-72.
11. Rajesh B, Jayachandran D, Mohandas G, Radhakrishnan K. A pilot study of a yoga meditation protocol for patients with medically refractory epilepsy. J Altern Complement Med. 2006;12(4):367-71.
12. Panjwani U, Selvamurthy W, Singh SH, Gupta HL, Mukhopadhyay S, Thakur L. Effect of Sahaja yoga meditation on auditory evoked potentials (AEP) and visual contrast sensitivity (VCS) in epileptics. Appl Psychophysiol Biofeedback. 2000;25(1):1-12.
13. Sirven JI, Drazkowski JF, Zimmerman RS, Bortz JJ, Shulman DL, Macleish M. Complementary/alternative medicine for epilepsy in Arizona. Neurology. 2003;61(4):576-7.
14. Lundgren T, Dahl JA, Yardi N, Melin L. Acceptance and commitment therapy and yoga for drug-refractory epilepsy: a randomized controlled trial. Epilepsy Behav. 2008;13(1):102-8.
15. Panebianco M, Sridharan K, Ramaratnam S. Yoga for epilepsy. Cochrane Database Syst Rev. 2017;10(10):CD001524.
16. Sathyaprabha TN, Satishchandra P, Pradhan C, Sinha S, Kaveri B, Thennarasu K, et al. Modulation of cardiac autonomic balance with adjuvant yoga therapy in patients with refractory epilepsy. Epilepsy Behav. 2008;12(2):245-52.
17. Mishra SK, Singh P, Bunch S, Zhang R. The therapeutic value of yoga in neurological disorders. Ann Indian Acad Neurol. 2012;15(4):247-54.
18. Deepak KK, Manchanda SK, Maheshwari MC. Meditation improves clinicoelectroencephalographic measures in drug-resistant epileptics. Biofeedback Self Regul. 1994;19(1):25-40.
19. Amudhan S, Gururaj G, Satishchandra P. Epilepsy in India I: Epidemiology and public health. Ann Indian Acad Neurol. 2015;18(3):263-77.
20. Streeter CC, Jensen JE, Perlmutter RM, Cabral HJ, Tian H, Terhune DB, et al. Yoga asana sessions increase brain GABA levels: a pilot study. J Altern Complement Med. 2007;13(4):419-26.
21. Desai R, Tailor A, Bhatt T. Effects of yoga on brain waves and structural activation: a review. Complement Ther Clin Pract. 2015;21(2):112-8.
22. Chen KM, Chen MH, Chao HC, Hung HM, Lin HS, Li CH. Sleep quality, depression state, and health status of older adults after silver yoga exercises: cluster randomized trial. Int J Nurs Stud. 2009;46(2):154-63.

SECTION 4

Other Important Aspects of Yoga

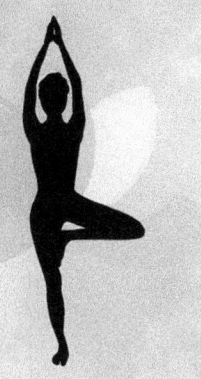

22. **Yoga for Caregivers**
    Aarti Jagannathan, Md Ameer Hamza, Naresh Katla

23. **Yoga and Positive Mental Health**
    Jyotsna Agrawal, Matthijs Cornelissen

24. **Looking Ahead: Tele-Yoga in Mental Health**
    Sanchari Mukhopadhyay, Nishitha Jasti, Venkataram Shivakumar, Aarti Jagannathan

CHAPTER 22

Yoga for Caregivers

Aarti Jagannathan, Md Ameer Hamza, Naresh Katla

INTRODUCTION

Role of the Caregivers

Majority of people with mental disorders in India live with their families,[1,2] and hence their family members become their primary caregivers. We define a caregiver as "A person between 18 and 75 years of age, who is the primary caretaker of the patient at home and who continues to care for the patient even after discharge from hospital".

Caregiving for people with mental disorders can be a chronic stressor and continued long-term care can have emotional and practical bearing on the caregivers. It often increases the caregiver's burden, anxiety, depression and influences their coping. It was noticed that caregivers who were in "high contact" with the patient in their daily life, often faced the highest burden.[3] Continued stress often makes them vulnerable to developing minor psychiatric disorders such as anxiety and depression. Coping with their family members' mental disorder is influenced by factors such as the availability of social support and network, opportunities, and their willingness to join various types of family support services and programs.[4]

Yoga for Caregivers

A number of interventions offered to family members of patients with schizophrenia have been developed with increasing sophistication, effectiveness, and cost-efficiency. Family interventions such as crisis-oriented family therapy, behavior family therapy, family psychoeducation, multiple family group intervention, relatives' groups, family consultation and yoga have shown positive outcomes both for patients and their families.[5-8]

The ultimate aim of the yoga program is to reduce the burden on caregivers either by addressing their needs or by developing a yoga program, which in turn would equip them with the ability and skills to reduce their burden. To achieve this aim, we developed a yoga program for caregivers based on the integrated approach to yoga therapy (IAYT) model developed by Swami Vivekananda Yoga Anusandhana Samasthana.[9] This model incorporated the "Self-Management of Excessive Tension (SMET)/Cyclic meditation" approach which helped to reduce burden and improve coping among the caregivers.

MECHANISM OF IAYT FOR CAREGIVERS

The main principle of IAYT is that "the root of all psychosocial problems is in the mind which causes imbalance or stress".[9] Excessive speed and demanding situations at the mental and physical levels *(Annamaya kosha* and *Pranamaya kosha)*, upsurges caused by strong likes and dislikes at emotional level *(Manomaya kosha)* and conflicts, egocentric behavior at the psychological level *(Vijnanamaya kosha)* are responsible for imbalances found at gross levels. IAYT through "successive stimulation-relaxation helps break the loop of uncontrolled speed of thoughts (stress)", "gains control over the mind", and harmonizes the disturbances at each of the five levels (*Panchakosha*) to tackle psychosomatic problems.[10]

Based on IAYT, yogic practices adopted to tackle psychosomatic problems at each level[11] that were used in the current study are detailed here.

Annamaya Kosha Practices

- *Asana*: A stable and comfortable posture, which gives deep relaxation to internal organs. All organs of the body start functioning in a harmonious manner and the mind becomes tranquil.
- *Diet*: Sattvic diet is recommended as it helps to maintain internal harmony in the body as well as mind.
- *Loosening exercises*: Loosens the joints and muscles of the body, and improves range of motion for performing postures effectively.

Pranamaya Kosha Practices

- *Breathing exercises*: Increases awareness about breathing and stimulates the autonomous nervous system.[12,13]
- *Pranayama*: Cleanses the lungs, corrects breathing, increases lung capacity, and slows down the breathing rate thereby calming and balancing the mind.[14]

Manomaya Kosha Practices

- *Cyclic meditation*: Practices with repeated stimulations and relaxation.
- Om meditation and chanting for creating awareness and slowing down self.
- *Devotional sessions*: Discussion on "*Bhakti yoga*" and science of emotional culture.

Vijnanamaya Kosha Practices

- Counseling/Lectures/Sharing of personal experience
- Satsanga

REVIEW OF LITERATURE

- Based on caregivers' need, literature review and expert opinion, a 10-day group yoga program was initially developed using the qualitative inductive method of inquiry. Each day's program included warm-up exercises, *yogic asanas*, *pranayama*, and *satsanga*. The yoga program was developed with the aim of reducing burden and improving coping of family caregivers of inpatients with schizophrenia in India.[15]
- In a randomized controlled study, caregivers of inpatients with schizophrenia were provided a yoga intervention. It was noticed that irrespective of the intervention, with reduction in patient symptoms, burden on caregivers also reduced leading to a plateau effect. It has to be noted that the yoga intervention was only provided for a period of 7 days, which experts in the field of yoga feel insufficient.[16]
- In another controlled study, it was noted that caregivers of outpatients with psychosis were able to learn and retain yoga practices for a period of 1 month leading to reduced burden and improved quality of life. However, a large proportion of caregivers were unable to enroll and adhere to the study protocol due to inability to attend yoga sessions which were provided at a geographically distant location from their homes.[17]
- A randomized controlled trial was conducted to study the effect of yoga therapy on anxiety and depressive symptoms, and quality of life among caregivers of inpatients with neurological disorders at a tertiary medical care center in India. Results showed significant reduction in anxiety and depression, and improved quality of life in the yoga group as compared with the control group ($p < 0.001$).[18]
- Gandhi et al. studied the effectiveness of caregivers' yoga module on psychological distress and mental well-being among caregivers of patients admitted to neuro-rehabilitation wards at NIMHANS. Findings showed that caregivers in the yoga group had reduced psychological distress and better mental well-being at the end of 1 month of yoga training.[19]

- The earlier-developed yoga program for caregivers of schizophrenia was remodeled into an audio-visual self-help manual format in three languages. Paired sample t-tests showed that at the end of 1 month, there was significant decrease in the burden on the caregivers who practiced the self-help manual as compared to the care as usual group. Caregivers who practiced yoga at home maintained an average of 50% attendance and "very well" level of yoga performance.[20]
- *Yoga module for caregivers*: A validated yoga module for caregivers of schizophrenia has been provided in **Appendix 1.15** at the end of the book. (The Yoga for Caregivers manual can be accessed at: https://nimhansyoga.in/books/)

IMPORTANT INSTRUCTIONS WHILE DOING PRACTICE

- This program is specially designed for caregivers. Persons with mental illness and physical ailments need to consult their yoga therapist before carrying out these practices.
- Do not push your body forcefully to attain the perfect pose.
- Do only what you can and do not compare your practices with anybody.
- Be aware of what you are doing and always pay attention to your breath.
- Be witness to the positive changes after practice of yoga.
- Surrender to the instruction of the instructor.

CONCLUSION

Yoga for caregivers of persons with mental and neurological disorders is observed to have qualitatively and quantitatively positive effects in improving well-being of caregivers. Yoga can be used as an effective intervention in the community for caregivers based on their adherence to yoga and its possible adoption as a lifestyle.

CASE VIGNETTES

Case 1

Mr X, a 60-year-old male farmer, caregiver of a patient with mental disorder, was referred to the NIMHANS Integrated Centre for Yoga (NICY), Bengaluru, for management of stress. He had a history of stress, headaches, and sleeping problems, as he was the sole caregiver of his wife who had been suffering from schizophrenia for the past 5 years. Mr X had the responsibility of taking care of the household, caring for the children, and earning an income for the family. Caregiving for his wife increased his stress levels, he often felt alone, burdened, and depressed, and had psychosomatic health issues. The expert doctor at the NICY taught him the caregivers' yoga module, which focused mainly on breathing exercises, loosening practices, cyclic meditation, Pranayama, and chanting. After each practice session, Mr X reported feeling calm and light in his head. He especially mentioned that the cyclic meditation techniques made him feel as relaxed as when he would get up after a good night's sleep.

Case 2

A 40-year-old lady caregiver of a patient suffering from epilepsy was referred to the NICY, Bengaluru, for management of her anxiety. She had a history of stress and anxiety about the future of her daughter's life as she had no support from her husband. She also suffered from knee pain and back pain. The NICY Yoga expert provided the caregivers' yoga module, with special emphasis on the caregivers' physical complaints design. The yoga module consisted of loosening practices, especially yogic sukshma vyayama (janu shakti vikasaka, anguli shakti vikasaka, and kati shakti vikasaka), breathing techniques, cyclic meditation, pranayama, chanting, and yogic counseling (jnana yoga—what do and what not do). After the Yoga session, the caregiver reported feeling less pain in her back and knee joints, and experienced peace of mind and complete silence. Of all the practices taught to her, she liked the deep relaxation technique part of cyclic meditation and yogic counseling the best.

CAREGIVERS' FEEDBACK

- "It is a very good initiative with easy and effective yoga techniques" (C1, 26 years, Female).
- "It helped relieve stress and tension, and made me feel healthy to take care of my patient" (C2, 55 years, Male).
- "I felt calm-peace of mind and had relief" (C3, 20 years, Male).
- "This program is very good. It totally relaxed me gave me more peace of mind" (C5, 42 years, Female).

REFERENCES

1. Thara R, Padmavati R, Kumar S, Srinivasan L. Burden assessment schedule: instrument to assess burden on caregivers of chronic mentally ill. Indian J Psychiatry. 199;40(1):21-9.
2. Murthy RS. Mental Health by the People. Bengaluru: Peoples Action for Mental Health; 2006. p. 335.
3. Winefield HR, Harvey EJ. Needs of family caregivers in chronic schizophrenia. Schizophr Bull. 1994;20(3):557-66.
4. Solomon P, Draine J. Examination of adaptive coping among individuals with a serious mentally ill relative. Unpublished paper, Philadelphia, Pennsylvania: Hanerman University, Department of Psychiatry and Mental Health Science. 1994.
5. Pekkala E, Merinder L. Psychoeducation for schizophrenia. Cochrane Database Syst Rev. 2002;(2):CD002831.
6. Barbato A, D'Avanzo B. Family interventions in schizophrenia and related disorders: a critical review of clinical trials. Acta Psychiatrica Scandinavica. 2000;102:81-97.
7. Leff J. Family work for schizophrenia: practical application. Acta Psychiatr Scand Suppl. 2000;(407):78-82.
8. Shinde SP. Short term effects of family psychoeducation in schizophrenia [PHD thesis]. Bengaluru: National Institute of Mental Health and Neurosciences; 2005.
9. Nagendra H, Nagarathana R. New Perspectives in Stress Management. Bengaluru: Swami Vivekananda Yoga Prakashana; 2010.
10. Krishnamoorthy. Concept of anxiety according to ancient Indian scriptures. Bengaluru: SYASA; 2007.
11. Nagarathna R, Nagendra HR. Combined Approach of Yoga Therapy for Positive Health. Bengaluru: Swami Vivekananda Yoga Prakashana; 2004.
12. Telles S, Nagarathna R, Nagendra HR. Breathing through a particular nostril can alter metabolism and autonomic activities. Indian J Physiol Pharmacol. 1994;38:133-7.
13. Raghuraj P, Telles S. Immediate effect of specific nostril manipulating yoga breathing practices on autonomic and respiratory variables. Appl Psychophysiol Biofeedback. 2008;33(2):65-75.
14. Muktibodhananda S. Hatha Yoga Pradipika. Munger, Bihar, India: Yoga Publications Trust; 2012. [online] Available from: http://buddhism.lib.ntu.edu.tw/BDLM/toModule.do?prefix=/search&page=/search_detail.jsp?seq=133882 [Last accessed October, 2020].
15. Jagannathan A, Thirthalli J, Nagarathna R, Hamza A, Nagendra H, Gangadhar B. Development and feasibility of need-based yoga program for family caregivers of in-patients with schizophrenia in India. Int J Yoga. 2012;5(1):42-7.
16. Jagannathan A, Hamza A, Thirthahalli J, Nagaendra HR, Kare M, Yadav M, et al. Efficacy of yoga and psychosocial training programme for caregivers of person with schizophrenia. Natl J Prof Soc Work. 2012;13(1-2):3-15.
17. Varambally S, Vidyendaran S, Sajjanar M, Thirthalli J, Hamza A, Nagendra HR. Yoga-based intervention for caregivers of outpatients with psychosis: a randomized controlled pilot study. Asian J Psychiatr. 2013;6(2):141-5.
18. Umadevi P, Ramachandra S, Varambally S, Philip M, Gangadhar BN. Effect of yoga therapy on anxiety and depressive symptoms and quality-of-life among caregivers of in-patients with neurological disorders at a tertiary care center in India: a randomized controlled trial. Indian J Psychiatry. 2013;55(Suppl 3):S385-9.
19. Gandhi S, Palled VK, Sahu M, Jagannathan A, Khanna M, Jose A. Effectiveness of caregivers' yoga module on psychological distress and mental well-being among caregivers of patients admitted to neurological rehabilitation wards of a tertiary care institute, Bengaluru, Karnataka, India. J Neurosci Rural Pract. 2019;10:657-65.
20. Hamza A, Jagannathan A, Hegde S, Katla N, U Bhide SR, Thirthallli J, et al. Development and testing of an audio-visual self-help yoga manual for Indian caregivers of persons with schizophrenia living in the community: a single-blind randomized controlled trial. Int J Yoga. 2020;13(1):62-9.

CHAPTER 23

Yoga and Positive Mental Health

Jyotsna Agrawal, Matthijs Cornelissen

INTRODUCTION

Although the definition of mental health includes positive mental health (PMH) and well-being,[1] its promotion requires consistent focused action, which has been missing over the years. This is especially unfortunate since promotion of PMH can benefit people anywhere on the mental health continuum, whether not at risk, at-risk, suffering, or recovering from mental health problems.[2] The limited resources which have been spent on mental health promotion in India have often been on programs originating in a Western culture, which are not always appropriate in an Indian context, due to low cultural and ecological validity. Since India has a rich philosophical-psychological heritage of its own, it would be apt to develop indigenous PMH programs. Apart from social structures like the extended family system as center of community support, one can think of the Yogic tradition, which has been honed and perfected in India over many centuries and which offers a rich source of psychological knowledge and know-how suitable for this purpose.

Current yoga research focuses predominantly on *asanas* (physical postures), *pranayama* (breathing practices) and brief meditation courses, and it looks at these either from within a physicalist-objective or a social-constructionist conceptualization of knowledge and reality. As a result, it misses out on what is most valuable in what the various yoga traditions can contribute to modernity.[3] The Indian civilization with its millennia-old focus on consciousness and inner development has a sophisticated and more integral understanding of reality and the human mind than modern science with its more limited focus on the physical and social domains. So, if we really want to know what the various yoga traditions can contribute to psychology, PMH and society in general, we must first study the various yoga traditions on their own terms and familiarize ourselves with the basic understanding of reality and knowledge that gave rise to them.

BASIC UNDERSTANDING OF REALITY BEHIND YOGA PRACTICE

There are many entirely different ways of "doing yoga" and so one may wonder where to start, but there is a way in which these different systems have been classified traditionally that leads to familiar terrain for psychologists. It is the *trimarga*, the three "paths" of *bhakti*, *jñāna*, and *karma yoga*, the yoga of devotion, knowledge and work, which is closely related to the division modern psychologists make between emotions, cognition and volition. Before we can go into the contributions yoga can make in these three specific areas, it may be useful to have a quick look at how the conception of reality that forms the basis of almost all systems of Indian thought differs from that of modern science.

In science, and in the new global civilization as a whole, it has become mainstream to look at the world as if it were primarily physical, with consciousness arising out of the complexity of the physical brain as if it were some kind of evolutionary afterthought. Though we tend to take this view of reality for granted, it is not only one-sided, but even in the West actually a rather recent development. The vast majority of well-known Western philosophers held that the universe was permeated with consciousness ("panpsychism" in European philosophy). In Indian thought, the modern, physicalist conception of reality is mainly mentioned as a beginners' error (*Chāndogyopaniṣhad,* viii, 8-12). Most major systems of yoga take the centrality of consciousness for granted, doubt the relevance if not the reality of the physical world, and have as their ultimate objective to achieve some aspect of pure consciousness: *kaivalya, mukti,* or *nirvaṇa.*[4,5]

It is crucial to keep all this in mind when we try to use practices from these ancient Indian systems within the modern materialistic setting. If we gloss over these basic differences, serious conceptual confusion is bound to arise. On the other hand, if we manage to find the right way to integrate the two ways of looking at reality, we may arrive at a deep and effective understanding of what it actually is in yoga that helps in curative, preventive, and positive approaches to mental health. In addition, we may find a more integral understanding of reality as a whole that goes at least in some respects beyond what either approach can offer on its own.

ESSENTIAL CORE OF WHAT BHAKTI, JÑĀNA AND KARMA YOGA CAN CONTRIBUTE TO PSYCHOLOGY

Bhakti yoga: The path of *bhakti* is centered around love for the Divine and ultimately leads to *ananda,* pure bliss, whether experienced as a bliss of union or a bliss of oneness. There is no upper limit to the intensity of this joy other than the bearing capacity of the practitioner, and as it appears to be independent of circumstances and the path followed, the Indian tradition came to the conclusion that *ananda* is one of the essential qualities of reality itself. Though it is hard—and as a consequence rare—for people to arrive at a state in which the higher intensities of inner joy are entirely uninterrupted and independent of circumstances, every step on the way helps the seeker to get closer to this ideal. As the unconditional nature of the happiness removes the urgency of personal, egoistic satisfaction, progress in this dimension facilitates more "objective", less biased observation, as well as action which is in harmony with the interests of the whole. This not only helps in the other two paths, but provides a major support for any effort at therapy and self-development and enhances personal qualities that are invaluable for all those working and doing research in the field of mental health.

Jñāna yoga: The processes and end result of the yoga of knowledge are in appearance quite different but in essence the same. While in *bhakti yoga,* "the Divine" is generally—though not always—experienced in a personal form, in *jñāna yoga* it is generally—though again not always—conceptualized in a more abstract manner, for example, as the consciousness which has manifested the world out of itself. When one realizes this consciousness in its absolute purity, whether transcendent, beyond the manifest world, or cosmically, as a "secret ingredient" pervasive throughout every part of the creation, one realizes, just like in *bhakti yoga,* that in the end all is well, and that there is nothing personal to gain or to lose. This, once again, not only helps one to move happily and unperturbed through all the vicissitudes of life, but it also allows an unbiased and "objective" vision of subjective realities, and especially of consciousness and all that happens inside of it. It may be clear how valuable this could be for the in-depth study of psychological processes.

Karma yoga: The third path, *karma yoga*, is by some authorities (e.g. Shankara and Patañjali) looked at only as a crucial preparation during the early stages of the specific path they advocate. In the *Bhagavad Gītā* (and in modern times in the work of Sri Aurobindo) it is, however, honored as a path in itself that can lead to *sādharmyamukti*, "the acquisition of the divine nature by the transformation of this lower being into the human image of the divine".[6] Though one could argue that absolute perfection on this path is not humanly feasible, any progress in this direction will clearly be useful for anyone interested in Maslow's "self-actualization" and for PMH in general.

A WORD OF CAUTION: THE NEED FOR THERAPISTS TO HAVE THEIR OWN YOGA PRACTICE

It may be clear, even from this nano-overview of the three paths of *bhakti, jñāna*, and *karma yoga*, that the differences between yoga and modern society in terms of their basic outlook on life and the possibilities for human growth and development are considerable. The Indian tradition goes far beyond what even the most positive of modern psychologies would dare to aim at, and, if used well, this may lead to as yet unprecedented progress both in theoretical as well as applied psychology, but there are also considerable dangers. The mood disorders, delusions and self-aggrandizement that can follow from misguided efforts on any of these paths are well-known. These risks make it essential for counselors and therapists to be well grounded in their own path of yoga before they use it with their clients. This may seem an unreasonable demand that could postpone the use of yoga-based therapies far into the future, but we hope a time will come when people may look at psychology without an understanding of yogic principles as we now would look at physics without mathematics.

YOGA AND POSITIVE MENTAL HEALTH

After this brief overview of the yogic *trimarga*, we can proceed with a few pointers for PMH based on the psychological aspects covered by them, i.e., emotion, cognition, and intentional action, which, as we already saw, are not watertight compartments but closely interwoven in human nature. Empirical studies based on psychological aspects of the yoga tradition have reported positive outcomes for mental health.[7,8] Two widely considered core yoga texts, the *Bhagavad Gītā* and Patañjali's *Yoga Sūtras* give a foundation upon which many new PMH modules can be developed and tested.

Emotion: Happiness is an important emotion linked with PMH. As mentioned earlier, the yogic pathway of *bhakti* emphasizes the *ananda* of a liberated person. Apart from this, the *Bhagavad Gītā* has differentiated between three common varieties of *sukha* on the basis of the *triguṇa*, the three principle strands of nature, in a descending order of psychological health. *Sattvic sukha* is the result of a healthier living approach, taking the good path (*śreyas*) of values, of developing one's potentials and working for social and universal well-being. It requires self-discipline and giving up of egocentric pleasures, and therefore may be difficult initially, but it has beneficial results in terms of long-lasting, calm happiness, and it may take one closer to *ānanda* (*Bhagavad Gītā; Kaṭhopaniṣhad*).[9] On the other hand, *rajasic* and *tamasic sukha* are based on desire fulfillment and maximization of pleasure by taking the pleasant path (*preyas*)[10,11] leading to short term happiness, and suffering in the medium to long term. These ideas are also in consonance with the Greek ideas of eudemonic (Aristotle, Nicomachean Ethics, 1985) versus hedonistic approaches (Aristippus, 4th century) to happiness from which modern positive psychology has borrowed heavily, and which have been supported empirically in modern times.[12]

Cultivation of other-directed positive emotions and attitudes such as *maitri* (friendliness, loving kindness), *karuṇa* (compassion), *mudita* (appreciative, sympathetic joy) and *upekṣhā* (equanimity), collectively known as *Brahmavihara*, are similarly important for PMH. In the yogic traditions, there is a sense of the inherent oneness of all beings, interconnected and emerging as we are from the same original divine consciousness. From this perspective one can cultivate feelings of friendliness for all beings, along with softness (*mārdava*), straightforwardness (*ārjava*), non-hurting and nonviolence (*ahiṃsā*). Further, on the foundation of *maitri*, one needs to develop *mudita*, an ability to be happy for other's well-being while overcoming jealousy; *karuṇa* for someone who is suffering along with kindness (*daya*) and giving (*dāna*); and *upekṣhā* along with forgiveness (*kṣēma*) for the ones whom one may consider as difficult (*Bhagavad Gītā*; Patañjali's *Yoga Sūtras*).

Cognition: Clear perception of reality, without the interplay of cognitive errors is important for mental health, therapy, as well as research. The Vedantic perspective of reality as discussed in the beginning, is based on the idea that the entire universe is permeated with consciousness. Before one has direct perception of that, one can try to work on diminishing the separative ego-sense along with concomitant cognitive errors, as per the yogic perspective.

One such important error is that of attachment (*asakti*, or *raga*), discussed both in the *Bhagavad Gītā* and in Patañjali's *Yoga Sūtras*. To find freedom, one needs to contemplate (*manana, nidhidhyāsana*) on the idea that material things are temporary and they may not be as important as we may tend to treat them in our priority list. Whatever we consider as "good" has its limitations and what we consider as "not good" has its strengths. One can try to develop nonattachment and equality of ideas by trying to find something useful in all events and ideas (Sri Aurobindo).[13] Some amount of desirelessness can also lead to growth in equality (*samatā*). Sri Aurobindo has differentiated this equality into passive and active types, which may start from tolerance (*titikṣhā*), go on to an active acceptance and appreciation, and culminate in a complete surrender (*nati*).[13] There are also ideas in the *Bhagavad Gītā*, which overlap with modern definitions of wisdom such as rich knowledge about life, emotional regulation, insight, and a focus on the common good.[14] Cultivating such qualities may cumulatively contribute to PMH.

Intentional action: Goals and related activities constitute a large part of human life; however, the way people approach them can lead to a variety of problems, from excessive worry about the outcome, to performance-related anxiety, to disappointment or boredom. Instead of withdrawal from all actions to avoid such psychological difficulties, the *Gītā* has given the option of *Karma yoga*, which is a healthier process of engaging in intentional actions. It has multiple aspects from: (1) selection of goals, not for materialistic benefits but for inner perfection or larger social well-being; (2) initially not clinging to preferred outcomes and later, as one develops, not clinging to the process of action itself; (3) treating all outcomes and then all moments, good and bad, with a sense of equality; and (4) offering all one's work to the highest consciousness, the Divine or the wisdom and optimal order inherent in things.[9] We may notice that the connection between *karma yoga/niṣhkāma karma* and *samatā* is a mutually interactive relationship, since desirelessness can lead to equality, while on the other hand seeing all outcomes with equal-mindedness can lead to desirelessness.

However, another note of caution is required here, so that nonattachment and equanimity do not lead to a *tamasic* withdrawal from all action, where the desire is present to avoid all actions. If understood correctly, nonattachment gives up desire but not action, and equality involves treating all situations without personal preference. This will not lead to an unhappy life since one finds a greater happiness within, irrespective of the external rewards and deprivations.

Similar to character strengths as studied in positive psychology, the *Bhagavad Gītā* and Patañjali's *Yoga Sūtras* have emphasized cultivation of positive traits which may contribute to PMH. In the *Gītā*, these traits range from nonattachment, perseverance, nonviolence and nongreed to modesty, stability, forgiveness, fearlessness, self-control, etc. Similarly, Patañjali's Yoga Sūtras have given a set of five *yamas* to be cultivated as the first step in yoga, such as practicing non-violence (*ahiṃsā*), truthfulness (*satya*), non-stealing (*asteya*), non-possessiveness (*aparigraha*), and restraint (*brahmacharya*). Self-control is one of the most emphasized traits, to the point where the entire *"aṣṭāṅgayoga"* of Patañjali has been considered as an integrated program of self-regulation, bringing together top-down and bottom-up pathways.[15-17] These positive qualities are easily tied within the model of *triguṇa*, whereby they generally belong to the *sattvic* meta-trait (of light and harmony), which is related to better mental health.[18,19]

How to Develop These Qualities?

The qualities related to PMH we have discussed so far, are in the yogic literature sometimes mentioned as outer changes that will bring about a desirable inner change, and sometimes as the spontaneous outer result of what begins as an inner realization. We have suggested some broad attitudinal changes and inner gestures that can help with their development here.

1. The first step on the path is wanting something different, an aspiration to grow from one's present stage of development.
2. In this aspiration, one will need to bring together all the different voices within oneself, resolve any lingering conflict or divided sincerity, remove mental or emotional barriers, and finally make it a deep commitment (*sankalpa*).
3. The next step is to keep reminding oneself of one's commitment (*smṛti*) and go on practicing (*abhyāsa*), without worrying much about immediate outcomes.
4. One may require a feedback loop by regular self-observation and reflection to remove immediate or distant barriers to the path and not to give in to undesirable impulses (*śuddhi*).
5. Cultivating the discipline of attention, of speech and of mind is another helpful step. Being able to hold attention on something is necessary in daily life and the Aṣṭāṅga yoga of Patañjali emphasizes this training in terms of *pratyahara* (bringing one's attention back to the present moment); *dhāraṇā* (holding it on an object of attention) and *dhyāna* (continuous flow of unbreakable attention). This also has been discussed in terms of a constant remembrance (*smṛti*) of one's original nature and/or the Divine. Further, one is expected to have discipline of speech.
6. Finally, having a deep faith in divine guidance (*śraddhā*), along with surrender to Divine will (the *Īśhvarapraṇidhāna* in Patañjali's *Yoga Sūtras*), and active offering of one's actions and experiences (*Gītā*) is a required component for progress on the path. It can have two ongoing processes, of accepting everything as a blessing (*prasad buddhi*) and offering everything (*arpan buddhi*).

■ CONCLUSION

To conclude, we would like to stress once more the desirability of a deeper theoretical as well as practical understanding of yoga among mental health professionals. If the practice of yoga can make a major contribution to PMH, then it makes sense to promote yoga education first among those working in the field. There are several reasons why this should be considered a public mental health priority. The first is simple: one cannot teach yoga, or even convincingly advocate its practice, unless one has made at least some progress on one's own path first. The second is that given the large influence therapist-variables have on the outcome of therapy and counseling,[20,21] any positive influence of yoga on mental health professionals should logically multiply in the population they serve. As such, it should prove cost-effective in the long run. The third is an area that is as yet only beginning to receive the attention it deserves. The emotional detachment and mental clarity that yoga engenders, together with the attention to minute inner movements and gestures which the practice of yoga demands, provide an excellent training ground for anyone who wants to get a deeper understanding of how the human mind actually works. This is not only invaluable for psychotherapists, counselors and others in the helping professions, but potentially even more so for researchers in psychology and other human sciences. The qualities that according to the tradition are promoted by the practice of yoga come strikingly close to those that are needed for good qualitative research in the field of psychology.[22]

Though the increasing appreciation of yoga in the treatment of mental health problems is without the slightest doubt a positive development, we should not forget that in the culture of origin, it developed not only to cope with suffering, but also to go beyond humanity's normal capacities.[23] In the words of the *Bṛhadāraṇyaka Upaniṣad* (1.3.28), it aims to develop in us an inalienable, unconditional happiness, an absolutely perfect knowledge, and a direct realization of the immortality of our soul.

REFERENCES

1. World Health Organization. The World health report 2001: mental health: new understanding, new hope. World Health Organization; 2001. p. 208.
2. World Health Organization. World report on knowledge for better health: strengthening health systems. World Health Organization; 2004. p. 162.
3. Varambally S, Gangadhar BN. Current status of yoga in mental health services. Int Rev Psychiatry. 2016;28(3):233-5.
4. Kuppuswamy B. Elements of Ancient Indian Psychology. New Delhi: Vikas Publishing House; 1985.
5. Rao KR. Scope and substance of India psychology. In: Rao KR, Marwaha SB (Eds). Towards a Spiritual Psychology: Essays on Indian Psychology. New Delhi: Samvad India Foundation; 2005.
6. Aurobindo S. The Life Divine. Pondicherry: Sri Aurobindo Ashram Publication Dept.; 2005.
7. Meissner M, Cantell MH, Steiner R, Sanchez X. Evaluating emotional well-being after a short-term traditional yoga practice approach in yoga practitioners with an existing western-type yoga practice. Evid Based Complement Altern Med. 2016;7216982.
8. Dabas P, Singh A. Bhagavad Gita teachings and positive psychology: efficacy for semi-urban Indian students of NCR. Cogent Psychol. 2018;5:1467255.
9. Aurobindo S. Essays on the Gita. Pondicherry: Sri Aurobindo Ashram Publication Dept.; 1997.
10. Salagame KK. Psychology of Meditation: A Contextual Approach. New Delhi: Concept Publishing Company; 2002.
11. Mishra S. Two Paths: Shreyas and Preyas. 2018. [online] Available from: http://bhagavadgita.org.in/Blogs/5ab0b9b75369ed21c4c74c01 [Last accessed October, 2020].
12. Agrawal J. Ananda and Sukha: Indian Model of Happiness and Its Mental Health Implications. 2020. [online] Available from: https://doi.org/10.31231/osf.io/g6msr [Last accessed October, 2020].
13. Banerji D. Seven Quartets of Becoming: A Transformative Yoga Psychology Based on the Diaries of Sri Aurobindo. LA, USA: Nalanda International; 2016.
14. Jeste DV, Vahia IV. Comparison of the conceptualization of wisdom in ancient Indian literature with modern views: focus on the Bhagavad Gita. Psychiatry. 2008;71(3):197-209.
15. Gard T, Noggle JJ, Park CL, Vago DR, Wilson A. Potential self-regulatory mechanisms of yoga for psychological health. Front Hum Neurosci. 2014;8:770.
16. Schmalzl L, Powers C, Blom EH. Neurophysiological and neurocognitive mechanisms underlying the effects of yoga-based practices: towards a comprehensive theoretical framework. Front Hum Neurosci. 2015;9:235.
17. Pascoe MC, Bauer IE. A systematic review of randomized control trials on the effects of yoga

on stress measures and mood. J Psychiatr Res. 2015;68:270-82.
18. Sharma MP, Salvi D, Sharma MK. Sattva, rajas and tamas factors and quality of life in patients with anxiety disorders: a preliminary investigation. Psychological Studies. 2012;57:388-91.
19. Chandana N, Agrawal J, Sharma MP, Murthy P. Triguna, anasakti, personality, and subjective well-being: a comparison of healthy males with males having alcohol dependence (MPhil dissertation). Bengaluru: NIMHANS; 2018.
20. Stubbs JP, Bozarth JD. The dodo bird revisited: a qualitative study of psychotherapy efficacy research. Appl Prev Psychol. 1994;3(2):109-20.
21. Norcross JC, Lambert MJ. Psychotherapy relationships that work II. Psychotherapy. 2011;48(1):4-8.
22. Petitmengin-Peugeot C. The intuitive experience. In: Varela FJ, Shear J (Eds). The View from Within: First-person Approaches to the Study of Consciousness. London: Imprint Academic; 1999. pp. 43-77.
23. Braud W. Integrating yoga epistemology and ontology into an expanded integral approach to research. In: Cornelissen M, Misra G, Varma S (Eds). Foundations of Indian Psychology. New Delhi: Pearson; 2010.

CHAPTER 24

Looking Ahead: Tele-Yoga in Mental Health

Sanchari Mukhopadhyay, Nishitha Jasti, Venkataram Shivakumar, Aarti Jagannathan

YOGA AND MENTAL HEALTH

Yoga has emerged as an important adjunctive treatment modality in a number of medical, psychiatric, and neurological illnesses. In the last three to four decades, there has been an increased scientific interest in yoga. Research in this area has generated evidence in favor of its benefit in improving mental health and in managing psychiatric illnesses such as depression, anxiety disorders, bipolar disorder, schizophrenia, obsessive compulsive disorder, alcohol dependence, childhood disorders like attention-deficit/hyperactivity disorder (ADHD), etc.[1,2] Yoga increases awareness, acceptance, adaptability, and attention and has a calming effect.[3] Yogic practices are shown to have certain neurobiological effects which include the reductions in proinflammatory markers, sympathetic overdrive, levels of serum cortisol and adrenocorticotropic hormone (ACTH), and enhancement in gamma-aminobutyric acid (GABA), neurotrophic factors such as brain-derived neurotrophic factor (BDNF), neurophysiological markers like P300 amplitude.[1,4] Effect of yoga on depressive disorders has been extensively studied. It is found to be useful as an add-on treatment and also as a stand-alone one.[1,5] Clinical trials have confirmed the beneficial effect of yoga in anxiety.[6,7] In schizophrenia, it has been proved as an effective adjunct treatment with benefits in areas of general psychopathology, positive and negative symptoms, quality of life and social cognition.[1] Randomized controlled trials (RCTs) affirmed the effect of Kundalini yoga on obsessive compulsive disorder, alongside antiobsessive medication.[8,9] While there is sufficient evidence for integrated yoga therapy in mood, anxiety, and psychotic disorders,[6,7] preliminary evidence exists for most of the other illnesses including somatoform disorders, autism, ADHD, alcohol and opioid dependence.[4,10]

However, there are several barriers that prevent easy access to yoga therapy for patients with both physical and mental health conditions. For example, an article by Baspure et al.[11] enumerates several of these barriers in patients with schizophrenia, the primary one being the need to come frequently to hospitals or yoga centers located in cities for prolonged periods of time. This is in spite of the fact that most patients with schizophrenia felt that yoga could help them and wanted to attend the yoga sessions.[12] These barriers become even more critical in crisis situations such as the current one caused by coronavirus disease 2019 (COVID-19). One of the methods of reaching yoga to patients who really need it is tele-yoga.

WHAT IS TELE-YOGA?

Telemedicine and telehealth are upcoming concepts to facilitate accessibility of health care across the world.[13] The Institute of Medicine defined "Telemedicine" as "the use of electronic information and communications technologies to provide and support health care when distance separates participants (1996)".[14] The American Telemedicine Association, in 2012, distinguished telemedicine and telehealth stating that the former is sometimes associated with direct patient clinical services and the latter with a broader definition of remote health care services.[15]

The Ministry of Health and Family Welfare, Government of India released telemedicine practice guidelines in March, 2020. Here too, telehealth is defined as a broader concept of health care including medical care, information, education and self-care by telecommunication and digital communication.[16]

With the advent of digital platforms for several aspects of medical care, a similar approach for yoga therapy is also required. In the advisory released by the Ministry of Ayurveda, Yoga and Naturopathy, Unani, Siddha and Homoeopathy (AYUSH), Government of India in July, 2020, tele-yoga has been defined as delivery of yoga practices including yoga postures (*asanas*), breathing practices (*pranayamas*), meditation, relaxation techniques, and counseling through virtual video platforms for therapeutic purpose.[17]

Yoga therapy involves physical postures and breathing exercises which require keen supervision and training. This might be difficult to achieve through tele-yoga. However, there is evidence for the efficacy and acceptability of tele-physiotherapy, which also requires in-person supervision and training. In fact, tele-physiotherapy has been shown to provide equivalent benefit as compared to the physical sessions.[18] Psychotherapy via tele-mode was evaluated and found to have good results in terms of benefit and acceptance. Although these studies have demonstrated good acceptance and benefits similar to in-person sessions, the challenges associated with tele-therapy need further systematic evaluation.[18,19]

Tele-yoga is a bottom-up approach like telemedicine which can help a substantial section of the population access this specialized service beyond the geographical barriers. Access to quality care which is also cost-effective can be achieved through this approach. To bring health care to people on a large scale, tele-yoga can be an effective mode.[20]

In this chapter, we aim to provide a brief overview of research on tele-yoga in general and mental illnesses, its feasibility, acceptance and reported benefits. In addition, this chapter also aims at presenting some recommendations related to tele-yoga services for mental health.

■ OVERVIEW OF AVAILABLE RESEARCH ON TELE-YOGA: BENEFITS AND FEASIBILITY

Over the past few years, tele-yoga has been studied for different conditions such as chronic pain, cardiac illnesses, respiratory problems, depressive disorders, post-traumatic stress disorder (PTSD) and general stress management, where its feasibility, acceptability, and benefits have been studied. Most of the studies on tele-yoga have focused on medical disorders and psychological symptoms secondary to a medical problem or stressors. There are very few systematic studies in the area of tele-yoga for mental health conditions systematically. We would like to discuss a few relevant studies to ascertain the beneficial effects of tele-yoga.

Preliminary data confirm the feasibility and safety of tele-yoga for chronic pain.[21] There is some evidence of tele-yoga being as effective as in-person Yoga sessions. However, larger head-to-head comparative trials are needed to establish the efficacy of tele-yoga.[21]

Home-based tele-yoga classes administered for 8 weeks to patients with heart failure and chronic obstructive pulmonary diseases were found to have beneficial physical effects in the form of reduced muscle tension and improvement in body flexibility. Safety was monitored by a research-registered nurse. Several psychological benefits were also reported in areas of sleep, anxiety, stress, and motivation. Further, tele-yoga was found to be acceptable and appropriate by the participants.[22] Tele-yoga in a group format, with flexible schedule has been found feasible and acceptable in a study on patients undergoing breast cancer treatment.[23]

One of the very few studies evaluating the comparative efficacy of tele-yoga and in-person Yoga therapy for reducing stress levels in case of in vitro fertilization failure demonstrated a significant reduction in stress and anxiety level after the Yoga sessions for 6 months. There was no difference in the outcome between the two groups. This shows that tele-sessions can be as effective as in-person sessions.[24] Similarly, tele-yoga was found to have equivalent effect as in-person Yoga, on war veterans, on the symptoms of pain, energy level, irritability, sleep problems, depression, and anxiety. About 80% of the participants reported improvement irrespective of the mode of Yoga delivery. The subjective satisfaction level of participants in both the groups was also comparable.[15]

A study of tai chi and tele-yoga in adult informal caregivers of patients with any disability or disease including mental illnesses or old age showed significant increase in muscle strength, muscle endurance, functionality, and flexibility. The tele-yoga group had better improvement in chest press endurance and abdominal endurance.[25]

Effect of synchronous yoga over video-chat with partner or close friend has been studied and it was found that most of the participants felt a sense of belonging and a sense of community with both audio and video modes. Yoga teachers who were a part of the study reported no significant difficulty in conducting tele-yoga as compared to in-person yoga. A few problems that arose with tele-yoga were consciousness regarding the camera, lack of enough space and frequent adjustments required in the camera to see the yoga poses.[26]

Tele-yoga session of 30 minutes' duration in patients with mood disorders showed positive results in the domains of feasibility, acceptability, and affect. Among the participants, 57% gave positive feedback and 28% gave suggestions for improvement. The acceptability was high (67.9%). There was a statistically significant reduction in the negative affect with a large effect size after the intervention.[27]

Home-based tele-yoga sessions, in 90 women who had experienced stillbirth, for 12 weeks were found to result in significant decrease in symptoms of PTSD and depression, and improvement in sleep, and subjective health rating. These women were randomized into low dose (60 min/week) and moderate dose (150 min/week) yoga groups, and stretch-and-tone control group. Perinatal grief was significantly reduced in the intervention group as compared to the control group. There were no significant differences between the low and moderate dose groups. Feasibility was ascertained and low dose session fared slightly better than the moderate dose one in participants' opinion. About 70% of the participants reported 75% satisfaction after the therapy, and acceptability was reported by 50% of them.[28]

In a project to evaluate the feasibility and pilot testing of tele-yoga for individuals with mental health disorders in the community, undertaken by the National Institute of Mental Health and Neuro Sciences (NIMHANS), Bengaluru, a Yoga training checklist was developed and validated in the first phase and feasibility and pilot test were done in the second phase. It showed improvement in the well-being and satisfaction of the participants over a period of 1 month. This study concluded that tele-yoga is feasible with minimum technological requirements and is effective. It also recommended that tele-yoga trainers must be trained and assessed for providing these services.[29]

With the evidence into consideration, we would like to propose a few recommendations that need to be followed for tele-yoga services.

RECOMMENDATIONS FOR THE PRACTICE OF TELE-YOGA

Based on our clinical experience and in line with the advisory released by the Government of India, certain recommendations can be made regarding the precautions to be taken in imparting tele-yoga.[17]

The Yoga professional must try to ensure privacy, security, and confidentiality of data of all patients. No recording of yoga sessions should be done or shared with others without prior permission of both the patient and the therapist. These points are to be discussed and ensured while obtaining the informed consent which is necessary before starting tele-yoga. All recordings of sessions, if retained during the course, must be destroyed after the course is complete. Yoga professionals are to make themselves familiar with the relevant Acts and laws in India such as those related to yoga and tele-yoga, tele-medicine, use of technology in service, etc. Professional boundaries and ethics are to be maintained. Details of the practices and protocols related to tele-yoga can be accessed from the advisory.[17]

Do's and Don'ts in Tele-Yoga

1. Record the entire case proforma of the patient in order to understand the overall clinical picture including comorbid illnesses. This will enable the therapist and clinical yoga expert to advise the patient to avoid certain yoga postures (e.g., avoiding *Padahastasana* from the yoga module for patients with schizophrenia with comorbid hypertension).
2. Improper practice of yoga can lead to many physical and psychological problems. Hence it is important to assess the patient's previous knowledge and practice of yoga to understand the source of his/her learning (books/Youtube videos/guru/school of yoga). This will help the therapist and the clinical yoga expert advice improvisations in their practices.
3. The therapist as well as the patient should practice in a quiet room with proper lighting and ventilation.
4. Advise the patient to adjust the camera such that his/her entire body is visible to the therapist. The therapist also needs to focus the camera on the parts of the body that are involved in practicing a certain posture.
5. The first session can be a direct in-person or one-on-one tele-yoga session based on the discretion of the therapist (nonmedical graduation/postgraduation in yoga) and clinical yoga expert (medical graduate with postgraduation in yoga).
6. In the first session, the therapist must teach and demonstrate each yoga practice of the yoga module in great detail. The decision to admit a patient to any on-going group batch for the specific illness must be taken by the clinical yoga expert and yoga therapist, after discussion with the patient. The major aims of the one-to-one session are to evaluate the patient's clinical condition and ability to understand and perform the yoga postures and to educate the patient and the caregiver to avoid certain yoga postures from the yoga module that will be taught in the group therapy sessions, in view of comorbidity profile of the patient.
7. On the basis of patient's performance in the one-on-one session, if the therapist and the clinical yoga expert feel that a patient needs more than one session to learn the practices (particularly for patients with learning difficulties and severe mental illnesses), required number of individual tele-yoga sessions will be conducted.
8. Each group batch should not have more than 10 individuals. Caregivers may be allowed to participate in the session if the patient is comfortable with the same.
9. Duration of the group tele-yoga session should not exceed an hour. However, the first few individual tele-yoga sessions may

exceed an hour in order to incorporate detailed evaluation of the patient and teaching the specific yoga module with lucid instructions and corrections.
10. Two yoga therapists should be involved in delivering the group tele-yoga therapy sessions (maintaining a therapist to patient ratio of 1:5). The active therapist can impart yoga therapy with detailed instructions, precautions, common corrections, and modifications of certain yoga practices, considering the health profile of the patients admitted in the batch. The other therapist can scrutinize each person's practice and offer corrections at the end of the group session.
11. The yoga therapist needs to consult a clinical Yoga expert and the patient's doctor to shortlist the yoga practices that are safe and effective for the for a patient with particular disorder.
12. The practices in the module should be adapted to make it convenient to teach through virtual media and also to enable the patient to learn it easily and effectively.
13. A power-point presentation with detailed instructions of the yoga practice, pictures, and animations of the various steps in the practice and specific contraindications should be displayed on the screen while teaching.
14. The therapist should be available at the end of the session to answer patients' questions regarding the practices.
15. The following yoga practices are contraindicated due to associated risks and are not to be taught during tele-yoga sessions:
    a. Advanced yoga postures demanding enormous balance and core strength such as arm-balancing postures, hand-, shoulder- and headstands.
    b. Advanced postures requiring extreme stretching and flexibility of the body such as crossing the legs around the neck.
    c. Postures that alter the center of gravity such as forward and backward bending should be done with eyes open. However, avoid asanas requiring extreme backward bend (*Poorna chakrasana/Poorna ustrasana* or similar postures).
    d. Postures which require balancing on only one leg (*vrikshasana, garudasana*), particularly while teaching older adults and widely varying population.
    e. Yogic cleansing practices (*Shatkriyas*) except *Kapalabhati* and *Jatru Trataka*.
    f. *Bhastrika* with more than 20 strokes/min or *Kapalabhati* with more than 40 strokes/min.
    g. Maintaining any posture for more than 3 minutes except meditation and relaxation.
    h. Advanced meditative practices such as *Vipassana* and *Kundalini* yoga.
    i. In addition, there are several precautions and practices that are to be avoided in patients with neuropsychiatric disorders (see *Chapter 9* on "General Guidelines for Yoga Therapy" in clinical conditions in this textbook) which apply equally or even more so for tele-yoga.

■ IMPLICATIONS AND FUTURE DIRECTIONS

There is evidence to infer that tele-yoga can be a potential treatment approach to overcome healthcare accessibility issues due to distance, financial burden, physical problem or disability. With the COVID-19 pandemic resulting in restrictions on travel, mandatory social distancing and phased shutdown of facilities to prevent undue exposure, tele-yoga is the need of the hour.[30] Keeping in mind the possible negative impact on provision of health care services, especially the routine services,[31] tele-yoga can be an important alternative without breaching safety concerns.

The COVID-19 pandemic has resulted in stress, depressive, and anxiety symptoms in people across the world.[32] It has affected the stress levels of healthcare workers as well.[33] There has been a study of exacerbation of symptoms of preexisting obsessive compulsive disorder and anxiety in the patients.[34] The efficacy of yoga in stress management has been proven beyond doubt and certain studies have shown similar benefit with tele-yoga. In a recent study, the feasibility and efficacy of a 4-week tele-yoga program was examined on the perceived stress levels in the general public during the lockdown phase of COVID-19 pandemic. The participants were assessed on 10-item perceived stress scale (PSS-10), yoga performance assessment (YPA) scale, and visual analog scale (VAS) at the baseline and after 4-week yoga program. Participants reported moderate to high stress levels on PSS-10 at baseline. End-point assessment exhibited a significant reduction in the perceived stress levels. A significant improvement was observed in YPA scores which indicated that the participants could learn the yoga module effectively through the tele-mode; and VAS scores suggested an improvement in well-being and usefulness of the yoga program in reducing stress. No major side effects were reported by the participants, indicating the safety of tele-yoga intervention delivered in this study.[35] *The developed tele-yoga module for stress is provided in* **Appendix 1.16** of the book. The module is also accessible at: https://www.youtube.com/watch?v=n5tpM43wudA%26t=2s. However, to generalize these observations to the whole population, larger systematic RCTs are needed. Further, the feasibility of delivering yoga therapy through tele-mode for specific psychiatric illnesses such as depression, anxiety, obsessive compulsive disorder, psychoses, etc. should be evaluated.

Some important goals that can be attained through the implementation of tele-yoga include larger community outreach, simultaneous care of both patients and caregivers, possibility of flexible scheduling for better accessibility, healthcare cost reduction and the reduction in health care resource utilization. Limitations of tele-yoga services may include technological difficulties, lack of access to technology, technological faults and privacy concerns, poor rapport between the therapist and the patient, problems with accurate learning of the postures, discomfort of patients in accepting tele-mode, etc.[27,28] However, the current pandemic is enforcing health care facilities to majorly shift to real-time virtual platform. Due to the current social distancing norms, delivering yoga therapy through tele-mode is likely to become a "new-normal" for the times to come. This warrants a detailed and systematic research into various factors related to tele-yoga to improve its acceptability and feasibility. With the overbearing pandemic scenario, tele-yoga can pave the way forward to effectively serve the mankind particularly in the domain of mental health.

CONCLUSION

Tele-yoga is a promising way to reach people, overcoming physical and other barriers, and maximizing healthcare provision. Evaluation, management, and monitoring of the possible barriers can take us a step ahead in ensuring quality specialized service provision. With appropriate clinical practice and scientific research, tele-yoga can be a very useful modality in revolutionizing healthcare services.

REFERENCES

1. Varambally S, Gangadhar BN. Yoga: a spiritual practice with therapeutic value in psychiatry. Asian J Psychiatr. 2012;5(2):186-9.
2. Sathyanarayanan G, Vengadavaradan A, Bharadwaj B. Role of yoga and mindfulness in severe mental illnesses: a narrative review. Int J Yoga. 2019;12:3-28.
3. Nagendra HR. Integrated yoga therapy for mental illness. Indian J Psychiatry. 2013;55 (Suppl 3):S337-9.

4. Naveen GH, Varambally S, Thirthalli J, Rao M, Christopher R, Gangadhar BN. Serum cortisol and BDNF in patients with major depression—effect of yoga. Int Rev Psychiatry. 2016;28(3):273-8.
5. Janakiramaiah N, Gangadhar BN, Naga Venkatesha Murthy PJ, Harish MG, Subbakrishna DK, Vedamurthachar A. Antidepressant efficacy of Sudarshan Kriya Yoga (SKY) in melancholia: a randomized comparison with electroconvulsive therapy (ECT) and imipramine. J Affect Disord. 2000;57(1-3):255-9.
6. Ravindran AV, da Silva TL. Complementary and alternative therapies as add-on to pharmacotherapy for mood and anxiety disorders: a systematic review. J Affect Disord. 2013;150(3):707-19.
7. Varambally S, Gangadhar BN. Current status of yoga in mental health services. Int Rev Psychiatry. 2016;28(3):233-5.
8. Shannahoff-Khalsa DS, Ray LE, Levine S, Gallen CC, Schwartz BJ, Sidorowich JJ. Randomized controlled trial of yogic meditation techniques for patients with obsessive-compulsive disorder. CNS Spectr. 1999;4(12):34-47.
9. Shannahoff-Khalsa D, Fernandes RY, Pereira CA, March JS, Leckman JF, Golshan S, et al. Kundalini yoga meditation versus the relaxation response meditation for treating adults with obsessive-compulsive disorder: a randomized clinical trial. Front Psychiatry. 2019;10:793.
10. Varambally S, George S, Gangadhar BN. Yoga for psychiatric disorders: from fad to evidence-based intervention? Br J Psychiatry. 2020;216(6):291-3.
11. Baspure S, Jagannathan A, Kumar S, Varambally S, Thirthalli J, Venkatasubramanian G, et al. Barriers to yoga therapy as an add-on treatment for schizophrenia in India. Int J Yoga. 2012;5(1):70-3.
12. Govindaraj R, Varambally S, Gangadhar BN. Yoga for schizophrenia: patients' perspective. Int J Yoga. 2015;8:139-41.
13. Schulz-Heik RJ, Meyer H, Mahoney L, Stanton MV, Cho RH, Moore-Downing DP, et al. Results from a clinical yoga program for veterans: yoga via telehealth provides comparable satisfaction and health improvements to in-person yoga. BMC Complement Altern Med. 2017;17(1):198.
14. Institute of Medicine (IOM). Telemedicine: A Guide to Assessing Telecommunications for Health Care. Washington, DC: National Academy Press; 1996.
15. Board on Health Care Services; Institute of Medicine. The role of telehealth in an evolving health care environment: workshop summary. Washington (DC): National Academies Press (US); 2012.
16. Board of Governors in supersession of the Medical Council of India. Telemedicine practice guidelines enabling registered medical practitioners to provide healthcare using telemedicine. 2020. [online] Available from: https://www.mohfw.gov.in/pdf/Telemedicine.pdf [Last accessed October, 2020].
17. Central Council for Research in Yoga and Naturopathy, Ministry of AYUSH, Government of India. Advisory on tele-yoga services: version 1.0. Government of India; 2020. pp. 9-27.
18. Odole AC, Ojo OD. A telephone-based physiotherapy intervention for patients with osteoarthritis of the knee. Int J Telerehabil. 2013;5(2):11-20.
19. Backhaus A, Agha Z, Maglione ML, Repp A, Ross B, Zuest D, et al. Videoconferencing psychotherapy: a systematic review. Psychol Serv. 2012;9(2):111-31.
20. World Health Organization (2010). Telemedicine opportunities and developments in Member States. [online] Available from: https://www.who.int/goe/publications/goe_telemedicine_2010.pdf [Last accessed October, 2020].
21. Mathersul DC, Mahoney LA, Bayley PJ. Tele-yoga for chronic pain: current status and future directions. Glob Adv Health Med. 2018;7:2164956118766011.
22. Selman L, McDermott K, Donesky D, Citron T, Howie-Esquivel J. Appropriateness and acceptability of a tele-yoga intervention for people with heart failure and chronic obstructive pulmonary disease: qualitative findings from a controlled pilot study. BMC Complement Altern Med. 2015;15:21.
23. Addington EL, Sohl SJ, Tooze JA, Danhauer SC. Convenient and live movement (CALM) for women undergoing breast cancer treatment: challenges and recommendations for internet-based yoga research. Complement Ther Med. 2018;37:77-9.
24. Martini AE, Hammer K, Heller B, Hirshfeld-Cytron JE. The impact of in-person and online structured yoga programs on anxiety levels in patients after in vitro fertilization (IVF) failure: a preliminary analysis. Fertil Steril. 2017;108(3):e301.
25. Martin AC, Candow D. Effects of online yoga and tai chi on physical health outcome measures of adult informal caregivers. Int J Yoga. 2019;12:37-44.
26. Muntean R, Neustaedter C, Hennessy K. Synchronous Yoga and Meditation Over Distance using Video Chat. [online] Available from: http://clab.iat.sfu.ca/pubs/Muntean-VideoChatYoga-GI2015.pdf [Last accessed October, 2020].
27. Uebelacker L, Dufour SC, Dinerman JG, Walsh SL, Hearing C, Gillette LT, et al. Examining the

feasibility and acceptability of an online yoga class for mood disorders: a MoodNetwork study. J Psychiatr Pract. 2018;24(1):60-7.
28. Huberty J, Sullivan M, Green J, Kurka J, Leiferman J, Gold K, et al. Online yoga to reduce post-traumatic stress in women who have experienced stillbirth: a randomized control feasibility trial. BMC Complement Med Ther. 2020;20(1):173.
29. Jagannathan A, Varambally S, Maharana S, Chandra PS. Feasibility and pilot testing of virtual-yoga sessions for individuals with mental health disorders in the community. Non-funded Project conducted at NIMHANS Bengaluru. 2018.
30. World Health Organization (2019). Coronavirus. [online] Available from: https://www.who.int/emergencies/diseases/novel-coronavirus-2019. [Last accessed October, 2020].
31. Kavoor AR. COVID-19 in people with mental illness: challenges and vulnerabilities. Asian J Psychiatr. 2020;51:102051.
32. Rajkumar RP. COVID-19 and mental health: a review of the existing literature. Asian J Psychiatr. 2020;52:102066.
33. Bohlken J, Schömig F, Lemke MR, Pumberger M, Riedel-Heller SG. COVID-19 pandemic: stress experience of healthcare workers—a short current review. Psychiatrische Praxis. 2020;47(4): 190-7.
34. Kumar A, Somani A. Dealing with corona virus anxiety and OCD. Asian J Psychiatr. 2020;51: 102053.
35. Jasti N, Bhargav H, George S, Varambally S, Gangadhar BN. Tele-yoga for stress management: need of the hour during the COVID-19 pandemic and beyond? Asian J Psychiatr. 2020;54:102334.

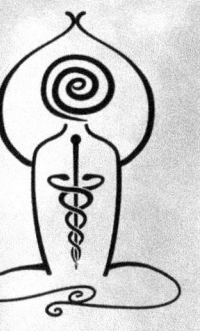

APPENDIX 1

Yoga Therapy Modules for Common Neuropsychiatric Disorders

- 1.1 Validated Yoga Module for Depression
- 1.2 Validated Yoga Module for Generalized Anxiety Disorder
- 1.3 Validated Yoga Module for Obsessive Compulsive Disorder
- 1.4 Validated Yoga Module for Schizophrenia
- 1.5 Validated Yoga Module for Bipolar Affective Disorder
- 1.6 Validated Yoga Module for Older Adults
- 1.7 Yoga Module for Attention Deficit Hyperactivity Disorder
- 1.8 Yoga Module for Autism Spectrum Disorder
- 1.9 Validated Yoga Module for Opioid Use Disorder/ Substance Use Disorders
- 1.10 Validated Yoga Module for Somatoform Pain Disorder
- 1.11 Validated Yoga Module for Low Back Pain
- 1.12 Validated Yoga Module for Migraine
- 1.13 Validated Yoga Module for Parkinson's Disease
- 1.14 Validated Yoga Module for Epilepsy
- 1.15 Validated Yoga Module for Caregivers of Patients with Schizophrenia
- 1.16 Tele-Yoga Module for Stress Reduction
- 1.17 Guided Yogic Relaxation (GYR)

INTRODUCTION TO YOGA MODULES FOR SPECIFIC NEUROPSYCHIATRIC DISORDERS

The yoga modules given in this section which are in use at the NIMHANS—Integrated Centre for Yoga for the respective neuropsychiatric disorders have been derived by a process of development and validation which is briefly described here.

DEVELOPMENT PHASE

The objectives to be addressed through yoga therapy in the particular condition were identified by approximating the description and application of the practices for various physical or psychological problems as given in the traditional yogic texts. For this purpose, a thorough literature review of traditional and contemporary yoga texts such as *Hatha Yoga Pradipika, Gheranda Samhita, Patanjali Yoga Sutras*, and scientific search engines such as PubMed, Google Scholar and PsychInfo in the respective domain was conducted. Subsequently, the yoga practices indicated for the particular objective were pooled and a draft module was developed following a general scheme: initial *sukshma vyayama* followed by *asanas, pranayama* and relaxation/meditative practices ending with *sankalpa*. Particular yogic counseling techniques were also added if appropriate for the condition.

VALIDATION PHASE

A number of yoga experts (a minimum of 10) with experience in treating the respective ailment with yoga therapy were invited to help validate the module. The experts had a minimum of 5 years of experience after Doctorate degree/Doctor of Medicine in Yoga or 7 years of experience after Master's in Yoga therapy/Bachelor's in Yoga and Naturopathic Sciences.

The list of yoga practices pooled from the literature review was presented to the experts selected along with case vignettes of the particular condition. The experts were requested to rate the practices on a 3-point Likert scale: (1) Not essential; (2) Useful but not essential; and (3) Essential. Each yoga practice was rated for its usefulness in treating the respective neuropsychiatric condition and the feasibility of the practice to suit the learning ability of subjects with the condition based on the experience of the yoga expert. The experts were also requested to opine on the dose of each practice and ideal duration of each session. They were also asked to suggest any other practice(s) that they would recommend for the condition. The agreement between the experts was assessed by calculating the content validity ratio (CVR) for each practice using Lawshe's formula.[1] Further, a cut-off value for CVR is decided on the basis of number of experts involved in validation process.[1] Only practices with a CVR equal to or more than the cut-off value were selected for the final module.

The validated yoga modules were then subjected to pilot feasibility testing in patients with the respective disorders and then finalized (see Hariprasad et al., 2013).[2]

> **Use of the Suggested Yoga Modules and Disclaimer**
>
> *The given yoga modules are designed to be learnt and practiced under the supervision of a trained yoga therapist only. The authors/publishers of the book will not be responsible for any untoward effects resulting due to unsupervised self-practice.*

REFERENCES

1. Lawshe CH. A quantitative approach to content validity. Personnel Psychology. 1975;28(4):563-75.
2. Hariprasad VR, Varambally S, Varambally PT, Thirthalli J, Basavaraddi IV, Gangadhar BN. Designing, validation and feasibility of a yoga-based intervention for elderly. Indian J Psychiatry. 2013;55(Suppl 3):S344–9.

APPENDIX 1.1

Validated Yoga Module for Depression

(Developed by Dr Naveen GH et al., 2013 at NIMHANS)

1. Preparation (Sukshma and Sthula Vyayama):

S. No.	Practice (Sanskrit)	Practice (English)	Rounds	Time (minutes)
a.	Griva shakti vikasaka-I	Neck sideward movement	5	1
b.	Griva shakti vikasaka-II	Neck forward and backward bending	5	1
c.	Manibandha shakti vikasaka	Wrist movement	10	1
d.	Kaphoni shakti vikasaka	Elbow flexion and stretching	3	1
e.	Bhuja valli shakti vikasaka	Arms movement	3	1
f.	Janu shakti vikasaka	Knee stretching	5	1
g.	Gulpha, pada pristha, pada tala shakti vikasaka	Ankle rotation (clockwise and anticlockwise)	5	1
h.	Kati shakti vikasaka	Twisting	10	1
i.	Jogging	• Slow jogging • Forward jogging • Backward jogging • Sideward jogging	10	2
j.	Mukha Dhauti	Cleaning through single blast breath	5	15 seconds

2. Surya namaskar:

S. No.	Practice (Sanskrit)	Practice (English)	Rounds	Time (minutes)
a.	Surya namaskar	Sun salutation—12 steps	3	15

3. Specific relaxation:

S. No.	Practice (Sanskrit)	Practice (English)	Rounds	Time (minutes)
a.	Shavasana (with chanting of "A")	Relaxation in corpse pose	1	2

4. Specific standing asanas for depressive disorder:

S. No.	Practice (Sanskrit)	Practice (English)	Rounds	Time (minutes)
a.	Ardha chakrasana	Backward bending pose	5	2

5. Specific sitting asanas for depressive disorder:

S. No.	Practice (Sanskrit)	Practice (English)	Rounds	Time (minutes)
a.	Ardha ustrasana	Camel pose	5	2
b.	Paschimottanasana	Seated forward bending pose	5	2

6. Specific prone asanas for depressive disorder:

S. No.	Practice (Sanskrit)	Practice (English)	Rounds	Time (minutes)
a.	Bhujangasana	Serpent pose	5	2

7. Specific supine asanas for depressive disorder:

S. No.	Practice (Sanskrit)	Practice (English)	Rounds	Time (minutes)
a.	Pawanamuktasana	Wind releasing pose	5	2
b.	Viparitakarani mudra	Legs-up-the-wall pose	5	2
c.	Setu bandhasana	Bridge pose	5	2

8. Specific relaxation:

S. No.	Practice (Sanskrit)	Practice (English)	Rounds	Time (minutes)
a.	Shavasana	Relaxation in corpse pose/Yoga nidra	1	4

9. Specific kriya practices for depressive disorder:

S. No.	Practice (Sanskrit)	Practice (English)	Rounds	Time (minutes)
a.	Kapalabhati	Breath of fire/Skull shining breath	2 (40–60 strokes/min)	2

10. Specific pranayama practices for depressive disorder:

S. No.	Practice (Sanskrit)	Practice (English)	Rounds	Time (minutes)
a.	Surya anuloma viloma	Right nostril breathing	21	3
b.	Ujjayi	Victorious breath	9	2
c.	Bhastrika	Bellows' breathing	3 (20 strokes per cycle with 30 sec rest after each cycle)	3

11. Meditation practice:

S. No.	Practice (Sanskrit)	Practice (English)	Rounds	Time (minutes)
a.	Nadanusandhana	Sound resonance technique: • AA kara • UU kara • MM kara • AUM kara	9 9 9 9	5

12. *Yogic counseling for depressive disorder:* Understanding of kleshas according to Yoga and ways to overcome them according to *Patanjali*.

APPENDIX 1.2

Validated Yoga Module for Generalized Anxiety Disorder

(Developed by Dr Pooja More et al., 2020 at NIMHANS, Bengaluru)

1. Specific loosening practices for generalized anxiety disorder (GAD):

S. No.	Practice (Sanskrit)	Practice (English)	Rounds	Time (minutes)
a.	Griva sithilikarana	Neck exercise	5	1
b.	Bahumula sithilikarana	Shoulder rotation	5	1
c.	Kaphoni sithilikarana	Elbow movement	5	1
d.	Manibandha sithilikarana	Wrist rotation	5	1
e.	Anguli sithilikarana	Loosening of fingers	5	1
f.	Kati sithilikarana	Waist rotation	5	1
g.	Janu sithilikarana	Knee rotation	5	1
h.	Gulpha sithilikarana	Ankle rotation	5	1

2. Specific breathing practices for GAD:

S. No.	Practice (Sanskrit)	Practice (English)	Rounds	Time (minutes)
a.	Shvasa kriya	Hand stretch breathing	3	3
b.	Shvasa kriya	Hands in and out breathing	1	2
c.	Tadasana shvasa kriya	Ankle stretch breathing	1	1
d.	Shashankasana shvasa kriya	Hare pose/Moon pose breathing	1	2
e.	Marjariasana shvasa kriya	Tiger breathing	1	2
f.	Setu bandhasana shvasa kriya	Bridge pose breathing	1	2

3. Specific surya namaskar practices for GAD:

S. No.	Practice (Sanskrit)	Practice (English)	Rounds	Time (minutes)
a.	Surya namaskar (12-step practice to be done slowly)	Sun salutations	3 (Maintain each step for 5 breaths)	5

4. Specific standing asanas for GAD:

S. No.	Practice (Sanskrit)	Practice (English)	Rounds	Time (minutes)
a.	Ardhakati chakrasana	Lateral arc pose (Right side and left side)	2	2
b.	Ardha chakrasana	Half wheel pose	2	2
c.	Padahastasana	Hand-to-feet pose	2	2

5. Specific sitting asanas for GAD:

S. No.	Practice (Sanskrit)	Practice (English)	Rounds	Time (minutes)
a.	Shashankasana	Rabbit pose	1	2
b.	Vakrasana	Sitting twisted pose	2	2
c.	Paschimottanasana	Back stretch pose	1	2

6. Specific supine asanas for GAD:

S. No.	Practice (Sanskrit)	Practice (English)	Rounds	Time (minutes)
a.	Pawanamuktasana	Wind releasing pose (both legs)	1	2
b.	Setu bandhasana	Bridge pose	1	2

7. Specific prone practices for GAD:

S. No.	Practice (Sanskrit)	Practice (English)	Rounds	Time (minutes)
a.	Bhujangasana	Serpent pose	2	2
b.	Parvatasana	Mountain pose	1	2

8. Specific pranayama practices for GAD:

S. No.	Practice (Sanskrit)	Practice (English)	Rounds	Time (minutes)
a.	Chandra bhedana	Single nostril breathing	9	3
b.	Nadi shuddhi	Alternate nostril breathing	9	3
c.	Chandra anuloma viloma	Left nostril breathing	21	5
d.	Sheetali	Cooling pranayama	9	3
e.	Bhramari	Humming bee breath	9	3
f.	Ujjayi	Ocean breath	9	3

9. Specific relaxation techniques for GAD:

S. No.	Practice (Sanskrit)	Practice (English)	Rounds	Time (minutes)
a.	Sampurna vishranti paddati in Shavasana	Deep relaxation technique	1	5
b.	Sheeghra shitilikaran upaya in Shavasana	Quick relaxation technique	1	3

10. Specific meditation techniques for GAD:

S. No.	Practice (Sanskrit)	Practice (English)	Rounds	Time (minutes)
a.	Om dhyana/Japa	Om meditation	1	5
b.	Nadanusandhana	A, U, M and AUM chanting	1	5

11. Specific counseling for GAD:

S. No.	Practice (Sanskrit)	Practice (English)	Rounds	Time (minutes)
a.	Panchakosha model	Five sheaths of existence	1	5
b.	Sattvic ahara	Balanced diet	1	5
c.	Yama and Niyama	Do's and don'ts, conduct	1	5
d.	Pratipaksha bhavana	Principle of opposite	1	5
e.	Jnana, Bhakti, Raja, and Karma yoga	Concept of four streams of yoga	1	5

APPENDIX 1.3

Validated Yoga Module for Obsessive Compulsive Disorder

(Developed by Mrs Shubha Bhat et al., 2016 at NIMHANS, Bengaluru)

1. Specific breathing practices for obsessive compulsive disorder (OCD):

S. No.	Practice (Sanskrit)	Practice (English)	Rounds	Time (minutes)
a.	Shvasa kriya	Hand stretch breathing	3	3
b.	Shvasa kriya	Hands in and out breathing	1	2
c.	Shvasa kriya	Ankle stretch breathing	1	2
d.	Marjariasana shvasa kriya	Tiger breathing	1	2
e.	Shashankasana shvasa kriya	Hare pose/Moon pose breathing	1	2
f.	Setu bandhasana	Bridge pose	1	2
g.	Pada uttanasana	Single leg raising	2	2

2. Specific surya namaskar practices for OCD:

S. No.	Practice (Sanskrit)	Practice (English)	Rounds	Time (minutes)
a.	Surya namaskar	Sun salutations	3	5

3. Specific standing asanas for OCD:

S. No.	Practice (Sanskrit)	Practice (English)	Rounds	Time (minutes)
a.	Ardhakati chakrasana	Lateral arc pose (Right side and left side)	2	3
b.	Ardha chakrasana	Half wheel pose	2	2

4. Specific sitting asanas for OCD:

S. No.	Practice (Sanskrit)	Practice (English)	Rounds	Time (minutes)
a.	Vajrasana	Diamond pose	1	2
b.	Vakrasana	Sitting twisted pose	2	3
c.	Ustrasana	Camel pose	2	2

5. Specific supine asanas for OCD:

S. No.	Practice (Sanskrit)	Practice (English)	Rounds	Time (minutes)
a.	Pawanamuktasana	Wind releasing pose (both legs)	2	2

6. Specific supine practices for OCD:

S. No.	Practice (Sanskrit)	Practice (English)	Rounds	Time (minutes)
a.	Bhujangasana	Serpent pose	2	2

7. Specific pranayama practices for OCD:

S. No.	Practice (Sanskrit)	Practice (English)	Rounds	Time (minutes)
a.	Nadi shuddhi*	Alternate nostril breathing	21	5
b.	Sheetali	Cooling pranayama	10	5
c.	Bhramari	Humming bee breath	10	5

8. Relaxation techniques for OCD:

S. No.	Practice (Sanskrit)	Practice (English)	Rounds	Time (minutes)
a.	Sampurna vishranti paddati in Shavasana with A, U, M chants	Deep relaxation technique	1	5

Note: Left nostril breathing has also been found useful in recent studies on OCD and can be added to the practices.

APPENDIX 1.4

Validated Yoga Module for Schizophrenia

(Developed by Dr Ramajayam Govindaraj et al., 2016 at NIMHANS)

1. Specific loosening practices for schizophrenia:

S. No.	Practice (Sanskrit)	Practice (English)	Counts	Time (seconds)
a.	Sithilikarana vyayama	Slow jogging	10	20
b.	Sithilikarana vyayama	Fast jogging	10	25
c.	Sithilikarana vyayama	Forward jogging	10	25
d.	Sithilikarana vyayama	Backward jogging	10	25
e.	Sithilikarana vyayama	Side jogging	10	25
f.	Mukha dhauti	Mouth washout breathing	10	30

2. Specific breathing practices for schizophrenia:

S. No.	Practice (Sanskrit)	Practice (English)	Rounds/Counts	Time
a.	Shvasa kriya	Twisting	20 counts	30 seconds
b.	Shvasa kriya	Hand stretch breathing	3 rounds	5 minutes
c.	Hastottanasana padahastasana shvasa kriya	Forward and backward bending	20 counts	1 minute
d.	Vyaghra shvasa kriya	Tiger breathing	20 counts	1 minute
e.	Trikonasana shvasa kriya	Side bending	20 counts	1 minute
f.	Shashankasana shvasa kriya	Hare pose/Moon pose breathing	20 counts	1 minute

3. Surya namaskar:

S. No.	Practice (Sanskrit)	Practice (English)	Rounds	Time (minutes)
a.	Surya namaskar	Sun salutations—10 steps	4 rounds slow and 4 rounds fast	10

4. Specific relaxation after breathing and surya namaskar:

S. No.	Practice (Sanskrit)	Practice (English)	Rounds	Time (minutes)
a.	Sheeghra shitilikaran upaya in Shavasana	Quick relaxation technique	1	4

5. Specific sitting asanas for schizophrenia:

S. No.	Practice (Sanskrit)	Practice (English)	Rounds	Time
a.	Vakrasana	Twisted sitting pose	1 round right, 1 round left	10 seconds each side
b.	Ustrasana	Camel pose	2 (1st half camel pose and 2nd full camel pose)	10 seconds each

6. Specific prone asanas for schizophrenia:

S. No.	Practice (Sanskrit)	Practice (English)	Rounds	Time (seconds)
a.	Bhujangasana	Serpent pose	2	10 each

b.	Ardha shalabhasana and shalabhasana	• Half locust pose:
		  – Right leg
		  – Left leg
		• Locust pose: Both legs
			
			1
			1
			1
				
				10
				10
				10

c.	Dhanurasana	Bow pose	1	10

7. Specific supine practices for schizophrenia:

S. No.	Practice (Sanskrit)	Practice (English)	Rounds	Time (seconds)
a.	Viparita Karani Mudra	Legs-up-the-wall pose	1	10
b.	Ardha matsyasana	Half fish pose	1	10
c.	Matsyasana	Fish pose	1	10

8. Specific pranayama for schizophrenia:

S. No.	Practice (Sanskrit)	Practice (English)	Rounds	Time (minutes)
a.	Bhastrika	Bellows breathing	2	4
b.	Nadi shuddhi	Alternate nostril breathing	9	5

9. Specific meditative practices for schizophrenia:

S. No.	Practice (Sanskrit)	Practice (English)	Rounds	Time (minutes)
a.	Nadanusandhana	Sound resonance technique while lying down: • AA kara • UU kara • MM kara • AUM kara	 9 9 9 9	 5

10. *Yogic counseling for schizophrenia:* Understanding the disease from yoga perspective and ways to overcome.

APPENDIX 1.5

Validated Yoga Module for Bipolar Affective Disorder

(Developed by Dr Hemant Bhargav et al., 2020 at NIMHANS)

1. Bipolar affective disorder (BPAD) module for those in remission

1.1. Relaxation technique:

S. No	Practice (Sanskrit)	Practice (English)	Rounds	Time (minutes)
a.	Tatkshan shitilikaran upaya in Shavasana	Instant relaxation technique	1	1

1.2. Sithilikarana vyayama (loosening exercises):

S. No	Practice (Sanskrit)	Practice (English)	Rounds	Time (minutes)
a.	Vyaghrasana shvasa kriya	Tiger stretch breathing	10	1

1.3. Specific standing asanas:

S. No	Practice (Sanskrit)	Practice (English)	Rounds	Time (minutes)
a.	Ardhakati chakrasana	Sideward bending pose	2	1
b.	Ardha chakrasana	Backward bending pose	3	1
c.	Vrikshasana	Tree pose	2	1

1.4. Surya namaskar:

S. No	Practice (Sanskrit)	Practice (English)	Rounds	Time (minutes)
a.	Surya namaskar	Sun salutation—12 steps	8 (Maintain each step in the last round for 5 breaths)	15

1.5. Specific relaxation:

S. No	Practice (Sanskrit)	Practice (English)	Rounds	Time (minutes)
a.	Sheeghra shitilikaran upaya in Shavasana	Quick relaxation technique in corpse pose	1	1

1.6. Specific supine asanas:

S. No	Practice (Sanskrit)	Practice (English)	Rounds	Time (minutes)
a.	Pavanmuktasana kriya	Wind relieving pose	10 rounds clockwise, 10 rounds anticlockwise with each leg	2
b.	Ardha halasana	Half plough pose	1	1

1.7. Specific relaxation:

S. No	Practice (Sanskrit)	Practice (English)	Rounds	Time (minutes)
a.	Makarasana	Relaxation in crocodile pose	1	1

1.8. Specific prone asana:

S. No	Practice (Sanskrit)	Practice (English)	Rounds	Time (minutes)
a.	Bhujangasana	Cobra pose	5	1

1.9. Specific pranayama:

S. No	Practice (Sanskrit)	Practice (English)	Rounds	Time (minutes)
a.	Vibhagiya pranayama	Sectional breathing in three mudras: • Chin • Chinmaya • Ādi	Abdominal breathing: 5 Thoracic breathing: 5 Clavicular breathing: 5	3
b.	Nadi shuddhi pranayama	Alternate nostril breathing	9	3

1.10. Meditation practice:

S. No	Practice (Sanskrit)	Practice (English)	Rounds	Time (minutes)
a.	Nadanusandhana (Feel the vibrations on different body parts with one hand during chants: AA—Chest; UU—Neck and MM–Head)	Sound resonance technique • AA kara • UU kara • MM kara • AUM kara	9 9 9 9	5
b.	Gayatri mantra Mahamrityunjaya mantra	Energizing and calming mantra chants as per cultural inclination (Loud chant with eyes closed, focus on vibrations)	5	2

2. BPAD module for current episode depression

2.1. *Additions in BPAD remission module:*

2.1.1. Sithilikarana vyayama (loosening exercises):

S. No	Practice (Sanskrit)	Practice (English)	Rounds	Time (minutes)
a.	Kati chakrasana	Spinal twist	10	2
b.	Padahastasana and ardha chakrasana shvasa kriya	Forward and backward bending	10	2
c.	Parivrtta trikonasana shvasa kriya	Alternate toe touching	10	2

2.1.2. Specific prone asana:

S. No	Practice (Sanskrit)	Practice (English)	Rounds	Time (minutes)
a.	Dhanurasana	Bow pose	5	2

2.1.3. Specific kriya practice:

S. No	Practice (Sanskrit)	Practice (English)	Rounds	Time (minutes)
a.	Kapalabhati	Breath of fire/ Skull shining breath	2 (40–60 strokes/min)	2

2.1.4. Specific pranayama:

S. No	Practice (Sanskrit)	Practice (English)	Rounds	Time (minutes)
b.	Bhastrika	Bellows breathing	2 cycles (20 strokes/cycle)	3

2.1.5. Meditation practice:

S. No.	Practice (Sanskrit)	Practice (English)	Rounds	Time (minutes)
a.	Gayatri mantra chanting	Energizing mantra chants as per cultural inclination	9	2

2.2. *Deletions in BPAD remission module:*

S. No.	Practice (Sanskrit)	Practice (English)	Rounds	Time (minutes)
a.	Mahamrityunjaya mantra chanting	Calming mantra chants as per cultural inclination (Loud chant with eyes closed, focus on vibrations)	9	2

3. BPAD module for current episode mania

3.1. *Additions in BPAD remission module:*

3.1.1. Sithilikarana vyayama (loosening exercises):

S. No.	Practice (Sanskrit)	Practice (English)	Rounds	Time (minutes)
a.	Alternate bhujangasana and parvatasana	Alternate snake and mountain pose	10	2
b.	Anantasana variation	Side leg raising	10	2

3.1.2. Specific sitting asana:

S. No.	Practice (Sanskrit)	Practice (English)	Rounds	Time (minutes)
a.	Shashankasana	Hare pose/Moon pose breathing	2	1
b.	Paschimottanasana	Seated forward bend	2	1

3.1.3. Specific kriya practice:

S. No.	Practice (Sanskrit)	Practice (English)	Rounds	Time (minutes)
a.	Kapalabhati	Breath of fire/Skull shining breath	2 (60–90 strokes/min)	2

3.1.4. Specific pranayama:

S. No.	Practice (Sanskrit)	Practice (English)	Rounds	Time (minutes)
b.	Bhastrika	Bellows breathing	3 cycles (30 strokes/cycle)	3

3.1.5. Meditation practice:

S. No.	Practice (Sanskrit)	Practice (English)	Rounds	Time (minutes)
a.	Shvasa prashvasa	Mindful breathing	9	2
b.	Mahamrityunjaya mantra chanting	Calming mantra chants as per cultural inclination	9	2

3.2. Deletions in BPAD remission module:

S. No.	Practice (Sanskrit)	Practice (English)	Rounds	Time (minutes)
a.	Gayatri mantra chanting	Energizing mantra chants as per cultural inclination (Loud chant with eyes closed, focus on vibrations)	5	2

Note:
1. First fast breathing practices (*Kapalabhati* and *Bhastrika*) should be performed followed by slow breathing practices (Sectional breathing and *Nadi shuddhi*) in both the modules.
2. Mantra should be chanted after *Nadanausandhana* practice (for both the modules).

APPENDIX 1.6

Validated Yoga Module for Older Adults

(Developed by Dr Hariprasad VR et al., 2013 at NIMHANS)

1. Specific loosening practices for older adults:

S. No.	Practice (Sanskrit)	Practice (English)	Rounds	Time (minutes)
a.	Griva sanchalana	Neck exercises	5	2
b.	Skandha sanchalana	Shoulder rotation	5	2
c.	Kati sanchalana	Waist rotation	5	3
d.	Pada sanchalana	Ankle and feet exercises	5	3

2. Specific standing asanas for older adults:

S. No.	Practice (Sanskrit)	Practice (English)	Rounds	Time (minutes)
a.	Tadasana	Standing stretch	1	1
b.	Kati chakrasana	Spinal twisting	5	2
c.	Konasana	Lateral arc pose • Right side • Left side	 1 1	 1 1

3. Specific sitting asanas for older adults:

S. No.	Practice (Sanskrit)	Practice (English)	Rounds	Time (minutes)
a.	Marjariasana	Cat stretch pose	5	2
b.	Vakrasana	*Seated twist pose:* • Right side • Left side	 1 1	 1 1

4. Specific prone practices for older adults:

S. No.	Practice (Sanskrit)	Practice (English)	Rounds	Time (minutes)
a.	Bhujangasana	Serpent pose	1	1
b.	Ardha shalabhasana	*Half locust pose:* • Right side • Left side	 1 1	 1 1

5. Specific supine practices for older adults:

S. No.	Practice (Sanskrit)	Practice (English)	Rounds	Time (minutes)
a.	Viparitakarani	Legs-up-the-wall pose	1	1
b.	Pawanamuktasana	Wind release pose	1	2
c.	Setu bandhasana	Bridge pose	1	2

6. Specific relaxation after asanas for older adults:

S. No.	Practice (Sanskrit)	Practice (English)	Rounds	Time (minutes)
a.	Shavasana	Relaxation in corpse pose	1	3

7. Specific kriya practices for older adults:

S. No.	Practice (Sanskrit)	Practice (English)	Rounds	Time (minutes)
a.	Kapalabhati	Breath of fire/Skull shining breath	3 rounds of 20–25 strokes	3

8. Specific pranayama practices for older adults:

S. No.	Practice (Sanskrit)	Practice (English)	Rounds	Time (minutes)
a.	Nadi shuddi	Alternate nostril breathing	9	3
b.	Surya anuloma viloma	Right nostril breath	10	2
c.	Chandra anuloma viloma	Left nostril breath	10	2
d.	Bhastrika	Bellows' breath	10	3
e.	Bhramari	Humming bee breath	5	2

9. Meditation practices for older adults:

S. No.	Practice (Sanskrit)	Practice (English)	Rounds	Time (minutes)
a.	Jyoti trataka	Light gaze technique		5
b.	Nadanusandhana	Sound resonance technique (with A, U, M chants)	AA kara: 9 UU kara: 9 MM kara: 9 AUM kara: 9	10

APPENDIX 1.7

Yoga Module for Attention Deficit Hyperactivity Disorder

(Feasibility tested by Dr Hariprasad VR et al., 2013 at NIMHANS)

1. Specific loosening practices for attention deficit hyperactivity disorder (ADHD):

S. No.	Practice (Sanskrit)	Practice (English)	Rounds	Time (minutes)
a.	Jogging	Jogging (slow, backward, forward, sideways, and jumping)	20 (for each)	5
b.	Mukha dhauti	Cleaning through a single blast breath (to relax)	5–10	1
c.	Kati chakrasana	Spinal twisting	10–20	1
d.	Kati shakti vikasaka	Backward and forward bending	20 (with increasing speed)	1
e.	Pada sanchalanasana	Cycling (forward and backward)	20 (for each)	1
f.	Pada uttanasana	Straight leg raise breathing	10 on each leg	2

2. Specific standing asanas for ADHD:

S. No.	Practice (Sanskrit)	Practice (English)	Rounds	Time (minutes)
a.	Tadasana (Variation I and II)	Mountain pose	1	1
b.	Ardha chakrasana	Half wheel pose	1	1
c.	Padahastasana	Forward bend pose	1	1
d.	Ardhakati chakrasana	Lateral arc pose	1 (each side)	1 (each side)

3. Specific sitting asanas for ADHD:

S. No.	Practice (Sanskrit)	Practice (English)	Rounds	Time (minutes)
a.	Vajrasana	Thunderbolt pose	1 (maintain for 10 rounds of deep breathing)	1
b.	Suptavajrasana	Sleeping thunderbolt pose	1 (maintain for about 10 breaths)	1
c.	Marjariasana	Cat stretch pose	20	2
d.	Paschimottanasana	Forward bend pose	1	1
e.	Shashankasana	Hare pose/Moon pose breathing	1	1
f.	Ustrasana	Camel pose	1	1

4. Specific prone asanas for ADHD:

S. No.	Practice (Sanskrit)	Practice (English)	Rounds	Time (minute)
a.	Bhujangasana	Serpent pose	1	1

5. Specific supine asanas for ADHD:

S. No.	Practice (Sanskrit)	Practice (English)	Rounds	Time (minutes)
a.	Pawanamuktasana	Wind-releasing pose	1	1
b.	Setu bandhasana	Bridge pose	1	1
c.	Shavasana	Corpse pose	1	2

6. Specific pranayama practices for ADHD:

S. No.	Practice (Sanskrit)	Practice (English)	Rounds	Time (minutes)
a.	Kapalabhati	Breath of fire/Skull shining breath	3 (30 strokes/min)	6
b.	Surya anuloma viloma	Right nostril yoga breathing	10	5
c.	Ujjayi	Ocean breath/Victory breath	10	5
d.	Chandra anuloma viloma	Left nostril yoga breathing	10	5
e.	Bhramari	Humming bee breath	10	3

7. Specific meditation practices for ADHD:

S. No.	Practice (Sanskrit)	Practice (English)	Rounds	Time (minutes)
a.	Nadanusandhana	Sound resonance technique: • AA kara • UU kara • MM kara • A-U-M kara	9 9 9 9	5

APPENDIX 1.8

Yoga Module for Autism Spectrum Disorder

(Based on Clinical Observations, Department of Integrative Medicine, NIMHANS)

1. Specific opening prayer for autism spectrum disorder (ASD):

S. No.	Practice (Sanskrit)	Practice (English)	Rounds	Time (minutes)
a.	Om chanting	Om chanting	3	1

2. Specific loosening practices for ASD:

S. No.	Practice (Sanskrit)	Practice (English)	Rounds	Time (minutes)
a.	Griva shakti vikasaka	Neck movements (forward and backward, turning and twisting, sideways)	5 (for each)	3
b.	Skandha chakra	Shoulder rotation	5 (clockwise and anticlockwise)	1
c.	Manibandha shakti vikasaka	Wrist joint rotation	5 (clockwise and anticlockwise)	1
d.	Kati sithilikarana	Waist rotation	5 (clockwise and anticlockwise)	1
e.	Janu shakti vikasaka	Knee stretching	5	1
f.	Gulpha pada-pristha pada-tala shakti vikasaka	Ankle joint rotation	5 (clockwise and anticlockwise)	1

3. Specific breathing practices for ASD:

S. No.	Practice (Sanskrit)	Practice (English)	Rounds	Time (minutes)
a.	Svana shvasa kriya	Dog breathing	10	2
b.	Vyaghra shvasa kriya	Tiger breathing	10	2
c.	Shashankasana shvasa kriya	Hare pose/Moon pose breathing	10	2

4. Specific balancing practices for ASD:

S. No.	Practice (Sanskrit)	Practice (English)	Rounds	Time (minutes)
a.	Tadasana stretching	Mountain pose stretching	10	1.5
b.	Walking in Tadasana stretch	Walking in mountain pose stretch	10	1.5

5. Specific standing asanas for ASD (Yogic postures in a *Mandalam* form):

S. No.	Practice (Sanskrit)	Practice (English)	Rounds	Time (minutes)
a.	Vrikshasana	Tree pose	1	1
b.	Trikonasana	Triangle pose	1 (each side)	2
c.	Veerbhadrasana	Warrior pose	1	1

6. Specific sitting asanas for ASD (Yogic postures in a *Mandalam* form):

S. No.	Practice (Sanskrit)	Practice (English)	Rounds	Time (minutes)
a.	Shashankasana	Moon/Hare pose	1	1
b.	Vajrasana	Thunderbolt pose	1	1
c.	Marjariasana	Cat stretch pose	1	1

7. Specific supine asanas for ASD (Yogic postures in a *Mandalam* form):

S. No.	Practice (Sanskrit)	Practice (English)	Rounds	Time (minutes)
a.	Pawanamuktasana	Wind-releasing pose	1	1
b.	Setu bandhasana	Bridge pose	1	1
c.	Ardha halasana	Half plough pose	1	1

8. Specific prone asanas for ASD (Yogic postures in a *Mandalam* form):

S. No.	Practice (Sanskrit)	Practice (English)	Rounds	Time (minutes)
a.	Bhujangasana	Serpent pose	1	1
b.	Navasana	Boat pose	1	1

9. Specific relaxation after asanas for ASD:

S. No.	Practice (Sanskrit)	Practice (English)	Rounds	Time (minutes)
a.	Sheeghra shitilikaran upaya in Shavasana (with chanting of "A")	Quick relaxation technique (QRT)	1	1

10. Specific *pranayama* practices for ASD:

S. No.	Practice (Sanskrit)	Practice (English)	Rounds	Time (minutes)
a.	Bhastrika	Bellows breath	2 cycles (1 cycle—20 rounds)	5
b.	Surya anuloma viloma	Right nostril yoga breathing	9	2.5
c.	Chandra anuloma viloma	Left nostril yoga breathing	9	2.5
d.	Nadi shuddhi	Alternate nostril yoga breathing	9	5
e.	Bhramari	Humming bee breath	9	2

11. Specific meditation practices for ASD:

S. No.	Practice (Sanskrit)	Practice (English)	Rounds	Time (minutes)
a.	Nadanusandhana	Sound resonance technique: • AA kara • UU kara • MM kara • A-U-M kara	9 9 9 9	5
b.	*Mantra* chanting (*Gayatri mantra* or any other *mantra* as per cultural background)	Mantra chanting (Loud chant with eyes closed, focus on vibrations)	9	5

12. Specific closing prayer for ASD:

S. No.	Practice (Sanskrit)	Practice (English)	Rounds	Time (minutes)
a.	Om Sarve Bhavantu Sukhinah Sarve Santu Niraamayaah Sarve Bhadraanni Pashyantu Maa Kashcid-Duhkha-Bhaag-Bhavet Om Shaantih Shaantih	Om, May all be happy, May all be free from illness, May all see what is auspicious, May no one suffer. Om Peace, Peace, Peace!!!	1	1

APPENDIX 1.9

Validated Yoga Module for Opioid Use Disorder/Substance Use Disorders

(Developed by Dr Hemant Bhargav et al., 2020 at NIMHANS)

1. Yoga module for substance use disorder: Acute withdrawal phase

1.1. Specific relaxation before breathing exercises for substance use disorder:

S. No.	Practice (Sanskrit)	Practice (English)	Rounds	Time (minutes)
a.	Tatkshan shitilikaran upaya in Shavasana	Instant relaxation technique (IRT)—rapid tightening of muscles from toes to head followed by relaxation	2	4

1.2. Specific breathing practices for substance use disorder:

S. No.	Practice (Sanskrit)	Practice (English)	Rounds	Time (minutes)
a.	Pawanamuktasana kriya	Wind releasing pose breathing	5 rounds clockwise, 5 rounds anti-clockwise	5
b.	Udara shvasana kriya	Deep abdominal breathing with prolonged exhalation (inhalation : exhalation = 1:2)	5	2
c.	Makarasana shvasana kriya	Crocodile pose breathing (Alternate legs followed by both legs)	5	2
d.	Bhujangasana shvasana kriya	Cobra pose breathing	5	2
e.	Naukasana shvasana kriya	Boat pose breathing (Alternate hands and feet followed by both)	5	2
f.	Marjariasana kriya	Tiger stretch breathing	5	2

1.3. Specific asanas for substance use disorder:

S. No.	Practice (Sanskrit)	Practice (English)	Rounds	Time (minutes)
a.	Uttanapadasana	Straight leg raising (Alternate legs followed by both legs)	5	2
b.	Titaliasana	Butterfly	100 strokes; 1 cycle	2
c.	Trikonasana	Side bending	5	2

1.4. Sectional breathing for substance use disorder:

S. No.	Practice (Sanskrit)	Practice (English)	Rounds	Time (minutes)
a.	Vibhagiya pranayama: First chin mudra (4:16:8—inhale:hold:exhale); Focus on the lower chest; maintain a ratio of 1:4:2 and reduce or increase the count depending on feasibility and practice	Sectional breathing: First chin mudra (4:16:8—inhale:hold:exhale)	5	2
b.	Vibhagiya pranayama: Second chinmaya mudra (4:16:8—inhale:hold:exhale); Focus on the middle chest	Sectional breathing: Second chinmaya mudra (4:16:8—inhale:hold:exhale)	5	2
c.	Vibhagiya pranayama: Third adi mudra (4:16:8—inhale:hold:exhale); Focus on the upper chest	Sectional breathing: Third adi mudra (4:16:8—inhale:hold:exhale)	5	2

1.5. Specific pranayama for substance use disorder:

S. No.	Practice (Sanskrit)	Practice (English)	Rounds	Time (minutes)
a.	Nadi shuddhi pranayama	Alternate nostril breathing	9	3
b.	Bhastrika pranayama	Bellows breath	2 × 20 counts	3
c.	Bhramari pranayama (Shanmukhi mudra)	Humming bee breath	9	2

1.6. Specific relaxation after pranayamas for substance use disorder:

S. No.	Practice (Sanskrit)	Practice (English)	Rounds	Time (minutes)
a.	Sampurna vishranti paddati in Shavasana	Deep relaxation technique with *Om* chanting or MMM chanting 9 rounds at the end with a positive affirmation "I am healthy, happy and satisfied"	–	9

2. Yoga module for substance use disorder: Maintenance stage

2.1. Specific relaxation before breathing exercises for substance use disorder:

S. No.	Practice (Sanskrit)	Practice (English)	Rounds	Time (minutes)
a.	Tatkshan shitilikaran upaya in Shavasana	Instant relaxation technique (IRT)	2	4

2.2. Specific breathing practices for substance use disorder:

S. No.	Practice (Sanskrit)	Practice (English)	Rounds	Time (minutes)
a.	Pawanamuktasana kriya	Wind releasing pose breathing	10 rounds clockwise and 10 rounds anticlockwise for each leg	4

Contd...

Contd...

S. No.	Practice (Sanskrit)	Practice (English)	Rounds	Time (minutes)
b.	Makarasana shvasana kriya (Alternate legs followed by both legs)	Crocodile pose breathing	5	2
c.	Bhujangasana shvasana kriya	Cobra pose breathing	5	2
d.	Naukasana shvasana kriya (Alternate sides followed by both sides)	Boat pose breathing	5	2
e.	Marjariasana kriya	Tiger breathing	5	2

2.3. Specific asanas for substance use disorder:

S. No.	Practice (Sanskrit)	Practice (English)	Rounds	Time (minutes)
a.	Uttanapadasana	Straight leg raising (Alternate legs followed by both legs)	5	2
b.	Patangasana	Butterfly	100 counts	2
c.	Surya namaskar (10 steps)	Sun salutation pose	8 rounds (4 slow: 4 fast)	8

2.4. Specific relaxation after asanas for substance use disorder:

S. No.	Practice (Sanskrit)	Practice (English)	Rounds	Time (minutes)
a.	Udara shvasana kriya	Deep abdominal breathing with prolonged exhalation (inhalation : exhalation = 1:2)	5	2

2.5. Sectional breathing for substance use disorder:

S. No.	Practice (Sanskrit)	Practice (English)	Rounds	Time (minutes)
a.	*Vibhagiya pranayama:* First chin mudra (4:16:8— inhale:hold:exhale); Focus on the lower chest	*Sectional breathing:* First chin mudra (4:16:8— inhale:hold:exhale)	5	2
b.	*Vibhagiya pranayama:* Second chinmaya mudra (4:16:8— inhale:hold:exhale); Focus on the middle chest	*Sectional breathing:* Second chinmaya mudra (4:16:8— inhale:hold:exhale)	5	2
c.	*Vibhagiya pranayama:* Third adi mudra (4:16:8— inhale:hold:exhale); Focus on the upper chest	*Sectional breathing:* Third adi mudra (4:16:8— inhale:hold:exhale)	5	2

2.6. Specific pranayama for substance use disorder:

S. No.	Practice (Sanskrit)	Practice (English)	Rounds	Time (minutes)
a.	Nadi shuddhi pranayama	Alternate nostril breathing	9	3
b.	Bhastrika pranayama	Bellows breath	2 × 20 counts	3
c.	Bhramari pranayama (Shanmukhi mudra)	Humming bee breath	9	2

2.7. Specific relaxation after pranayamas for substance use disorder:

S. No.	Practice (Sanskrit)	Practice (English)	Rounds	Time (minutes)
a.	Sampurna vishranti paddati in Shavasana	Deep relaxation technique with *Om* chanting or MMM chanting 9 rounds at the end with a positive affirmation "I am healthy, happy and satisfied"	-	9

APPENDIX 1.10

Validated Yoga Module for Somatoform Pain Disorder

(Developed by Dr Geetha Desai et al., 2020 at NIMHANS)

1. Specific loosening practices for somatoform pain disorder:

S. No.	Practice (Sanskrit)	Practice (English)	Rounds	Time (minutes)
a.	Padanguli naman	Toe bending	10	1
b.	Goolf naman	Ankle bending	10	1
c.	Goolf chakra	Ankle rotation	10	1
d.	Goolf ghoornan	Ankle crank	10	1
e.	Janu naman	Knee bending	10	1
f.	Poorna titali asana	Full butterfly	10	1
g.	Kati chakragati	Hip rotation	10 (5 clockwise and 5 anticlockwise)	1
h.	Kati sithilikarana	Waist rotation	10 (5 clockwise and 5 anticlockwise)	1
i.	Mushtika bandhana	Hand clenching	10	1
j.	Manibandha naman	Wrist bending	10	1
k.	Manibandha chakra	Wrist rotation	10 (5 clockwise and 5 anticlockwise)	1
l.	Kohani naman	Elbow bending	10	1
m.	Skandha chakra	Shoulder rotation	10 (5 clockwise and 5 anticlockwise)	1
n.	Griva sanchalana	Neck movements (forward and backward bending, side bending and rotations)	10 (for each practice)	2

2. Specific relaxation after loosening practices for somatoform pain disorder:

S. No.	Practice (Sanskrit)	Practice (English)	Rounds	Time (minute)
a.	Tatkshan shitilikaran upaya in Shavasana	Instant relaxation technique (IRT)	1	1

3. Specific breathing practices for somatoform pain disorder:

S. No.	Practice (Sanskrit)	Practice (English)	Rounds	Time (minutes)
a.	Shvasa kriya-2	Hand stretch breathing	10	1
b.	Marjariasana	Tiger breathing	10	1
c.	Suptaudarakarshanasana	Lumbar stretch breathing	10	2

4. Specific standing asanas for somatoform pain disorder:

S. No.	Practice (Sanskrit)	Practice (English)	Rounds	Time (minutes)
a.	Tadasana	Palm tree pose	5	2
b.	Padahastasana	Hand to foot pose/forward bending pose	5	2
c.	Ardha chakrasana	Half wheel pose	5	2

5. Specific sitting asanas for somatoform pain disorder:

S. No.	Practice (Sanskrit)	Practice (English)	Rounds	Time (minutes)
a.	Ustrasana	Camel pose	5	2
b.	Shashankasana	Hare pose	5	2

6. Specific prone asanas for somatoform pain disorder:

S. No.	Practice (Sanskrit)	Practice (English)	Rounds	Time (minutes)
a.	Bhujangasana	Cobra pose	5	2
b.	Navasana	Spinal column pose	5	2

7. Specific supine asanas for somatoform pain disorder:

S. No.	Practice (Sanskrit)	Practice (English)	Rounds	Time (minutes)
a.	Uttanapadasana/Viparitakarani	Raised legs pose/Inverted pose	5	2
b.	Pawanamuktasana	Wind relieving pose	5	2
c.	Setu bandhasana	Shoulder pose	5	2

8. Specific relaxation after asanas for somatoform pain disorder:

S. No.	Practice (Sanskrit)	Practice (English)	Rounds	Time (minutes)
a.	Sheeghra shitilikaran upaya in Shavasana (with chanting of "A")	Quick relaxation technique (QRT)	1	2

9. Specific pranayama practices for somatoform pain disorder:

S. No.	Practice (Sanskrit)	Practice (English)	Rounds	Time (minutes)
a.	Vibhagiya pranayama	Sectional breathing	5	3
b.	Nadi shuddhi	Alternate nostril breathing	9	3
c.	Bhramari	Humming bee breath	5	2

10. Specific meditation practices for somatoform pain disorder:

S. No.	Practice (Sanskrit)	Practice (English)	Rounds	Time (minutes)
a.	Nadanusandhana	Sound resonance technique • AA kara • UU kara • MM kara • A-U-M kara	9 9 9 9	5
b.	Sampurna vishranti paddati in Shavasana	Deep relaxation technique (DRT) with positive affirmations	1	5

APPENDIX 1.11

Validated Yoga Module for Low Back Pain

(Developed by Dr Nitin J Patil et al., 2015 at SVYASA University, adapted by NIMHANS)

1. Specific supine practices for low back pain (LBA):

S. No.	Practice (Sanskrit)	Practice (English)	Rounds	Time (minutes)
a.	Suptaudarakarshanasana	Folded legs lumbar stretch: • Right side • Left side	3 3	3
b.	Shava udarakarshanasana	Crossed legs lumbar stretch: • Right side • Left side	3 3	3
c.	Pawanamuktasana	Wind releasing pose: • Right side • Left side • Both legs	1 1 1	1 1 1
d.	Setu bandhasana breathing	Bridge pose lumbar stretch	3	2
e.	Uttanapadasana	Straight leg raise stretch: • Right side • Left side	3 3	3

2. Specific prone practices for LBA:

S. No.	Practice (Sanskrit)	Practice (English)	Rounds	Time (minutes)
a.	Bhujangasana	Serpent pose	3	2
b.	Shalabhasana breathing	Locust pose • Right side • Left side	3 3	3

3. Specific standing practices for LBA:

S. No.	Practice (Sanskrit)	Practice (English)	Rounds	Time (minutes)
a.	Ardhakati chakrasana	Lateral arc pose: • Right side • Left side	1 1	1 1
b.	Ardha chakrasana	Half wheel pose	3	1

4. Specific relaxation practices for LBA:

S. No.	Practice (Sanskrit)	Practice (English)	Rounds	Time (minutes)
a.	Tatkshan shitilikaran upaya in Shavasana	Instant relaxation technique	1	1

Contd...

Contd...

S. No.	Practice (Sanskrit)	Practice (English)	Rounds	Time (minutes)
b.	Sheeghra shitilikaran upaya in Shavasana (with chanting of "A")	Quick relaxation technique	1	3
c.	Sampurna vishranti paddati in Shavasana	Deep relaxation technique	1	5

5. Specific pranayama practices for LBA:

S. No.	Practice (Sanskrit)	Practice (English)	Rounds	Time (minutes)
a.	Vibhagiya pranayama	Sectional breathing: • Abdominal • Thoracic • Shoulder	3 3 3	4
b.	Nadi shuddi	Alternate nostril breathing	9	5
c.	Bhramari pranayama	Humming bee breath	9	4

6. Specific meditation practices for LBA:

S. No.	Practice (Sanskrit)	Practice (English)	Rounds	Time (minutes)
a.	Nadanusandhana	Sound resonance technique: • AA kara chanting • UU kara chanting • MM kara chanting • AUM kara chanting	9 9 9 9	5
b.	Om dhyana	Om meditation	1	5

7. Specific kriya practices for LBA:

S. No.	Practice (Sanskrit)	Practice (English)	Rounds	Time (minutes)
a.	Laghu shankhaprakshalana	Yogic colon cleansing	1	30 (to be done once weekly)

APPENDIX 1.12

Validated Yoga Module for Migraine

(Developed by Dr Usha Rani MR et al., 2020, NIMHANS, Bengaluru)

1. Specific loosening practices for migraine:

S. No.	Practice (Sanskrit)	Practice (English)	Rounds	Time (minute)
a.	Griva shakti vikasaka	Neck exercises (Forward, backward and sideward)	10	2
b.	Bhuja valli shakti vikasaka	Shoulder rotation (Clockwise and anticlockwise)	10	2
c.	Kaphoni shakti vikasaka	Elbow stretch	5	1
d.	Manibandha shakti vikasaka	Wrist bending	–	1
e.	Mushtika bandhana	Finger clench	–	1
f.	Janu shakti vikasaka	Knee tightening	5	1
g.	Gulpha sithilikarana	Ankle rotation	5	2
h.	Padanguli naman	Toe bending	5	1
i.	Pawanamuktasana kriya	Wind relieving pose (Rotation clockwise and anti-clockwise with each leg)	10	2

2. Specific breathing practices for migraine:

S. No.	Practice (Sanskrit)	Practice (English)	Rounds	Time (minutes)
a.	Uttanapadasana kriya	Stretched leg pose exercise: • Right side • Left side	 3 3	 1 1
b.	Marjariasana shvasa kriya	Cat stretch breathing	5	1
c.	Head rolling	Sideward, forward, backward and rotation	5 rounds each step	2

3. Specific standing asanas for migraine:

S. No.	Practice (Sanskrit)	Practice (English)	Rounds	Time (minute)
a.	Ardhakati chakrasana	Lateral arc pose: • Right side • Left side	 1 1	 1 1
b.	Trikonasana	Triangle pose: • Right side • Left side	 1 1	 1 1

4. Specific sitting asanas for migraine:

S. No.	Practice (Sanskrit)	Practice (English)	Rounds	Time (minute)
a.	Vakrasana	Half spinal twist posture: • Right side • Left side	 1 1	 1 1

5. Specific prone practices for migraine:

S. No.	Practice (Sanskrit)	Practice (English)	Rounds	Time (minute)
a.	Bhujangasana	Serpent pose	1	1

6. Specific supine practices for migraine:

S. No.	Practice (Sanskrit)	Practice (English)	Rounds	Time (minutes)
a.	Pawanamuktasana (Alternate and both legs)	Wind relieving pose: • Right side • Left side • Both	 1 1 1	 1 1 1
b.	Matsyasana	Fish pose	1	1

7. Specific relaxation after asanas for migraine:

S. No.	Practice (Sanskrit)	Practice (English)	Rounds	Time (minutes)
a.	Sheeghra shitilikaran upaya in Shavasana	Quick relaxation technique	1	5

8. Specific pranayama practices for migraine:

S. No.	Practice (Sanskrit)	Practice (English)	Rounds	Time (minutes)
a.	Vibhagiya pranayama	Sectional breathing: • Abdominal • Thoracic • Shoulder	 3 3 3	 4
b	Ujjayi	Victorious/Ocean breath	9	3
b.	Nadi shuddi	Alternate nostril breathing	9	5
c.	Bhramari pranayama (low pitch) with shanmukhi mudra with hand/elbow support (on a table/pillow)	Humming bee breath	9	3
d.	Sadanta	Cooling breathing technique	5	1

9. Specific meditation practices for migraine:

S. No.	Practice (Sanskrit)	Practice (English)	Rounds	Time (minutes)
a.	Nadanusandhana (Low pitch)	Sound resonance technique • AA kara • UU kara • MM kara • AUM kara	 3 3 3 3	 4

10. **Specific relaxation practice after pranayama for migraine:**

S. No.	Practice (Sanskrit)	Practice (English)	Rounds	Time (minutes)
a.	Sampurna vishranti paddati in shavasana	Deep relaxation technique/Yoga Nidra	1	10

Note: A brief introductory session to migraine (cause and risk factors, importance of adhering to a healthy lifestyle, yogic concept of disease, Panchakosha theory, concept of prana in relation to migraine and the role of yoga in restoring the prana imbalance) will be conducted on the first day followed by the practical yoga sessions.

APPENDIX 1.13

Validated Yoga Module for Parkinson's Disease

(Developed by Dr Kakde N et al., 2017 at SVYASA University)

1. Specific loosening practices for Parkinson's disease:

S. No.	Practice (Sanskrit)	Practice (English)	Rounds	Time (minute)
a.	Griva sithilikarana	Neck exercises	3	1
b.	Bhuja sithilikarana	Shoulder rotation	3	1
c.	Kati sithilikarana	Waist rotation	3	1
d.	Janu sithilikarana	Knee tightening	3	1
e.	Gulpha sithilikarana	Ankle rotation	3	1

2. Specific breathing practices for Parkinson's disease:

S. No.	Practice (Sanskrit)	Practice (English)	Rounds	Time (minutes)
a.	Shvasa kriya	Hands in and out	3	2
b.	Shvasa kriya	Hand stretch breathing	3	2
c.	Shashankasana (with "M" chants)	Hare pose/Moon pose breathing	3	2

3. Specific relaxation after breathing:

S. No.	Practice (Sanskrit)	Practice (English)	Rounds	Time (minutes)
a.	Sheeghra shitilikaran upaya in Shavasana (with chanting of "A")	Quick relaxation technique	1	3

4. Specific standing asanas for Parkinson's disease:

S. No.	Practice (Sanskrit)	Practice (English)	Rounds	Time (minute)
a.	Ardhakati chakrasana	*Lateral arc pose:* • Right side • Left side	 1 1	 1 1

5. Specific supine asanas for Parkinson's disease:

S. No.	Practice (Sanskrit)	Practice (English)	Rounds	Time (minutes)
a.	Setu bandhasana	Bridge pose	3	2
b.	Suptaudarakarshanasana	*Folded leg stretch:* • Right side • Left side	 3 3	3
c.	Ardha pawanamuktasana	*Half wind releasing pose:* • Right side • Left side	 1 1	 1 1

APPENDIX 1 | Yoga Therapy Modules for Common Neuropsychiatric Disorders

6. Specific supine practices for Parkinson's disease:

S. No.	Practice (Sanskrit)	Practice (English)	Rounds	Time (minutes)
a.	Bhujangasana	Serpent pose	3	2
b.	Ardha shalabhasana	Half locust pose: • Right side • Left side	 3 3	 1 1

7. Specific relaxation after asanas for Parkinson's disease:

S. No.	Practice (Sanskrit)	Practice (English)	Rounds	Time (minutes)
a.	Sampurna vishranti paddati in Shavasana	Deep relaxation technique	1	5

8. Specific kriya practices for Parkinson's disease:

S. No.	Practice (Sanskrit)	Practice (English)	Rounds	Time (minute)
a.	Kapalabhati	Skull brightening breath	Daily: 60 counts	1

9. Specific pranayama practices for Parkinson's disease:

S. No.	Practice (Sanskrit)	Practice (English)	Rounds	Time (minutes)
a.	Vibhagiya pranayama	Sectional breathing: • Abdominal • Thoracic • Shoulder	 3 3 3	 4
b.	Nadi shuddi	Alternate nostril breathing	9	4
c.	Bhramari pranayama	Bumblebee chant	5	2

10. Specific meditation practices for Parkinson's disease:

S. No.	Practice (Sanskrit)	Practice (English)	Rounds	Time (minutes)
a.	Nadanusandhana	Sound resonance technique • AA kara • UU kara • MM kara • AUM kara	 9 9 9 9	 5
b.	Om dhyana	Om meditation	–	5

APPENDIX 1.14

Validated Yoga Module for Epilepsy

(Clinically Found Useful by Dr Malla Bhaskara Rao at NIMHANS)

1. Specific breathing practices for epilepsy:

S. No.	Practice (Sanskrit)	Practice (English)	Rounds	Time (minutes)
a.	Shvasa kriya	Hand in and out breathing	5	1
b.	Shvasa kriya	Hand stretch breathing (in 3 variations)	5	2
c.	Vyaghra shvasa kriya	Tiger breathing	5	1
d.	Setu bandhasana breathing	Bridge pose breathing	5	1

2. Specific loosening practices for epilepsy:

S. No.	Practice (Sanskrit)	Practice (English)	Rounds	Time (minutes)
a.	Surya namaskar	Sun salutation	3	3

3. Specific standing postures for epilepsy:

S. No.	Practice (Sanskrit)	Practice (English)	Rounds	Time (minute)
a.	Tadasana	Palm tree pose	1	1
b.	Ardhakati chakrasana	Lateral arc pose	1	1
c.	Ardha chakrasana	Half wheel pose	1	1

4. Specific sitting postures for epilepsy:

S. No.	Practice (Sanskrit)	Practice (English)	Rounds	Time (minute)
a.	Vakrasana	Half spinal twist pose	1	1
b.	Vajrasana	Thunderbolt pose	1	1
c.	Shashankasana	Hare/Moon pose	1	1
d.	Paschimottanasana	Seated forward bend pose	1	1
e.	Ardha ustrasana	Half camel pose	1	1

5. Specific inverted practices for epilepsy:

S. No.	Practice (Sanskrit)	Practice (English)	Rounds	Time (minute)
a.	Ardha sirsasana	Half headstand pose	1	1
b.	Sirsasana	Headstand pose	1	1

6. Specific prone practices for epilepsy:

S. No.	Practice (Sanskrit)	Practice (English)	Rounds	Time (minute)
a.	Bhujangasana	Cobra pose	1	1
b.	Shalabhasana	Locust pose	1	1

7. Specific supine practices for epilepsy:

S. No.	Practice (Sanskrit)	Practice (English)	Rounds	Time (minute)
a.	Sarvangasana	Shoulder stand pose	1	1
b.	Halasana	Plough pose	1	1
c.	Viparitakarani	Legs-up-the-wall pose	1	1
d.	Matsyasana	Fish pose	1	1

8. Specific relaxation after postures for epilepsy:

S. No.	Practice (Sanskrit)	Practice (English)	Rounds	Time (minutes)
a.	Yoga nidra	Guided relaxation	1 (twice a week)	14

9. Specific pranayama practices for epilepsy:

S. No.	Practice (Sanskrit)	Practice (English)	Rounds	Time (minutes)
a.	Sampurna svasana kriya	Full yogic breathing and sectional breathing	5 rounds each	2
b.	Nadi shuddi	Alternate nostril breathing	9	2
c.	Chandra anuloma viloma pranayama	Left nostril breathing	9	2
d.	Sheetali pranayama	Cooling breathing technique-1	5	2
e.	Sitkari pranayama	Cooling breathing technique-2	5	2
f.	Sadanta pranayama	Cooling breathing technique-3	5	2
g.	Bhramari pranayama	Humming bee breath	5	2

10. Specific meditation practices for epilepsy:

S. No.	Practice (Sanskrit)	Practice (English)	Rounds	Time (minutes)
a.	Nadanusandhana	Sound resonance technique: • AA kara • UU kara • MM kara • AUM kara	5 5 5 5	3
b.	Om dhyana	Om meditation	1	5

APPENDIX 1.15

Validated Yoga Module for Caregivers of Patients with Schizophrenia

(Developed by Dr Aarti Jagannathan et al., 2012 at NIMHANS, Bengaluru)

1. Specific breathing practices:

S. No.	Practice (Sanskrit)	Practice (English)	Rounds	Time (minutes)
a.	Hasta shvasa kriya	Hand stretch breathing	3	1
b.	Bhujangasana shvasa kriya	Serpent pose breathing	3	1
c.	Salabhasana shvasa kriya	Locust breathing	3	1
d.	Surya namaskar	Sun salutations	5	10

2. Specific asanas and relaxation techniques:

S. No.	Practice (Sanskrit)	Practice (English)	Rounds	Time (minutes)
a.	Tatkshan shitilikaran upaya in Shavasana	Instant relaxation technique (IRT)	1	1
b.	Ardhakati chakrasana	*Lateral arc pose:* • Right side • Left side	1	1
c.	Sheeghra shitilikaran upaya in Shavasana	Quick relaxation technique (QRT)	1	3
d.	Ardha chakrasana	Half wheel pose	1	1
e.	Padahastasana	Hand to feet pose	1	1
f.	Vajrasana	Diamond pose	1	1
g.	Shashankasana	Rabbit pose	1	1
h.	Ardha ustrasana	Half camel pose	1	1
i.	Sampurna vishranti paddati in Shavasana	Deep relaxation technique (DRT)	1	10

3. Practices set 3:12 minutes:

S. No.	Practice (Sanskrit)	Practice (English)	Rounds	Time (minutes)
a.	Kapalabhati	Skull breathing	4	4
b.	Nadi shuddhi	Alternate nostril breathing	10	4
c.	Nadanusandhana	*Sound resonance technique:* • AA kara • UU kara • MM kara • AUM kara	1	4
d.	Jnana yoga	Yogic counseling	1	15

APPENDIX 1.16

Tele-Yoga Module for Stress Reduction

(Developed by Dr Nishitha Jasti et al., 2020 at NIMHANS)

1. Specific breathing practices for stress reduction:

S. No.	Practice (Sanskrit)	Practice (English)	Rounds	Time (minutes)
a.	Shvasa kriya-1	Hands in and out breathing	10	2
b.	Shvasa kriya-2	Hand stretch breathing	5 rounds each at 90°, 135°, and 180°	3
c.	Kati chakrasana shvasa kriya	Spinal twisting	10	2
d.	Ardha chakrasana padahastasana shvasa kriya	Forward and backward bending	10	3

2. Specific pranayama practices for stress reduction:

S. No.	Practice (Sanskrit)	Practice (English)	Rounds	Time (minutes)
a.	Vibhagiya pranayama	Sectional breathing: • Diaphragmatic • Chest • Clavicular	(Ratio: 6:4:8:4) 5 (Chin mudra) 5 (Chinmaya mudra) 5 (Adi mudra)	9
b.	Kapalabhati	Skull-shining breath	30 rounds, 2 cycles (Rest for 30 seconds in between)	3
c.	Bhastrika	Bellows breath	20 rounds, 3 cycles (Rest for 30 seconds in between)	5
d.	Ujjayi	Victorious breath	9	2
e.	Nadi shuddhi	Alternate nostril breathing	6	5

3. Specific meditation practices for stress reduction:

S. No.	Practice (Sanskrit)	Practice (English)	Rounds	Time (minutes)
a.	Nadanusandhana	Sound resonance technique/ Mantra chanting: • AA kara • UU kara • MM kara • AUM kara	(*Feel vibrations) 5 (*Chest region) 5 (*Throat region) 5 (*Head region) 5 (*Chest→throat→head)	5

Note: Available at https://www.youtube.com/watch?v=n5tpM43wudA&t=2s

APPENDIX 1.17

Guided Yogic Relaxation (GYR)

(Designed by Dr Hemant Bhargav et al., 2020 at NIMHANS)

- *Duration:* 20 minutes
- *Position:* It is advisable to perform in sitting position generally, but it can also be performed in lying down position especially at the bedtime.

INSTRUCTIONS

- Sit comfortably. Keep back and neck erect, whole body relaxed. Keep your palms on your thighs, palms facing upward and very gently bring your eyes to the state of 90% closure. Gently bring the awareness toward your breath.
- Just observe the incoming and outgoing breath without interfering with it. Try to feel the touch of the air in your nostrils as you breathe in and out. Cool air enters the nostrils as you breathe in and warm air goes out as you breathe out.
- Now, slowly shift your awareness to your feet and feel the touch of the ground on your feet. Take a deep breath in and hold your breath, tighten your feet, Tighten... Tighten... Tighten... As you breathe out, release and relax. Just observe your breath, allow it to settle down naturally.
- Now, bring the attention toward your calf muscles. Take a deep breath in and hold your breath, tighten your calf muscles, Tighten... Tighten... Tighten... As you breathe out, release and relax. Observe the breath.
- Try to tighten only the selected parts and keep the rest of the body relaxed. Now, bring your attention to the thigh muscles. Take a deep breath in and hold your breath, Tighten... Tighten... Tighten... As you breathe out, release and relax. Observe the breath.
- Attention on the buttocks. Take a deep breath in and hold your breath, Tighten... Tighten... Tighten... As you breathe out, release and relax slowly. Observe the breath.
- Gently shift your awareness toward your navel region. Become aware of the abdominal movements happening with your breath. Now, try to synchronize the abdominal movements with your breathing. As you breathe in, abdomen bulges out and as you breathe out, let it sink in. A beautiful synchronization of your abdomen with the breath. Try to take a deep breath in and try to bulge your abdomen as much as possible and completely breathe out sinking it deep in. Breathe in bulge up, breathe out sink in. Release and relax. Just observe the natural breath.
- Bring your attention to your chest. Take a deep breath in and hold, Tighten... Tighten... Tighten... As you breathe out, release and relax. Observe the breath.
- Become aware of your whole back region. Take a deep breath in and hold your breath, tighten your back, Tighten... Tighten... Tighten... As you breathe out, release and relax. Observe the breath.

- Next shoulders only, rest of the body relaxed. Take a deep breath in and hold, tighten both sides, Tighten... Tighten... Tighten... As you breathe out, release and relax. Observe the breath. Do not lose the thread of the breath.
- Next the arms and forearms only. Take a deep breath in and hold, Tighten... Tighten... Tighten... As you breathe out, release and relax. Observe the breath.
- Bring your attention to your palms, make a fist in both hands with thumb inside. Take a deep breath in and hold your breath, Tighten... Tighten... Tighten... As you breathe out, release and relax. Observe the breath.
- Attention on the neck. Take a deep breath in and hold, tighten only the neck, Tighten... Tighten... Tighten... As you breathe out, release and relax. Observe the breath.
- Now attention on the whole face and the head. Take a deep breath in. Make a fist with your hands and tighten. Clench your teeth, clench your eyes. Tighten your face and head. Take a deep breath in and hold your breath, Tighten... Tighten... Tighten... As you breathe out, release, open your fist and relax. Completely relax all the muscles of the body from head to toes.
- Take a deep breath in and as you breathe out, feel a wave of relaxation from the head to the toes. Take another breath in and this time relax even more from the head to the toes as you breathe out. One more round, take a deep breath in and this time let the relaxation be total as you breathe out.
- Gently bring the attention back to the breath. Just observe as an uninvolved witness doing nothing, but merely observing.
- Bring your attention between your eyebrows and feel a small bright white light between your eyebrows. Feel the rays of this light spreading throughout the body. Feel that this light diffuses and spreads the lightness throughout your body making it bright and light. Your whole body glowing with brightness and this glow spreads within and a few inches around your body; on the front and back, right and left, above and below. As you become more and more relaxed, with each exhalation, the glow expands around your body to 1 meter (m) all around and within the body, above and below, front and back, right and left. With further relaxation as you breathe out, it expands to 10 m within and around the body. Observe the lightness and the glow all around.
- Now expand further, let go completely by repeating the aphorism and feeling it. "I do nothing", as you let go, you expand more and more... "I do nothing". Observe the complete relaxation. Let the body function, let the breath flow, let the thoughts come and go as an uninvolved witness while you keep repeating "I do nothing". Complete silence, limitless expansion, inherent bliss.
- Slowly, bring the awareness back to your breath. Just observe the breath without interfering, as you observe the breath and you breathe in, the consciousness develops a center and a boundary and starts contracting more and more with each inhalation 10 m around your body, becoming more and more dense, filling your body with brightness and glow. Next 1 m around the body, more and more dense, a few inches above and below, front and back, right and left, within the body. Feel the harmony of energies within your body, relaxation of all the cells in the body, rhythm and gentleness in your breath, untouched peacefulness in your mind.
- Now, very gently become aware of your body by moving your fingers and your toes. Keep on observing the breath and whenever you feel comfortable, gently open your eyes with a few blinks. GYR, available at: https://youtu.be/SdXiUD87vuU?t=2.

Index

Page numbers followed by *f* refer to figure and *t* refer to table.

A

Aberrant immune system 69
Abhinivesha (fear) 111, 153
Abhyasa yoga 14
   regulations of 14
Acetaminophen 186
Acharya charaka 101
Activated B-cells 200
Acupuncture, use of 187
Acute migraine 186
Acute panic and depression, state of 13
Adhi 165, 167
Adhija 9, 165, 166
   vyadhi 9, 88, 166, 187, 188
Adrenocorticotropic hormone 228
Agnisara kriya 182
Agoraphobia 101, 137
Ahamkara, levels of 10
Ahara 18, 25
Ahimsa 3, 17
Ahirbudhnya Samhita 79
ākaśa 25
Akathisia 198
Alcohol dependence 228
Alocasia macrorrhizos 28
Alternanthera sessilis 28
Alzheimer's disease 62, 200
Amaranthus polygonoides 28
Anadhija 9, 165, 166
   disorders 165
   vyadhis 9, 10, 187
Ananda 222, 223
Anandamaya kosha 8, 9, 17, 166, 188
Anapana-sati 45
Annamaya kosha 8, 9, 17, 88, 166, 167, 187, 201, 217
   practices 218
Antarayaha 153
Antiemetics 186
Anxiety 51, 119 197, 198, 217, 208
   emerging therapy for 105
   literature review of 102
   state of 15
   symptom 128, 233

Anxiety disorder 27, 82, 100, 101, 138, 209, 228
   generalized 100, 243
   neurobiology of 101
   prevalence of 100
   treating 101
   validated yoga module for generalized 243
   yoga for 100, 103, 144
Aparigraha 17
   practice of 17
Apoptotic machinery 69
Ardha chakrasana 145, 169
Ardha pawanamuktasana 270
Ardha salabhasana 182
Ardha shirshasana 145
Ardhakati chakrasana 192
Arizona 206
Arjuna Vishada yoga 13, 87
Arjuna's depression, yoga of 13
Arpan buddhi 225
Arthritis 132
Asana 4, 7 11, 83, 190, 04, 105, 119, 127, 132, 145, 199, 201, 206, 218, 221, 229, 239
   postures 200
Ashtanga yoga 3, 4, 7
   limbs of 17
Ashtayoga 3
Asmita 111, 153
Aṣṭāṅgayoga 225
Asteya 3, 17, 18
Astika 3
Atharva veda 3, 118
Attention deficit hyperactivity disorder 83, 137, 145, 228, 255
   yoga for 141
   yoga module for 255
Attentional performance, test of 142
Auditory reaction time 144
Aura 186
Aushadhi 10
Autism 83
   high-functioning 144
   spectrum disorder 137, 145, 257

   yoga for 143
   yoga module for 257
   symptoms 143*f*
Autonomic disturbances 198
Autonomic dysfunction 102
Autonomic function tests 206
Autonomic nervous system 27, 33, 139, 141, 207
   functioning, modulation of 40
Autonomic system through pranayama, balance of 138
Avidya 111, 153
Ayurveda 18, 24-26, 137, 199
   characteristics of 26*t*
   classification of 27
   focus 25
AYUSH 229

B

Back pain
   chronic 176
   yoga for 179*t*
Baroreflex sensitivity 40
Behavior family therapy 217
Behavioral addictions 83
Benzodiazepines, administration of 100
Beta-blockers 186
Bhagavad Gita 4, 9, 13-16, 29, 87, 91, 126, 154, 222-225
Bhajans 11
Bhakti 14, 221
   path of 222, 223
   yoga 14, 16, 218, 222
Bhastrika 80, 94, 120, 159, 182, 211, 232
Bhramari 145
   pranayama 112
Bhujangasana 94, 159, 182
   simplified version of 182
Bhunamanasana 159
Biological rhythms, modulation of 72
Biomedicine 26
Bipolar disorder 72, 82, 94, 228, 249

Blood
  flow 181
  oxygen level dependent 53
B-lymphocytes 69
Body pain 89
Brahma Kumaris Rajayoga 46
Brahmacharya 3, 17, 225
Brahmana 16, 101
  varna 16
Brahmavihara 224
Brain
  computer interface 56
  derived neurotrophic factor 36, 69, 94, 131, 200, 228
  injury, traumatic 209
  networks, higher-level 140
  template 53f, 55f
Breath awareness 189
Breathing exercises 218
Brihadaranyaka upanishad 118, 226

C

Calcium-channel blockers 186
Caloric restriction 212
Canadian Network for Mood and Anxiety Treatments 94
Cardiac autonomic control 102
Cardiac illnesses 229
Cardiorespiratory system 139
Cardiovascular diseases 127
Cardiovascular disorders 37, 39
Caregivers
  role of 217
  yoga for 217
  yoga module for 219
Cauda equina syndrome 177
Cellular aging 68
Cellular mechanisms 68
Cellular pathways 68
Central nervous system 70, 139, 201
Cerebellum 131
Cerebral cortex, magnetic stimulation of 61f
Chakra 119, 169
Chāndogyopaniṣhad 222
Chandra anuloma viloma pranayama 112, 159
Chandra nadi 112
Charaka Samhita 25
Chemical neuroimaging 53

Chenopodium album 28
Childhood autism rating scale 144, 146
Childhood disorders 228
Childhood psychiatric disorders 141
Chitta udvega 101
Chitta vritti nirodaha 51
Chittavikshepa 88, 90
Chronic pain 165-167, 170, 229
  perception of 167
  syndromes 82, 167
  yoga in 165
Chronic primary pain 165
  syndrome 165
Cingulate cortex, anterior 113, 158f
Circadian rhythm 134
Clinical conditions, yoga for 77
Clinical global impression 116
Cognition 208, 223, 224
Cognitive behavioral therapy 100, 128, 187
  yoga-enhanced 103
Cognitive deficits 198
Cognitive impairment, mild 82, 126, 198
Cognitive remediation 198
Cognitive stimulation 212
Cognitive therapy, mindfulness-based 65, 103
Complementary therapy 189
Compression fracture 177
Computed tomography scan 52, 177
Consciousness
  complexity measure of 63
  layers of 8f, 9, 17
  neural correlates of 63
Constipation 186
Contemplative meditation 45
Core strength 181
Coronary artery disease 189
Cortical silent period 63
Cortical thickness 131
Counselling, basic concepts of 13
COVID-19 228
C-reactive protein 69
Crisis-oriented family therapy 217
Cyclic meditation 36, 218

D

Deep brain stimulation 197
Dehydroepiandrosterone-sulfate 70
Dementia 82
  praecox 118
Dendritic cells 69
Dentate gyrus, excitability of 211
Deoxyhemoglobin 55
Deoxyribonucleic acid 69
Depression 51, 87, 89, 94, 95, 102, 119, 186, 208, 217
  conventional management of 90
  moderate-to-severe 82
  monotherapy for 92
  pathogenesis of 88
  pathological conception of 89f
  pathophysiology of 89f
  research with 65
  validated yoga module for 241
  yoga for 90, 91, 92t, 144
  yoga-based management of 90
  yogic understanding of 87
Depressive disorder 87, 229
  yogic counseling for 242
Depressive symptom 233
Devotional sessions 218
Dharana (concentration) 4, 7, 11, 45, 225
Dhatus (bodily tissues) 127
Dhyana (meditation) 4, 7, 11, 45, 127, 200, 206, 225
Diet 218
Diffusion tensor imaging 53
Digestive disturbances 89
Disability, developmental 144
Disability-adjusted life years 51
Disabling disorder 186
Divergence index 64
Dog breathing 182
Dopamine
  dysregulation 122
  replacement therapy 197
Doshas 18, 21, 29, 118, 137
  predominance 18
  terms of 27
Drugs
  antiepileptic 205

antipsychotic 68
antiseizure 212
Duḥkha, types of 25
Dwesha (hatred) 25, 111, 153
Dyskinesias 197
Dysthymia 87

E

Eating disorders 138
Ego 166
Ekagrata 45
Electrocardiogram 33
Electroconvulsive therapy 90
Electroencephalogram 61, 208
Electroencephalography 33, 44, 52, 56, 206
Electromyography 33, 61
Elimination disorders 138
Emotion 223
Emotional disturbances 198
Endocrine system 139, 193
Energy metabolic pathway, regulation of 73
Epidural abscess 177
Epigenetic modulation 71
Epilepsy 102, 205
   chronic drug-resistant 205
   foundation 206
   primary 209
   supine practices for 273
   treatment of 211
   validated yoga module for 272
   yoga for 205, 211
Ergot alkaloids 186
Evidence-based medicine 144
Excessive rajasic energy 119
Excessive tamasic energy 119
Excessive tension, self-management of 217

F

Fatigue 186
Fear, state of 15
Feeding disorders 138
Fractional anisotropy 54
Functional near-infrared spectroscopy 55, 55f
Functional neuroimaging 53

G

Gabaergic inhibitory 41
Galvanic skin resistance 40, 208

Gamma-aminobutyric acid 37, 62, 113, 170, 205, 228
   system 69
Garudasana 232
Gayatri Mantra 258
Gender dysphoria 138
Geriatric psychiatric disorders
   management of 127
   yoga for 126
Geriatric psychiatry 126
Gheranda Samhita 5, 27, 126, 239
Glaucoma 105, 132
Global cortical excitability 62
Glucocorticoid receptor 37
Glutamate neurotransmission 62
Goraksha samhita 5
Gray matter volume, age-related 36
Group tele-yoga therapy 232
Guided yogic relaxation 276
Gunas 15, 16, 25, 27, 29, 87, 91
   composition of 21
Gunatita 15, 17

H

Hamilton Anxiety Scale 130
Hamilton Depression Rating Scale 92, 130
Hand muscle 61
Hatha rathnavali 5
Hatha yoga 5, 93, 113, 155, 178
   practice of 104
   pradipika 5, 27, 126, 139f, 239
Hatkarma practices 127
Head pain, pulsating 186
Headache 83, 89, 186
   disorders, primary 186
Health
   and disease, yogic model for 8
   care, yoga in 1
   psychological dimensions of 127
   social dimensions of 127
Healthy volunteers, research on 64
Heart
   problems 132
   rate variability 35, 49, 102, 171, 201, 205

Hemoglobin 52
Hering-Breuer reflex 193
Herniated disk 132
Himalochika 28
Hippocampus 131
Holistic adjunct therapy 160
Hormonal imbalances, correcting of 139
Human body tries 33
Human immunodeficiency virus 155
Human leukocyte antigen-G, levels of 71
Humming sound, use of 91
Hydrogen peroxide 70
Hyperactivity disorder 142, 142t
Hypertension 127
Hypomanic episode 82
Hyponatremia 105
Hyposmia 198
Hypothalamic-pituitary-adrenal axis 51, 69, 113, 122, 201

I

Ichchha shakti 187
Illness, yoga-based model of 9
Immune
   function-related genes 73
   mediators 73
   pathways 69
Indian National Mental Health Survey 87
Inflammatory cytokines, regulation of 193
Inflammatory gene 200
Inflammatory marker interleukin-6 37
Information integration theory 64
Injuries, reports of 80
Integrative medicine 24
   department of 106
Intellectual disability 137, 144
Intelligence quotient 144, 208
Interferon-gamma 69
Interim analysis 210
Interleukin 69, 170
Intermittent fasting 121
Intracortical facilitation 63
Intracortical inhibition, long-interval 63
Invasive neuromodulation treatments 187

Irritability 186, 208
Ishvara pranidhana 3, 11, 18, 166
Iyengar's yoga 93, 105, 178
  therapy 167

J

Jatru Trataka 232
Jñāna 221
  yoga 16, 222

K

Kakkola 28
Kapalabhati 27, 57, 80, 82, 94, 120, 145, 154, 159, 182, 192, 211, 232
Kapha 18, 118, 137
  dosha 18, 137
Karana sharira 188
Karma 14
  yoga 14, 16, 221-224
    philosophy of 16
Kathopanishad 3, 13
Kleshas 153
Klishta chitta vrittis 88
Kripalu yoga, effect of 104
Kriya 4, 154
  shakti 187
  yoga 166
Kshatriya 16
  varna 16
Kumbhaka 80
Kundalini 103
  yoga 54, 104, 112, 232

L

Lifestyle advice 211
Lifestyle intervention, yoga-based 208
Limbic system 207
Low back pain 82, 176, 178, 265
  chronic 176, 177
  validated yoga module for 265
  yoga for 176, 177

M

Magnetic resonance spectroscopy 54, 62
Magnetoencephalography 52, 64, 210

Manah prashamanopayah yoga ityabhidhiyate 4, 101, 112
Manas 25
Mandala yoga 144*f*
Mandalam 258
Mandukya
  karika 11, 17, 94
  upanishad 19, 91
Manic episode 82
Manodoṣas 25
Manomaya kosha 8, 9, 17, 88, 119, 154, 166, 167, 187, 188, 201, 217
  level of 88
  practices 218
Manovaha srotas 137
  hyperactivity of 138
Mantra 10, 139
  chanting 90
Matsyendrasana 127
Medical disorders 229
Medical illnesses, number of 228
Medicine
  alternative 101, 137, 206
  complementary 101, 137, 206
Meditation 154
  neurophysiology of 44
  practice, neurocognitive effects of 47
  states 45
Memory 208
  disturbances 197
  enhancing 139
  functions 131
Mental disorder 25, 68, 217
  manual of 137
  range of 72
Mental distraction 154
Mental health 24, 51, 139, 221, 228
  positive 221
  yoga in 51
Mental state shifts, neurophysiology of 46
Mesial temporal
  lobe epilepsy 210
  sclerosis 210
Metta-bhavana 46
Migraine 83
  asanas for 268

chronic 186
headaches 186
meditation practices for 268
phases of 186
pranayama for 269
prone practices for 268
sitting asanas for 268
standing asanas for 267
supine practices for 268
symptoms of 186
validated yoga module for 267
yoga for 186, 188, 190*t*
yogic understanding of 187
Mind-body
  interventions 167
  therapies 143
Mindfulness 189, 200
Mirror neuron system 61, 64
Mitāhārah 28
M-kara 112
Modulate psychological disorders 102
Mokṣha 25
  attainment of 26
Molecular processes 70
Monocausal theories 29
Mood disorders 138
Mood swings 208
Motion, cervical range of 168
Motivation 208
Motor symptoms, onset of 198
Motor-evoked potential 62
Mudras 154
Mukha bhastrika 144
Mukha dhouti 182
Muscle 192
  strength 181
Musculoskeletal pain disorders 167
Musculoskeletal system 139

N

Naada 199
Nada yoga 199
  sadhana 199
Nadanusandhana 120, 145, 258
Nadi 139, 139*f*
Nadi shuddhi 120
  pranayama 112
Naiṣthiki chikitsa 26
Naltrexone 152
National Comorbidity Replication Survey 100

National Institute for Mental Health and Neuro Sciences 35, 44, 90, 106, 111, 145, 159, 192, 230
National Mental Health Survey 79, 137
Natural killer cells 69
Naukasana 159
Navasana 169
Near-infrared spectroscopy 52
Neck pain 82, 192
Negative syndrome scale 121
Neocortex 131
Nerve conduction 193
Nervous system 139
Neural bodies, loss of 131
Neural pathway 69
Neurobiological dimensions 31
Neurochemicals pathway 69
Neurodevelopment disorders 138
Neuroendocrine
 axis 33
 systems 134
Neurological disorders 219
 yoga for 79
Neurological illnesses, number of 228
Neurological motor disorder, complex 197
Neurophysiological markers 228
Neurophysiology 34
Neuropsychiatric disorders 73, 239
 common 237
 yoga for 81
Nidra 166
Nimhans Integrated Centre for Yoga 114, 182, 219
Niṣkāma karma 224
Niyama 4, 7, 17, 154
 level of practice of 18
 practice of 18
 status of 21
Noncommunicable disorders 8
 emergence of 24
 pathogenesis of 10f
Noncommunicable lifestyle-related disorders 26
Noninvasive neuromodulation treatments 187
Nonmotor symptoms 197, 198
Nonrapid eye movement 48

Nonsteroidal anti-inflammatory drugs 186
Nonviolence 17
Norepinephrine 34
 dopamine reuptake inhibitor 153
Numeric Pain Rating Scale 168
Nutritional deficiencies 165
Nyaya 3

O

Obsessive compulsive disorder 80, 82, 111, 112f, 138, 228, 245
 validated yoga module for 245
 yoga in 111
Obsessive related disorders 138
Obstacles distraction 154
Occupational therapy 198
Ojas (immunity) 130
Opioid antagonist 152
Opioid dependence syndrome 159
Opioid use disorder, validated yoga module for 260
Orbitofrontal cortex 113
Orthodox 3
Osteoarthritis 127
Oxyhemoglobin 55
Oxytocin 73

P

Padahastasana 169, 231
Pain 197, 198
 yogic understanding of 165
Panchabhutas 118
Panchakosha 17, 88, 132, 166, 187, 201
 model 8f, 17, 88, 89f, 154
 theory 154
 viveka 187
Panchamahabhutas 18
Panic disorder 101
Paramahansa yogananda 5
Parasympathetic nervous system 37, 208
Paresthesia 198
Parivrtta trikonasana 145
Parkinson's disease 197, 200, 270
 validated yoga module for 270
 yoga for 197, 199

Paschimottanasana 94, 127
Patangasana 159
Patanjali's yoga sutras 87, 88, 126, 153, 166, 225, 239
Patient-therapist interactions 81
Pawanamuktasana 94, 192
 kriya 159
Peripheral nervous system 201
Personality traits, basis of 20f
Perturbation complexity index 63
Pharmacological treatments 186
Pharmacotherapy 198
Phobias 100
Phobic anxiety disorder 137
Physical body 8
Physical disorders 68
 comorbid 74
Physical function 168
Physiotherapy 198
Piper cubeba 28
Pitta 18, 118
Polysomnography 45
Poorna chakrasana 232
Poorna ustrasana 232
Positive syndrome scale 121
Post-headache 186
Post-traumatic stress disorder 51, 102, 119, 205, 229
Post-yoga practice 189
Pracchardana vidharanabhyam va pranasya 154
Prajna purusha 19, 20
Prakriti 18, 25
Prakriti types 26t
Pramana 19, 166
 vritti 112
 dominance 112
Prana (breath), flow of 41
Pranamaya 9, 201
Pranamaya kosha 8-10, 17, 119, 166, 167, 187, 188, 217
 practices 218
Pranava japa 94
Pranayama (breath control) 4, 7, 20, 83, 102, 104, 120, 127, 139, 145, 154, 167, 200, 201, 206, 210, 218, 221, 229, 239
 and kriyas 11
 meditation 181

neurophysiology of 39
on metabolism, effect of 41
on psychophysiology, effect of 40
on respiratory system, effect of 40
practice of 206
practices 193
Prasad buddhi 225
Prasada kapha 138
Pratyahara 4, 7, 127
  terms of 225
Proinflammatory cytokines 193
Promises and challenges 73
Prone asana 250
Psychiatric disorders 27, 51, 52, 72, 81, 82t, 89
  causes of 24
  minor 217
  yoga for 54, 79, 137
Psychiatric illness 128
  number of 228
Psychiatry, branch of 126
Psychological distress, prevalence of 209
Psychological symptoms 229
  reduction of 181
Psychosocial interventions 153
Psychosomatic disease 166, 188
Psychosomatic disorders 187
Psychotic disorder 82, 137
Psychotic symptoms 122, 198
Puberty, delaying 138
Purva mimamsa 3

Q

Quality of life 168, 197
  health-related 206

R

Radicular pain 177
Radiculopathy 177
Raja yoga 4, 14, 16
Rajas guna 88, 154
Rajasic activities 91
Rajo guna 112
Randomized controlled trial 40, 80, 92, 103, 112, 113t, 120, 154, 168, 178, 179
Rapamycin, mammalian target of 70
Rasayana 127
Recreation and activities 91

Recurrent depressive disorder 137
Relaxation 90, 104
  effect 181
  technique 181
  yoga-based 120
Reproductive system 139
Respiratory problems 229
Resting state networks 54
Rhythmic auditory stimulation 199
Riboflavin 187
Riddhavastha 127
Rod and frame test 41

S

Ṣaḍdarśanas 3
Sādharmyamukti 223
Sahaja yoga 91, 93, 206, 208
  effect of 206
Salabhasana 182
  breathing 182
Samadhi 7, 11, 45, 127
Sankalpa 239
Sankhya 3
Sankhya School of Philosophy 27
Santosha (satisfaction) 11, 18
Sarvangasana 119, 145
Satsanga 11, 218
Sattva 15, 17, 25, 88, 111
  guna 88
Sattvic 15, 91, 105, 225
  activity, promoting 91
  diet 218
  guna 119
  sukha 223
Satya 17, 225
Schizophrenia 80, 82, 118, 122, 123, 228, 274
  spectrum 138
  disorders 73
  symptoms of 119
  validated yoga module for 247
  yoga for 119
  yogic counseling for 248
Science of Emotional Culture 218
Science of Yoga Expounds 15
Sedatives hypnotics 153
Seizure disorders 83

Selective serotonin reuptake inhibitors 111
Sensory disturbances 198
Serum total glutathione 72
Sham yoga 207
Shanmukhi mudra 159
Shashankasana 119, 145, 192
Shatkriyas 232
Shatyoga 3
Shavasana 11, 94
Shithilikarana vyayama 104
Shiva Samhita 5
Short-interval intracortical inhibition 63
Shoucha 11
Shudra 16
  varna 16
Siddha Siddhanta Paddhati 5
Sitali pranayama 159
Sithilikarana vyayama 250, 251
Sitting asanas 264
Sleep 91, 197
  disturbance 208
  neurophysiology 48
Smrithi 19, 153, 166
Social anxiety disorder 100
Social cognition 73
Somatoform pain disorder 82, 169, 263, 264
  validated yoga module for 263
Spinal canal stenosis 177
Spinal gabaergic neurotransmission 63
Spondyloarthropathy 177
Sthula Sharira 187
Stress 89
  context of 141
  deep-rooted 17
  primes neuroinflammatory pathways 89
  reduction 181, 275
    mindfulness-based 103
  regulatory system 69, 72
  related disorders 102, 138, 187
  self-management of 209
  symptom 233
Substance use disorder 80, 83, 138, 152, 158f, 260
  yoga for 152
    module for 159
Subsyndromal disorders 134
Sudarshan kriya yoga 36, 91, 103

Suicidal ideations 208
Sukshma Sharira 188
Sukshma vyayama 132, 239
Superoxide dismutase, levels of 72
Suptaudarakarshanasana 263, 265, 270
Surya Bhedana 27
　　Pranayama 127
Surya Namaskar 94, 159, 182, 211
Suryanuloma 94, 145
Suryaviloma 94
Swabhavaja vyadhi 127
Sympathetic nervous system 37, 38, 51, 69, 201, 208
Sympathetic-adrenal-medullary axis 122

T
Tadasana 145
Taittiriya upanishad 8, 13, 17, 88, 154, 166, 187
Tamas guna 88
Tamasic
　　activities 91
　　sukha 223
Tamo guna 138
Tapas 3, 11, 18, 166
Teaching yoga therapy 94
Tejas purusha 19, 20
Tele-yoga 228, 229
　　module 275
　　practice of 231
　　settings 80
Telomere
　　activity 70
　　metabolism 69
Terminalia chebula 28
Therapeutic effect 153
Tinospora cordifolia 28
T-lymphocytes 69
Traditional Indian Medicine Perspective of Developmental Disorders 137
Trait anxiety 102
Transcendental meditation 34
　　effect of 44
Transcranial direct current stimulation 56
Transcranial magnetic stimulation 35, 56, 60, 187

coil 61*f*
machine 60*f*
safety of 65
Trataka 82, 90, 142, 192, 211
Trauma 138
Tremor 197
Tridoshas 18
Trigunas
　　play of 15
　　spectrum of 17
　　terms of 15
　　theory of 15
Trikonasana 145, 159
Trimarga 221
Triptans 186
Tumor necrosis factor-alpha 71
Turiya 19
Tyrosine kinase B 36

U
Ujjayi (breathing) 94, 145
　　pranayama 159
Uninostril breathing 40
Ustrasana 94, 145, 169
Uttanapadasana 169
Uttara mimamsa 3

V
Vaisheshika 3
Vaishvanara purusha 19, 20
Vaishya 16
　　varna 16
Vajrasana 145
Vanillylmandelic acid 208
Vardhakya 127
Varenicline 153
Varuna 13, 16, 166
Vascular disorders, risk for 189
Vascular endothelial growth factor 70
Vastaka 28
Vata 18, 118, 137, 138
　　governs 18
Vāyu 25
Vayu mahabhuta, derivatives of 138
Vedic 3
　　counseling 14
　　principle of 13, 14, 21*t*
　　literature 13, 20
　　Literature-based Counseling Program, development of 13

mantra 90
period 3
philosophy 15, 20, 21
principles 137
texts 14
tradition 25
Ventricular dilatation 131
Vichara 18, 188
Vijnanamaya 88
　　kosha 8, 9, 17, 88, 154, 166, 188, 201, 217
　　practices 218
Vikalpa 166
Viniyoga 178
Vinyasa yoga 105
　　therapy 167
Viparita karani 94, 127, 169
Viparyaya 19, 166
　　vritti 111, 112
Vipassana 232
　　bhavana 45
Virechana 18
Vishada 87
Visual acuity, impaired 198
Visual reaction time 144
Vital airs 187
Vrikshasana 159, 232
Vyadhi 9, 165
Vyaghrasana 159

W
Wear loose clothes 84
Wrinkles, appearance of 127

Y
Yale-brown obsessive compulsive scale 116
Yama 4, 7, 13, 17, 154, 225
　　level of practice of 18
　　practice of 17, 18
　　status of 21
Yoga 3, 4*t*, 6, 17, 18, 51, 70, 81, 92, 105, 138, 205, 212
　　ability of 131
　　adverse effects of 74
　　and anxiety neurosis 104
　　and body awareness 41
　　and cardiovascular disorders 37
　　and generalized anxiety disorder 103
　　and meditation 7

and mental health 228
and panic disorder 103
and performance anxiety 102
and phobia 104
and positive mental health 221, 223
and post-traumatic stress disorder 104
and state anxiety 103
and stress 37
aspects of 215
chair 132
class, precautions for 146
different streams of 14
discipline of 79
effectiveness of 155*t*
eight limbs of 5*t*
evolution of 3*f*
integration of 26
intervention, effect of 101
literature review of 102, 178
mechanisms of 128, 155, 200
    action of 158*f*, 167, 181, 181*f*, 192
mental health effects of 51
mode of action of 68
module 181, 189
music and nada 199
neurobiology of 113
neurophysiology of 33
neuroscience of 60
nidra 11, 20, 104, 200, 201, 210
on anxiety, effect of 102
on epilepsy, effect of 206
on gamma-aminobutyric acid, effect of 54
on mental disorders, effect of 68
on neuroplasticity, effect of 36
on pain pathway, effects of 171*f*
path of 153
performance assessment 81, 233
perspective 153
philosophy, attitude towards mind in 7
physiological benefits of 33
practice of 154
practitioner 28*t*
rahasya 126
research on 64
research, transcranial magnetic stimulation in 60
scientific generic 178
studies on 167
sūtras 6, 19, 126, 223
systems network model of 140*f*
therapist 160, 232
use of 127, 167
vāsiṣṭha 13, 88, 187
with intellectual disability 144
Yoga philosophy
    mentions 15
    perspective 112*f*
Yoga practices 82*t*, 208, 211
    adverse effects of 80
    duration of 192
    potential outcomes of 141*f*
Yoga therapy 8, 11, 29, 73, 79, 87, 101, 118, 123, 144, 145, 154, 189, 208
    approach to 143, 217
    effect of 139*t*, 218
    general guidelines for 79
    integrated 228
    modules 237
    practical tips for 145
    precautions for 81
    process of 10
Yoga Training Program 144
Yogasanas 206
Yogic asanas 218
Yogic concept 88
Yogic energetic perspective 119
Yogic path 16
Yogic practices 131
Yogic research, beginning of 34
Yogic texts 4*t*
Yogic trimarga 223
Yunajmi 3

EU GSPR Authorised Reprsentative
Logos Europe, 9 rue Nicolas Poussin
1700, La Rochelle, France
Phone: +33 (0) 6 67 93 73 78
E-mail: contact@logoseurope.eu

www.ingramcontent.com/pod-product-compliance
Ingram Content Group UK Ltd.
Pitfield, Milton Keynes, MK11 3LW, UK
UKHW060949220426
5322IPUK00033B/604

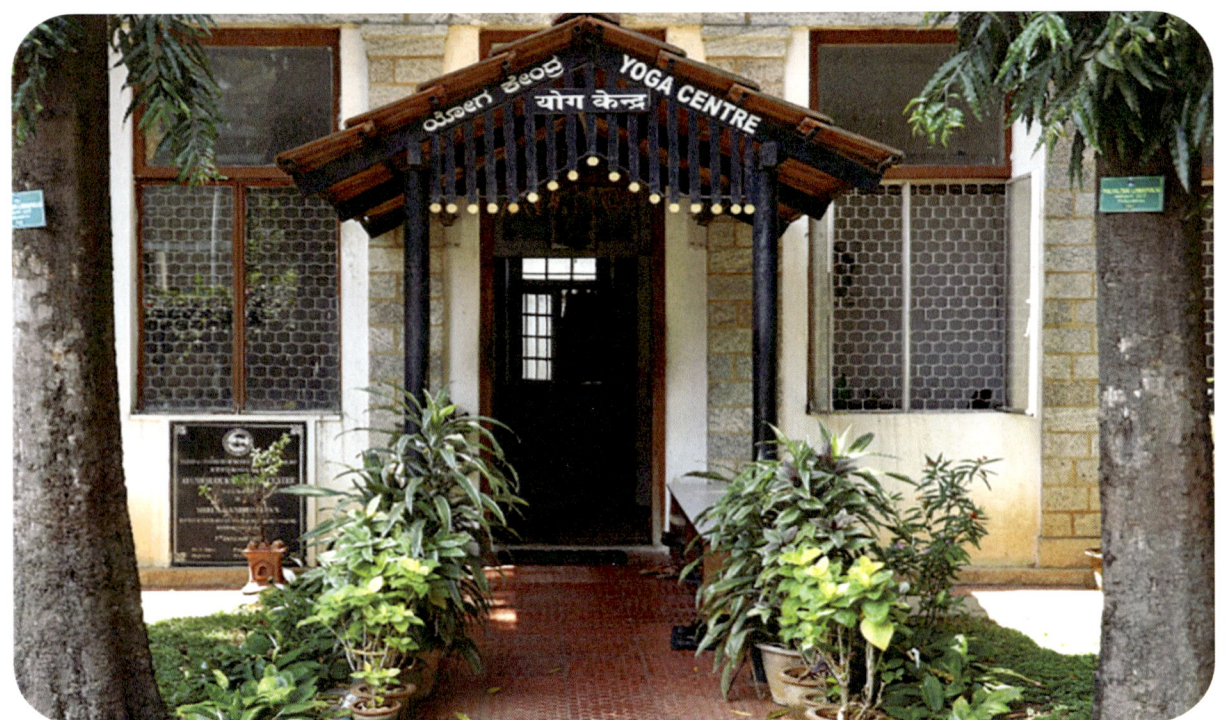

The National Institute of Mental Health and Neuro Sciences (NIMHANS) is an institute of national importance, recognized for its excellence in mental health and neuro sciences in terms of patient-care facilities, academics and research. The institute, under the directorship of Padmashri Dr BN Gangadhar has taken the initiative to incorporate Yoga in addition to conventional treatment options keeping in mind its potential to improve mental health. To achieve this, an Advanced Centre for Yoga–Mental Health and Neuro Sciences was established at NIMHANS in collaboration with Morarji Desai National Institute of Yoga (MDNIY) in November 2007. Later, the center was included in the Department of Psychiatry, NIMHANS, as the NIMHANS Integrated Centre for Yoga (NICY) in 2014. This center was dedicated to promote Yoga in therapeutics, academics and research. The center offered Yoga therapy to patients and their caregivers suffering from psychiatric and neurological conditions, and also carried out pioneering research into the use and efficacy of Yoga in these populations. Considering the untapped potential for integrative medicine in this area, NIMHANS established a full-fledged Department of Integrative Medicine in October 2019 incorporating Yoga, Ayurveda as well as Modern Medicine under the same umbrella to deliver the best in patient care. Generic validated Yoga modules have been designed and are being used for disorders such as Schizophrenia, Depression, Anxiety, Somatoform Pain Disorders, Substance Use Disorders, Obsessive-compulsive Disorder, Mild Cognitive Impairment, and Migraine. This department also extends its service to the vulnerable and stressed populations such as caregivers of the neuropsychiatric patients and people suffering from other lifestyle disorders. Apart from clinical services, the center also aims to promote academics and research activities to understand the mechanisms and role of Yoga in various neuropsychiatric and lifestyle disorders through modern research methodology and state-of-the-art research tools.

For further information, please visit our website www.nimhansyoga.in

The Science and Art of Yoga in Mental and Neurological Healthcare

Salient Features

- Compendium on Yoga therapy for common neuropsychiatric conditions
- Easy-to-understand practical guide for the students of Yoga therapy, Yoga therapists and Yoga clinicians treating neuropsychiatric conditions
- Each chapter involves a team of experts from the fields of modern medicine/psychology/Yoga
- Scientifically validated/clinically relevant Yoga modules for each neuropsychiatric disorder provided in the appendix
- Includes theoretical concepts from the perspective of Yoga philosophy, scientific mechanisms and compilation of research evidences
- Case vignettes have been provided to exemplify the practical applications of Yoga therapy for each neuropsychiatric condition described
- Special emphasis on practical application of Yoga in clinical conditions—provided as "Yoga Clinical Insights" by a clinical Yoga expert
- A useful guide for physicians, especially psychiatrists and neurologists interested in incorporating Yoga therapy into their clinical practice.

Shivarama Varambally MD MAMS DSc is a Professor of Psychiatry and Head, Department of Integrative Medicine, National Institute of Mental Health and Neuro Sciences (NIMHANS), Bengaluru, Karnataka, India. He has 20 years of experience in Psychiatry including 2 years of work in Australia. He has made original research contributions in the Neurobiology of Schizophrenia and the Applications of Yoga in Mental Health which have been internationally recognized.

Sanju George MBBS FRCPsych is a Senior Clinical Psychiatrist and Professor of Psychiatry and Psychology, Rajagiri College of Social Sciences, Kochi, Kerala, India. He worked in the UK for 15 years as an Academic and Consultant Psychiatrist. His areas of expertise include addictions, stress management and marital therapy.

TM Srinivasan PhD DSc is a Professor, Swami Vivekananda Yoga Anusandhana Samsthana (S-VYASA) University, Bengaluru, Karnataka, India. He was Professor of Biomedical Engineering at IIT, Chennai between 1972 and 1990. He was the Director of Research at Fetzer Institute, Michigan, USA during 1990–1995. He has edited and authored several books: *Energy Medicine around the World*, *Gita Sagara Saram*, *Yoga Sagara Saram* and *Model Methods and Perspectives in Yoga*.

Hemant Bhargav MBBS MD PhD (Yoga) is working as an Assistant Professor of Yoga, Department of Integrative Medicine, National Institute of Mental Health and Neuro Sciences (NIMHANS), Bengaluru, Karnataka, India. He has 10 years of experience as a Clinical Yoga Expert, particularly in the field of mental health and neurosciences. He has more than 60 research publications in these areas.

Available at all medical bookstores or buy online at www.jaypeebrothers.com

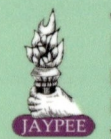

JAYPEE BROTHERS
Medical Publishers (P) Ltd.
EMCA House, 23/23-B, Ansari Road,
Daryaganj, New Delhi - 110 002, INDIA
www.jaypeebrothers.com

Join us on facebook.com/JaypeeMedicalPublishers

Shelving Recommendation
PSYCHIATRY

ISBN 978-81-948028-1-5